# Endocrinology

## *An Integrated Approach*

# Endocrinology

## *An Integrated Approach*

Stephen Nussey and Saffron Whitehead
*St. George's Hospital Medical School, London, UK*

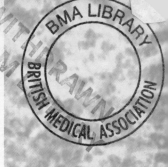

BIOS

© BIOS Scientific Publishers Limited, 2001

First published 2001
Reprinted 2002

A CIP catalogue record for this book is available from the British Library.

ISBN 1 85996 252 1

**BIOS Scientific Publishers Ltd**
**9 Newtec Place, Magdalen Road, Oxford OX4 1RE, UK**
**Tel. +44 (0)1865 726286. Fax +44 (0)1865 246823**
**World Wide Web home page: http://www.bios.co.uk/**

**Important Note from the Publisher**
The information contained within this book was obtained by BIOS Scientific Publishers Ltd from sources believed by us to be reliable. However, while every effort has been made to ensure its accuracy, no responsibility for loss or injury whatsoever occasioned to any person acting or refraining from action as a result of information contained herein can be accepted by the authors or publishers.

The reader should remember that medicine is a constantly evolving science and while the authors and publishers have ensured that all dosages, applications and practices are based on current indications, there may be specific practices which differ between communities. You should always follow the guidelines laid down by the manufacturers of specific products and the relevant authorities in the country in which you are practising.

Production Editor: Andrea Bosher
Typeset by Creative Associates, Oxford, UK
Printed by Polestar, Exeter, UK

# CONTENTS

# PREFACE

The challenge of writing a text for the medical curriculum at the beginning of the twenty-first century is not one to be under-estimated.

There are currently many different texts on endocrinology (some running to two or even three volumes), not to mention those restricted to diabetes mellitus or the more specialized areas of endocrinology. Many of these are edited multi-author works with up to 160 chapters. In addition, there are a number of slimmer volumes, often of the brief 'lecture note' variety for the student requiring only the 'essentials'. A number of these contain clinical cases or illustrative clinical vignettes, though these are usually adjuncts at the ends of chapters.

The style and approach of this book is not conventional. We set ourselves the task of producing a book in which actual clinical cases seen in recent years are integral to the text. The challenge of doing this in 8 chapters was entirely self-imposed. However, it reflected our existing integrated teaching style, the practical realities of clinical medicine (in which patients rarely fit completely into neat chapters) and our belief that the subject of endocrinology is best taught with an integrative rather than a divisive approach. We have attempted to avoid undue use of acronyms, eponyms, abbreviations and clinical jargon and have made extensive use of boxes to summarize information and to illustrate fundamental scientific and clinical principles. These are not only essential to the text but will hopefully provide useful summaries for revision purposes.

We regard it as an experimental text, based on the quirks of nature that give us clinical diseases. The majority of the material exists physically as a book. Further reading matter (including clinical case-based problems, references to pertinent reviews and multiple-choice questions) exists in a flexible and easily up-datable form on the BIOS website. It is anticipated that additional material will be added to the website if the approach is well-received. We hope that this approach is educative, but more than that we hope it is enjoyed.

It is impossible to acknowledge all the friends and colleagues who have contributed in various ways to this book as it developed. We would, however, particularly like to thank: Dr Philip Wilson for help with the histological illustrations; Drs Juliet Britton, Jane Adam, Sisa Grubnic and Rosemary Allen for help with radiological illustrations; Professor Alan Johnstone and Drs Guy Whitley, Helen Mason, Lindsay Bashford, Assunta Albanese, Murray Bain and Caroline Brain for helpful discussions and advice; the enthusiastic and energetic members of the clinical team, particularly Dr. Gul Bano; Dr Asjid Qureshi for help in designing the website material; the many unnamed students and other colleagues who gave helpful advice throughout the preparation; finally, the patience of our families.

## CHAPTER 1

# Principles of endocrinology

## Chapter objectives

*Knowledge of*

1. Classification of hormones and chemical signaling mechanisms
2. Hormone synthesis, secretion and transport
3. Hormone receptors and signal transduction processes
4. Interactions between the endocrine, nervous and immune systems
5. Genetics of endocrinology

*"The attempt and not the deed, Confounds us."*
*Macbeth, William Shakespeare.*

## Functions of hormones and their regulation

The word hormone is derived from the Greek *hormao* meaning 'I excite or arouse'. Hormones communicate this effect by their unique chemical structures recognized by specific receptors on their target cells, by their patterns of secretion and their concentrations in the general or localized circulation. The major hormones discussed in this book are listed in *Box 1.1*.

Their functions can be broadly grouped into several categories: reproduction and sexual differentiation; development and growth; maintenance of the internal environment; and regulation of metabolism and nutrient supply. A single hormone may affect more than one of these functions and each function may be controlled by several hormones. For example, thyroid hormone is essential in development as well as many aspects of homeostasis and metabolism, whilst glucocorticoids, such as cortisol, are important both in growth and nutrient supply and are also modulators of immune function. The roles several hormones play in one function is exempli-fied by the control of blood glucose which involves the pancreatic peptide insulin and its counter regu-latory hormone, glucagon, as well as cortisol, growth hormone and epinephrine. Hormones act in concert and thus, an abnormality in a controlled variable, such as blood glucose concentration may result from defects in the control of any one of several hormones.

The secretion of hormones is subject to negative feedback control, and there are several ways by which this is achieved (*Box 1.2*). Feedback loops may involve the hypothalamo–pituitary axis that detects changes in the concentration of hormones secreted by peripheral endocrine glands or a single gland may both sense and respond to changes in a controlled variable. The integration of feedback loops involving several hormones may be complex. Disturbances in feedback loops are clinically impor-tant and their significance in diagnosis is pivotal.

## Chemical signaling – endocrine, paracrine, autocrine and intracrine mechanisms

A chemical released by a specialized group of cells into the circulation and acting on a distant target tissue defines the 'classical' endocrine and neuroen-

1

Classification by structure of the major human hormones*

| Hormones | Peptide/protein | Steroid | Amino acid or fatty acid derived |
|---|---|---|---|
| Hypothalamic hormones | Thyrotrophin releasing hormone (TRH)<br>Corticotrophin releasing hormone (CRH)<br>Arginine vasopressin (AVP)<br>Gonadotrophin releasing hormone (GnRH)<br>Growth hormone releasing hormone (GHRH)<br>Somatostatin<br>Prolactin relasing factor (PRF)<br>Dopamine | | |
| Anterior pituitary hormones | Thyroid-stimulating hormone (TSH)<br>Adrenocorticotrophic hormone (ACTH)<br>Luteinizing hormone (LH)<br>Follicle-stimulating hormone (FSH)<br>Somatotrophin/growth hormone (GH)<br>Prolactin (PRL)<br>Melanocyte-stimulating hormone (MSH) | | |
| Posterior pituitary hormones | Oxytocin<br>Arginine vasopressin | | |
| Thyroid hormones | | | Thyroxine ($T_4$)<br>Triiodothyronine ($T_3$) |
| Pancreatic hormones | Insulin<br>Glucagon<br>Somatostatin<br>Pancreatic polypeptide | | |
| Calcium regulating hormones | Parathyroid hormone (PTH)<br>Calcitonin (CT)<br>Parathyroid hormone-related peptide (PTHrp) | 1,25-dihydroxyvitamin D | |
| Adrenal cortical steroids | | Cortisol<br>Aldosterone<br>Dehydroepiandrosterone | |
| Adrenal medullary hormones | | | Epinephrine<br>Norepinephrine |
| Male reproductive hormones | Inhibin | Testosterone<br>Dihydrotestosterone | |

contd

| Hormones | Peptide/protein | Steroid | Amino acid or fatty acid derived |
|---|---|---|---|
| Female reproductive hormones | Inhibin<br>Oxytocin<br>Human chorionic gonadotropin (hCG)<br>Human chorionic somatotrophin | Estradiol<br>Progesterone | |
| Plasma volume and sodium regulating hormones | Atrial natriuretic peptide (ANP)<br>Arginine vasopressin<br>Renin/angiotensin | Aldosterone | |
| Cardiovascular hormones | Atrial natriuretic peptide (ANP)<br>Endothelins<br>Erythropoietin<br>Bradykinin | | Nitric oxide |
| Pineal hormones | | | Melatonin<br>Serotonin |
| Growth factors or cytokines | Insulin-like growth factors (IGFs)<br>Epidermal growth factor (EGF)<br>Interleukins (ILs)<br>Tumor necrosis factor (TNF)-$\alpha$ | | |
| Eicosanoids | | | Prostaglandins<br>Thromboxanes<br>Prostacyclin<br>Leucotrienes<br>Lipoxins |

*Note that this list is not intended to be comprehensive

docrine signalling mechanism. A paracrine mechanism is defined as chemical communication between neighboring cells within a tissue or organ (*Box 1.3*). Autocrine signals are those in which a chemical acts on the same cell whilst an intracrine signal is generated by a chemical acting within the same cell.

## Chemical classification of hormones and their synthesis

Hormones are derived from amino acids, from cholesterol (*Box 1.4*) or from phospholipids (*Box 8.8*).

By far the most numerous are the protein or peptide hormones, ranging in size from just three to over 200 amino acids. Some hormones, such as insulin, are made up of two sub-units joined by disulfide bonds between two cysteine molecules whilst the glycoprotein hormones of the anterior pituitary gland are not only made up of two protein sub-units but also have complex sugar moieties attached.

The steroid hormones, which include vitamin D and those secreted by the adrenal cortex and gonads, are derived from cholesterol. All adrenal and gonadal steroids have the same basic ring

**Box 1.2:**
Principles of feedback control in the endocrine system

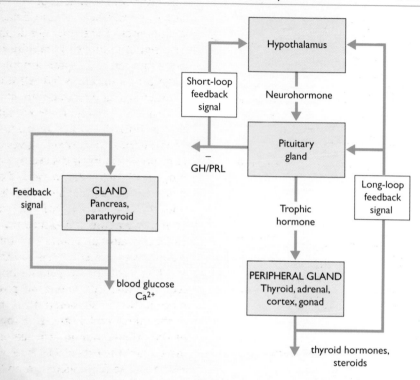

The activity of the thyroid gland, adrenal cortex and gonads is controlled by the feedback effects of their circulating hormones on the hypothalamic-pituitary axis. The secretory activity of glands not under direct control of the hypothalamic-pituitary axis i.e. endocrine pancreas and parathyroid gland is controlled by feedback signals of the regulated variable they control, blood glucose and calcium

Abbreviations: GH, growth hormone; PRL, prolactin.

structure (*Box 1.4*) and despite superficial 2D structural similarity, the side chains and spatial orientation generate specificity.

The third group of hormones are those derived either from tyrosine or from tryptophan. A single tyrosine molecule yields the catecholamines, epinephrine and norepinephrine, the latter being both a neurotransmitter and a hormone. In the endocrine system, these hormones are secreted by the adrenal medulla and are rapidly broken down once released into the circulation. The thyroid hormones are formed by the conjugation of two tyrosine molecules and resemble steroid hormones in binding

to serum proteins and in the mechanism of action. Tryptophan is the precursor of serotonin (5-hydroxytryptamine) and melatonin synthesis. Finally, hormones derived from lipids and phospholipids include the major classes of eicosanoids including prostaglandins, prostacyclins, thromboxanes and leukotrienes (*Box 8.8*).

## Hormone synthesis

Most protein and peptide hormones require the transcription of a single gene though the α and β

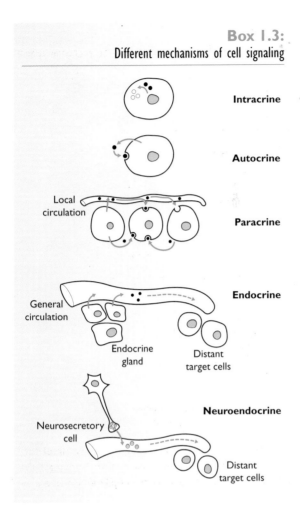

Intracrine

Autocrine

Local circulation

Paracrine

Endocrine

General circulation

Endocrine gland

Distant target cells

Neuroendocrine

Neurosecretory cell

Distant target cells

This signal sequence finds a docking protein, the signal recognition particle, on the rough endoplasmic reticulum so that as protein synthesis continues the assembled amino acids move into the membranes of the rough endoplasmic reticulum. The signal sequence is rapidly cleaved from the growing protein pre-prohormone and eventually a large pro-hormone is left within the membrane-bound rough endoplasmic reticulum (*Box 1.6*).

Inside the endoplasmic reticulum, the protein moves into the Golgi apparatus by fission and fusion of protein containing vesicles in which the large pro-hormone is cleaved by peptidases into the biologically active hormone and one or more fragments of the original molecule. Fragments are frequently co-secreted with the active hormone. Secretory granules are formed from budding of the Golgi apparatus and hormones and their associated fragments are stored in these prior to their release.

Thus, protein and peptide hormone synthesis requires transcription of gene, post-transcriptional modification by exision of the introns, translation of the mRNA and post-translational modifications of the original amino acid sequence. As a result, more than one pro-hormone may be derived from a single gene (e.g. calcitonin and calcitonin-gene related peptide, *Box 5.38*). Furthermore, post-translational processing of a pro-hormone may result in the formation of different biologically active peptide fragments (e.g. pro-opiomelanocortin). These processes are typically tissue-specific.

In contrast, the synthesis of steroid hormones (*Box 1.7*) that occurs in the mitochondria and rough endoplasmic reticulum does not require immediate gene expression. It requires the presence of specific enzymes that convert cholesterol into the appropriate steroid (*Box 4.5*). Different enzymes are expressed in different steroid secreting cells and their expression is controlled by trophic hormones and/or other factors. Cholesterol for steroid synthesis and the amino acid, tyrosine, for thyroid hormone synthesis are ubiquitous, but synthesis of thyroid hormones (*Box 1.4*) requires both specific enzymes (containing selenium) and iodine, both of which are trace elements (*Box 3.5*).

The amine hormones such as the catecholamines, melatonin and serotonin are formed by

subunits of the glycoprotein hormones (TSH, LH and FSH) are derived from different genes. The initial RNA undergoes modifications such that the introns are excised from the molecule and there are modifications to the 3′ and 5′ ends of the messenger (m) RNA. The mature mRNA, containing only the exons, is then used as the template for the assembly of amino acids, through transfer (t) RNA, on the rough endoplasmic reticulum (*Box 1.5*).

Since protein and peptide hormones are stored in, and secreted from, secretory granules it is necessary for their synthesis and packaging to take place within membrane-bound structures of the cell. For this reason, the first amino acids that are translated from the mRNA template form a signal sequence.

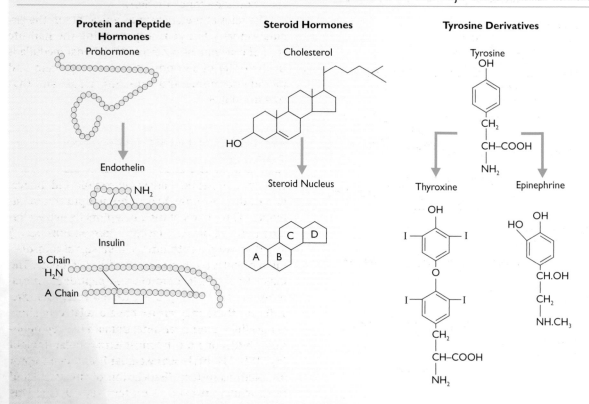

**Protein and Peptide Hormones** — Prohormone, Endothelin, Insulin (B Chain, A Chain)

**Steroid Hormones** — Cholesterol, Steroid Nucleus

**Tyrosine Derivatives** — Tyrosine, Thyroxine, Epinephrine

Other hormones include those derived from tryptophan (serotonin and melatonin, *Boxes 7.33* and *8.12*) and those derived from fatty acids (eicosanoids, *Box 8.8*).

side-chain modifications of either a single tyrosine or tryptophan molecule while the eicosanoid family of hormones are formed from lipids (*Box 8.8*).

## Transport of hormones in the circulation and their half-lives

Steroid and thyroid hormones are less soluble in aqueous solution than protein and peptide hormones and over 90% circulate in blood as complexes bound to specific plasma globulins or albumin. Bound and free hormones are in equilibrium (*Box 8.28*). More recently, binding proteins for several protein and peptide hormones (e.g. CRH, GH) as well as growth factors (e.g. IGF) have also been identified.

It is generally accepted that it is the unbound or free hormone that is biologically active and that hormone binding delays metabolism and provides a circulating reservoir of hormones. More recently, it has been suggested that the specific binding globulins are not just passive transporters but may interact with membrane receptors and that hormone binding to the globulins initiates a signal transduction pathway.

Most binding proteins are synthesized in the liver and alterations in the serum concentrations of these proteins alter total serum concentrations of a

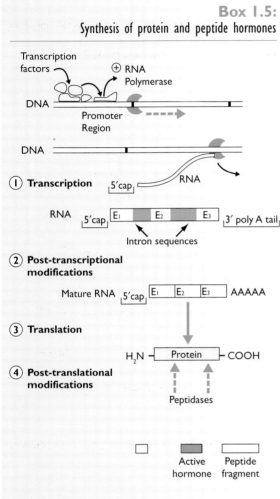

Transcription
factors

$\oplus$ RNA
Polymerase

DNA

Promoter
Region

DNA

① **Transcription** — 5'cap — RNA

RNA — 5'cap | E₁ | E₂ | E₃ | 3' poly A tail

Intron sequences

② **Post-transcriptional modifications**

Mature RNA — 5'cap | E₁ | E₂ | E₃ | AAAAA

③ **Translation**

$H_2N$ — Protein — COOH

④ **Post-translational modifications**

Peptidases

☐ ▨ ☐
Active  Peptide
hormone  fragment

① Transcription of the DNA sequence into RNA
② Excision of sequences (introns) from the initial DNA transcript and modifications of the 3' and 5' terminals
③ Translation of the mRNA into a protein (the signal sequence is rapidly cleaved)
④ The prohormone (*Box 1.6*) is cleaved into fragments, a process that normally occurs prior to secretion

hormone but may have much less effect on the concentrations of free hormone. As a result, situations may arise in which assays of total hormone concentrations do not reflect changes in free hormone concentrations. Measurement of biologically relevant free hormone concentrations (*Box 3.30*), however, is generally more difficult than measuring total hormone concentrations.

The rates of metabolism of hormones in the circulation vary but generally speaking the half life ($t_{1/2}$) of catecholamines from the adrenal medulla is in the order of seconds, minutes for protein and peptide hormones and hours for steroid and thyroid hormones.

## Hormone receptors – cell surface

Proteins and peptides are water soluble and, hence, do not diffuse across hydrophobic lipid cell membranes. Thus, parts of their receptors lie extracellularly (where hormone-receptor interactions occur) and they couple with intracellular signal transducing molecules by traversing the cell membrane. The majority of classical protein and peptide hormone receptors are the G-protein linked receptors (*Box 1.8*) and these may either have a relatively short extracellular amino terminal domain (e.g. epinephrine, GnRH) or a much longer extracellular domain (e.g. TSH, LH, PTH). Extracellular hormone-receptor interactions induce dissociation of the associated intracellular trimeric G protein (*Box 1.10*). This may either open ion channels in the membrane or activate a membrane bound enzyme that stimulates (or inhibits) the production of a second messenger such as cyclic AMP or diacylglycerol and inositol trisphosphate (*Box 1.10*). These second messengers then activate serine/threonine kinases (*Box 1.9*) or phosphatases.

Activation of these protein kinases may have three consequences. It can lead to alterations in specific cytosolic enzyme activity, activation of nuclear transcription factors (*Boxes 1.10 and 1.13*) or initiation of a cascade of subsequent phosphorylations on the serine or threonine residues of protein kinases that can also regulate transcription (*Box 1.10*).

The second most common type of cell surface receptors is that used in the signaling of insulin, growth hormone, prolactin, most growth factors and cytokines. This type is a transmembrane receptor with either inherent protein tyrosine kinase

**Box 1.6:**

## Synthesis of protein and peptide hormones within the endoplasmic reticulum and the process of post-translational modification

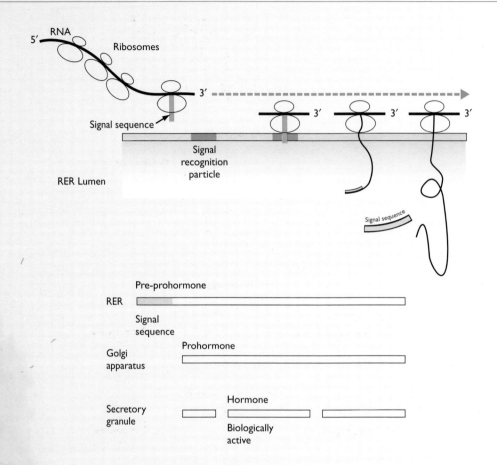

The initial amino acid sequence to be translated is the signal sequence that finds a signal recognition particle on the membrane of the rough endoplasmic reticulum (RER). Synthesis is thus directed into the RER lumen. The entire transcript of the mRNA is known as a pre-prohormone but usually the signal sequence is cleaved rapidly before the end of transcription. In the Golgi apparatus, the large prohormone is cleaved into smaller peptides and stored as such in secretory granules.

activity on the intracellular domain (e.g. insulin and growth factor receptors) or associated intracellular molecules (*Box 1.9*) that have this activity (e.g. receptors for growth hormone, prolactin and cytokines). Binding of the hormone or growth factor to the extracellular domain results in receptor dimerization with an adjacent receptor initiating either autophosphorylation (*Box 1.10*) or phosphorylation of an associated enzyme. Subsequently, there are similar signal transduction events to those described above that involve both cytoplasmic and nuclear events.

#### Simplified diagram of the major pathways of steroid synthesis from cholesterol

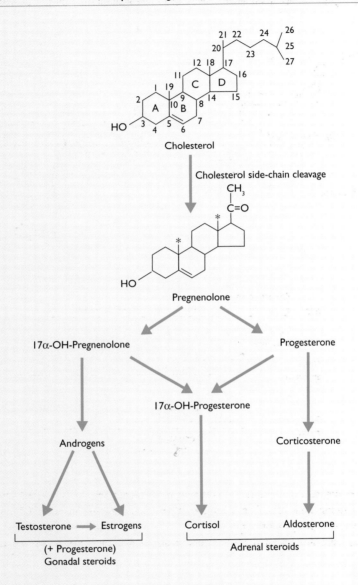

The numbers shown on the structure of cholesterol indicate the position of the carbon atoms.

*Conventionally a single line indicates the attachment of a methyl ($CH_3$) group but is not shown.

The two main classes of protein and peptide hormone receptors

G-protein linked receptors that frequently activate serine/threonine kinases through second messengers such as cAMP, diacylglycerol, calmodulin

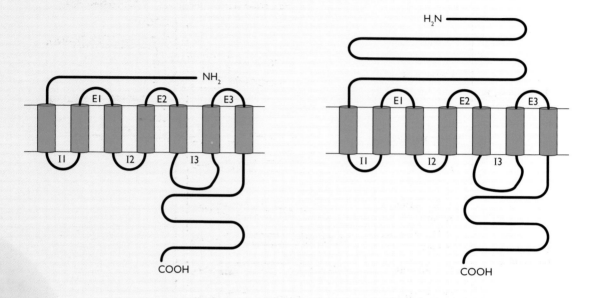

Receptors with inherent tyrosine kinase activity or associated with intracellular molecules possessing tyrosine kinase activity. Some intracellular kinases are attached to the membrane.

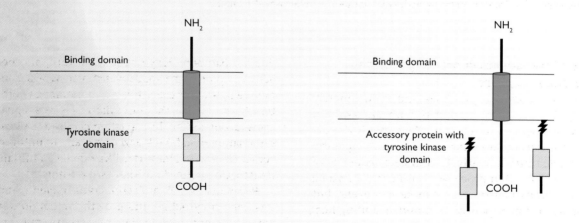

Box 1.9:

Kinases associated with signal transduction mechanisms of protein and peptide hormone receptors

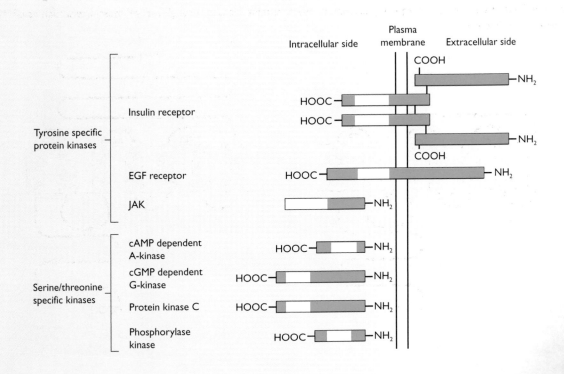

Some receptors possess inherent tyrosine kinase activity or are associated with intracellular molecules (e.g. JAK) that are activated upon hormone binding. G-protein linked receptors activate intracellular serine/threonine kinases via second messengers. The location of kinase activity is indicated by open (white) frames.

## Signal transduction pathways for cell surface receptors

These are complex processes and unfortunately dogged by terminology that is confusing and not always logical – a legacy from the periodic discovery of intracellular factors that were subsequently assembled into a relatively complete sequence of signal tranduction processes. It is not in the scope of this book to pursue all the molecular events but a broad outline is pertinent to understanding hormone action and genetic mutations that can cause endocrine disorders.

Receptors that have inherent tyrosine kinase activity bind molecules that have a specific SH2 domain (src homology domain). In turn, another accessory protein may be activated such as SOS (son-of-sevenless). This can activate a monomeric G-protein known as Ras that essentially acts as a signal transduction switch. Its activation can lead to phosphorylation of Raf, MEK and eventually to mitogen activated protein kinase (MAPK) which can initiate transcription (termed the MEK-MAPK pathway).

Receptors for GH, prolactin, erythropoietin, and a variety of cytokines and growth factors do not have inherent protein kinase activity but are associated with a protein that has tyrosine kinase activity. One of these proteins, known as JAK (just another kinase) may activate downstream effectors

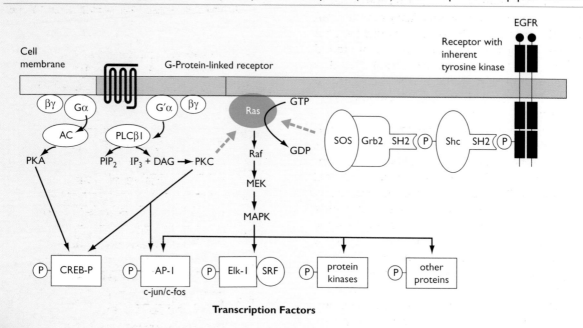

**Box 1.10:**
Signal transduction pathways and transcriptional (nuclear) actions of protein and peptide hormones

Protein and peptide hormones can activate a number of transcriptional factors by phosphorylation. This may involve the MEK-MAP pathway (serine-threonine kinases) or direct activation of transcription factors by protein kinase (PK) A, PKC or the $Ca^{2+}$-calmodulin activated CaM protein kinase (not shown).

Abbreviations: EGFR, epidermal growth hormone receptor; AC, adenylate cyclase; PLC, phospholipase C; $PIP_2$, phosphatidylinositol 4,5-bisphosphate; $IP_3$, inositol 1,4,5-trisphosphate; DAG, diacylglycerol; Shc/Grb, accessory proteins with SH2 (src homology) domains; SOS, son-of-sevenless; Ras, monomeric G-protein; Raf/MEK, kinases; MAPK, mitogen activated protein kinase (serine/threonine kinase); CREB-P, cyclic AMP response element binding protein; SRF, serum response factor.

that include the STAT proteins – the JAK-STAT pathway. Binding of insulin to its receptor induces phosphorylation of insulin receptor substrate proteins (IRS) which activates further signal transduction pathways including activation of nuclear transcription factor κB (NF-κB). In essence, there is a cascade of protein phosphorylations that ultimately end in the nucleus to induce transcription.

The transcription factor targets for kinases that are activated by protein and peptide hormones include c-jun and c-fos which make up the heterodimeric AP-1 complex, the serum response factor (often targeted by the MAP kinase dependent pathway), and nuclear CREB-P (cAMP response element binding protein) which is phosphorylated by protein kinase A and enhances transcriptional activity of closely positioned promoters (*Box 1.10*).

## Hormone receptors – intracellular

Steroid and thyroid hormones are lipophilic and readily diffuse across cell membranes. Their receptors are typically intracellular and are classified according to their cellular location, their dimerization and the sequences of DNA to which they bind. There is a large family of steroid receptors, all of which are transcription factors. They bind to DNA and with other transcription factors initiate RNA synthesis. Whilst receptors for the major steroid hormones have been identified (*Box 1.11*) other structurally similar molecules have been identified though their ligands have not. These have been termed orphan receptors.

The characteristic single polypeptide chain is structurally and functionally divided into six domains. At the amino terminus are the A/B domains that are variable both in sequence and length. The C domain, also called the DNA binding domain (DBD), is a highly conserved sequence across all steroid receptors and is characterized by possessing two zinc fingers which readily slot into the helix of the DNA molecule. The D domain is thought to represent a hinge region in the molecule whilst E represents the ligand binding domain and F a variable region in the carboxyl terminus. This end of the molecule is also the region where the heat shock proteins (hsps) are bound and where dimerization occurs.

Receptors that exist predominantly in the cytoplasm are classified as Type 1 receptors and these include the glucocorticoid, mineralocorticoid, androgen and progesterone receptors. They are bound to heat shock proteins (e.g. hsp 90, hsp70 and hsp 56). Upon steroid binding the hsp complex is released and the receptor forms a dimer with another identical receptor (*Boxes 3.9 and 5.7*). The homodimer translocates to the nucleus where it binds to a specific base sequence on the DNA. The estrogen receptor is also associated with hsps and whilst this receptor shuttles between the nucleus and cytoplasm, most are confined to the nuclear compartment. Type 2 receptors are typically located in the nucleus and may be bound to DNA. They characteristically form heterodimers (e.g. thyroid hormone receptor and retinoid X receptor) or may initiate transcription as monomers upon ligand binding.

The specific amino acid sequence of the zinc fingers in the DNA binding domain is important for determining the bases in the DNA helix to which the receptor binds and, thus, the specificity of the

**Box 1.11:**

### Structures of the main steroid hormone receptors showing their domains and numbers of amino acids

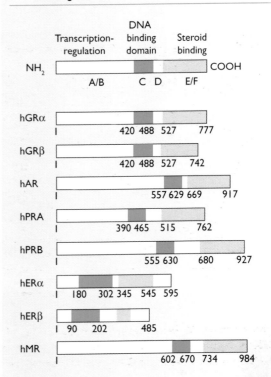

The DNA binding domain (C) is highly conserved in all steroid receptors. The two types of the human glucocorticoid receptor (hGRα and hGRβ) arise from alternate splicing of the same mRNA transcript; the two progesterone receptors (hPRA and hPRB) result from alternate sites of transcription initiation; the two estrogen receptors (hERα and hERβ) are coded by different genes. Only one type of androgen receptor (hAR) and mineralocorticoid receptor (hMR) have been described.

transcriptional activity of the receptor. This is determined through what is called the recognition helix that lies at the end of the first zinc finger and part of the amino acid sequence between the two zinc fingers. Amino acids in the second zinc finger make specific contacts with the phosphate backbone of the DNA.

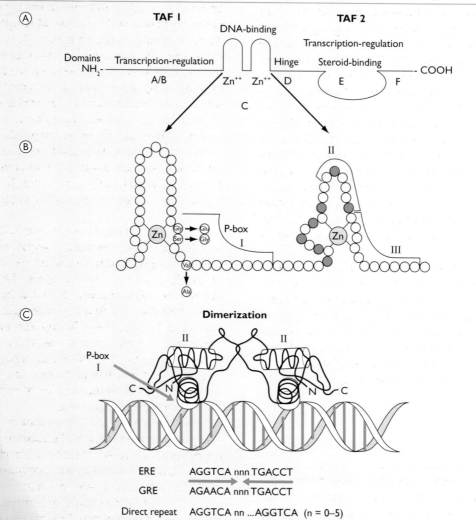

(A) Generalized structure of all steroid hormone receptors showing the different domains, location of the zinc fingers and the regions of the receptor responsible for transcriptional activity (TAF).

(B) Two-dimensional structure of the zinc fingers of the DNA binding domain (DBD) in a single receptor. I, II and III indicate the helical regions of the DBD. The first helix contains the P box which determines the specificity of the DNA binding. The 3 amino acids that determine whether the receptor will combine with a glucocorticoid response element (GRE) or an estrogen response element (ERE) on the DNA are indicated. Arrows indicate the different amino acids that convert GRE specificity to ERE specificity. Amino acids shown as solid circles indicate those that are important for dimerization of two receptors.

(C) Diagram showing dimerization of two receptors and helix I of each receptor slotting into the helix of the DNA. The base sequences of the ERE and GRE are shown plus the palindromic sequence. An example of a direct repeat sequence is also shown.

Type 1 receptors recognize a base sequence AGAACA whilst Type 2 receptors and the estrogen receptors recognize a base sequence AGGTCA. These are known as hormone response elements on the DNA and can be further defined as a glucocorticoid response element (GRE) or estrogen response element (ERE), respectively (*Box 1.12*). These, however, are half-site specificities of hormone receptors; the other half-site forms an inverted palindrome, as recognized by Type 1 and the estrogen receptors, or by a direct repeat of bases with variable number of bases between the half-site specificity. These are generally recognized by thyroid hormones, vitamin D, and retinoid receptors. The other way in which steroid hormones can alter transcription is not via interaction with a GRE or ERE on the DNA but by binding to and activating/repressing other transcription factors that recognize a particular site on DNA (*Box 1.13*).

Many steroids and thyroid hormones can stimulate rapid responses in target cells that are clearly non-genomic and may be explained by interaction with cell surface receptors. Such receptors may initiate the opening of ion channels or activate classical second messenger systems. The difficulty of isolating such receptors has hampered their investigation but it is clear that steroids exert membrane effects.

## Hormones and gene transcription

The receptors of all classes of hormones may regulate gene transcription either by activating transcription factors or by acting as transcription factors in their own right. Transcription is not, however, a simple process of a factor or receptor binding to DNA and activating RNA polymerase at an initiation site. It also requires a complex of enzymes, referred to as the holo-enzyme complex, before transcription is initiated down-stream of the factors and promoters. Thus, for example, a steroid receptor may have transcriptional activity but only when promoters (or repressors) bind with a particular part of the molecule. Sometimes these factors may act independently of ligand binding, others require ligand binding before they can be activated.

## Hormone receptor regulation

Receptor regulation is an important part of endocrine function and this occurs through up or down-regulation of the number of receptors and by desensitization of the receptors. This occurs by increasing or decreasing receptor synthesis, by internalization of membrane receptors after ligand binding, or by uncoupling of the receptor from its signal transduction pathway (desensitization). The latter usually involves phosphorylation of the receptor. Some hormones may regulate their own receptors (homologous regulation) such as GnRH on the pituitary gonadotrophs whilst other receptors are regulated by other hormones (heterologous regulation) e.g. estrogen regulating oxytocin receptors.

Interaction between hormones and their receptors depends on the number of receptors, the concentration of circulating hormone and the affinity of the hormone for the receptor. The latter is defined as the concentration of a hormone at which half the total number of receptors is occupied (*Box 1.14*) and the higher the affinity the lower the concentration of hormone required. Generally speaking the affinity of hormone receptors does not change and thus the biological response depends on the number of receptors and the concentration of hormone.

Usually less than 5% of hormone receptors are occupied at any one time and maximum biological responses are achieved when only a fraction of the total number of receptors are occupied. Thus, it might be questioned why a small reduction in receptor number or a change in hormone concentration should make much difference to the overall biological response. This is governed by the law of mass action. If receptor numbers are reduced then the chances of a hormone binding to a receptor are decreased. Thus, a higher concentration of hormone is required to achieve a similar receptor occupancy. A similar argument may be applied when hormone concentrations are reduced. Together these two parameters are important in determining the target cell's response to a hormone despite low occupancy of receptors (*Box 1.14*).

Signal transduction pathways of a peptide hormone and a steroid hormone that control gene expression by activating or inhibiting the activity of the transcription factor, nuclear factor-κB (NF-κB)

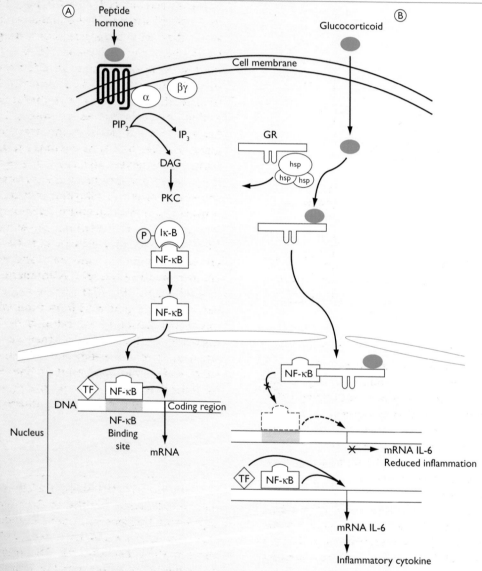

(A) Protein kinase C (PKC), activated by a peptide hormone via the inositol pathway, releases the transcription factor, NF-κB from its inhibitory subunit through phosphorylation. NF-κB moves into the nucleus where, along with other transcription factors (TF), initiates transcription.

(B) The binding of an anti-inflammatory glucocortocoid to the glucocorticoid receptor (GR) induces release of the heat shock proteins and the hormone/receptor complex translocates to the nucleus. It binds with NF-κB preventing its transcriptional activity for pro-inflammatory proteins such as interleukin-6 (IL-6). This forms part of the anti-inflammatory effects of glucocorticoids.

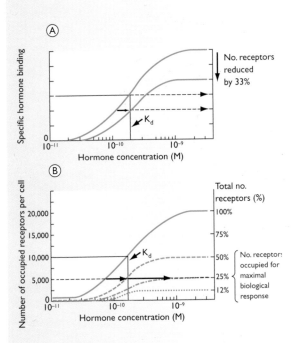

Ⓐ Relationship between specific hormone binding and total number of receptors. The $K_d$ is the concentration of hormone required to occupy 50% of the receptors. When the total number of receptors is reduced by a third, $K_d$ remains the same but the concentration of hormone required to achieve a certain level of hormone binding is increased (arrow).

Ⓑ These curves demonstrate the consequences of reducing the number of receptors when only 25% occupancy is required for maximal biological response. Again $K_d$ remains unchanged but the concentration of hormone required to achieve the occupancy of 5000 receptors per cell increases (arrows).

## Neuroendocrine interactions

All endocrine glands are innervated by autonomic nerves and these may either directly control their endocrine function and/or regulate blood flow (and hence function) within the gland. Hormones, in turn, may affect central nervous system functions such as mood, anxiety and behavior.

Neurosecretory cells (*Box 1.3*) may directly convert a neural signal into a hormonal signal. In other words they act as transducers converting electrical energy into chemical energy. Thus, activation of neurosecretory cells leads to secretion of a hormone into the circulation. These neurosecretory cells include: those that secrete hypothalamic releasing and inhibiting hormones controlling TSH, ACTH, LH and FSH release from the anterior pituitary gland; the hypothalamic neurons the axon terminals of which secrete oxytocin and vasopressin from the posterior pituitary gland; the chromaffin cells of the adrenal medulla (embryologically modified neurons) that secrete epinephrine and norepinephrine into the general circulation. The significance of these neurosecretory cells is that they allow the endocrine system to integrate and respond to changes in the external environment. Thus, for example, the CRH-ACTH-cortisol axis can be activated by stress generated from external cues as is oxytocin secretion by a suckling baby. The recent discovery that the nervous system itself can synthesize neurosteroids has added new dimensions to the concept of neuroendocrine integration. With regard to endocrine function *per se*, the significance of these discoveries remains to be elucidated.

## Hormones and the immune system

Since the discovery that surgical ablation of the pituitary gland caused atrophy of the thymus gland, experimental evidence from animal studies has indicated that there is a complex network of interactions between these two systems. The thymus gland, which is essential for orchestrating immune responses, has two regions – one in which T cell precursors from bone marrow mature and the other that secretes thymic hormones (*Box 1.15*). The physiological role of thymic hormones is not clear but they are postulated to promote T cell maturation (*Box 1.15*).

The immune system can be considered a sensory system as it responds to stimuli such as bacteria,

Simplified overview of the organization of the immune system

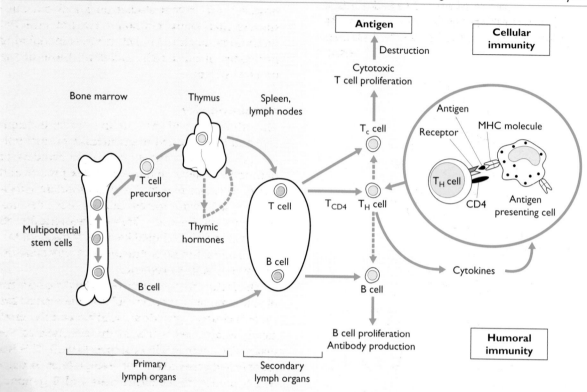

*The interaction of antigen-presenting cells (these include monocytes, macrophages and dendritic cells) that present peptide antigens bound to class II MHC molecules to T cells that express CD4 co-receptors is shown in detail (see text).

viruses, tumors and other antigens. When stimulated, cell-mediated or humoral immune responses are activated and this information is sent to the hypothalamus (via the circumventricular organs) by cytokines and peptide hormones secreted from cells of the immune system. In addition neural and non-neural cells in the brain also synthesize cytokines. The neuroendocrine system responds to these signals which, in many ways, may be considered a stress response.

Both cytokines and thymic hormones may influence the release of hypothalamic neurohormones and, hence, pituitary secretions; overall, immune activation is stimulatory to the release of pituitary hormones (Box 1.16). There is also evidence that cytokines act directly on endocrine glands such as the pituitary, thyroid, pancreas, adrenals and gonads and alter their secretions. Pituitary hormones and the secretions of their peripheral target endocrine glands may modulate immune function. Thus, for example, ACTH/glucocorticoids are immunosuppressants as are progesterone and testosterone whilst the action of estrogens is both stimulatory and inhibitory. GH and prolactin may also potentiate immune responses through a variety of effects and can stimulate growth and activity of the thymus gland (Box 1.16).

Thymic hormones and immunomodulators may alter endocrine function and hormones may modu-

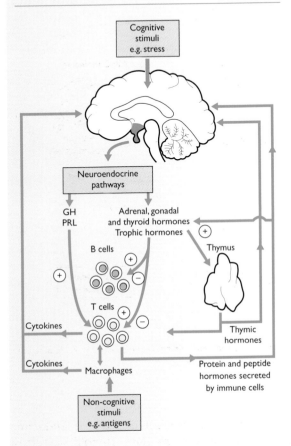

late immune responses. Cross-talk between the systems also occurs because immune cells release peptides that are identical to those produced by the hypothalamus and pituitary gland. They are released in response to stimulation from both antigens and hypothalamic hormones. For example, immune cells release ACTH that can stimulate the release of glucocorticoids and thus, to some extent over-ride the negative feedback effects of stress-induced increases in cortisol secretion on the hypothalamo-pituitary axis. Furthermore, interleukin-1,

released by macrophages, stimulates the secretion of hypothalamic CRH release. Thus, high cortisol secretion rates are maintained. It should be noted, however, that recent studies on knock-out mice suggest that many hormones are not essential immunomodulators but act as stress-modulating hormones in most cells, including those of the immune system.

## Autoimmunity

The primary role of the immune system is defensive and it is required to distinguish normal self-components from those of foreign invaders or pathogens. Tolerization is a complex process and loss of tolerance may lead to inappropriate activation of the immune system causing tissue destruction and autoimmune disease. Theoretically all tissues in the body should be equally frequent targets for autoimmune destruction but endocrine tissues appear more susceptible.

The factors that predispose to the development of autoimmunity are not completely understood but there is clearly a genetic association and the most clearly established is that of the genotype of the major histocompatability complex (MHC). This is a set of linked genes coding for glycoproteins through which monocytes/dendritic cells and B lymphocytes present antigens to receptor molecules on T cells (*Box 1.15*). In humans, the MHC is referred to as human leukocyte antigen (HLA) and the HLA region, located on the short arm of chromosome 6, contains at least 50 genes extending over 4 million base pairs.

Whilst genetic linkages in the HLA complex and autoimmune disease have been established, how they contribute to the pathogenesis of autoimmunity remains unknown. The strongest linkage has been with certain HLA-DQ β-chains (specifically the presence of aspartic acid at position 57). Since this is involved in the peptide binding cleft of the molecule it has been thought that it involves an error in antigen presentation. However, the exact mechanism remains uncertain.

The same can be said of the role of T and B cells in the pathogenesis of autoimmunity. T cells maturing in the thymus gland can certainly be deleted to prevent autoimmune disease (if they react too strongly to the MHC complex) and the same may be true of B cells. Whatever the mechanism of autoimmunity, there is no simple explanation of the sequence of events. Human autoimmune diseases only become clinically evident after considerable tissue damage or disruption has occurred and this makes it difficult to establish the course of pathogenesis and particularly its initiation. There are clearly familial traits of inheritance that can predispose to autoimmune disease, but the fact that only 30–50% of identical twins develop the same autoimmune disease suggests that other factors are involved, including those of the environment.

## Hormones, growth promotion and malignancy

Many hormones and growth factors promote growth in fetal and post-natal life and, thus, it has been suggested that they may also promote tumorigenesis. Whilst it is known that many growth factors such as the insulin-like growth factors induce proliferation in both normal and malignant cells, their precise role in the development of malignancy is unknown. There is, however, substantial evidence that human cancers do not result from a single genetic event but from stepwise genetic changes that result in the activation of proto-oncogenes and the inactivation of so-called anti-oncogenes or tumor suppressor genes.

Proto-oncogenes are cellular (c) genes that are thought to have been captured and recombined into transforming (viral) oncogenes (v) by certain retroviruses. Such genes code for growth factors or their receptors that are homologous or identical to the proteins coded by the normal cellular proto-oncogenes. For example c-erb B-1 codes for the EGF receptor whilst its transformed oncogene v-erb B-1 codes for a truncated form of the EGF receptor. Similarly c-src which codes for the IGF-1 receptor, can be tranformed into v-src that codes for a modified protein kinase. These receptors may be constitutively active, not requiring the presence of a ligand. Similarly, genes for the growth factors, e.g. c-sis and c-int that code for platelet derived growth factor beta chain and basic fibroblast factor, respec-

tively, can be transformed and inappropriately expressed in tumor cells. The importance of growth factors and their receptors in the phenotype of many malignancies makes them potential therapeutic targets.

Sex steroids are well known to cause or promote tumor growth in target tissues such as breast, endometrium and prostate. Thyroid, testicular and ovarian tumors, occurring in glands controlled by the trophic hormones TSH, LH and FSH may also be putatively included in the list of endocrine-dependent cancers. Two final points need to be noted with regard to growth factors, hormones and cancer. First, transformed cells may produce protein and peptide hormones providing an ectopic source of a hormone that is not under the regulatory feedback control of normally functioning endocrine glands. Second, tumors or their treatment may cause long-term endocrine complications.

## Genes, mutations and endocrine function

It has been said that the practice of clinical genetics has always been facilitated by the fact that those carrying mutations always present to clinicians. Clearly this is not always true as some mutations in crucially important genes will be uniformly fatal *in utero* and never present clinically. The genetic study of such, albeit rare, patients presenting clinically has provided an enormous amount of knowledge in endocrinology. When such mutations are in the germ line, such conditions present as familial diseases. Novel somatic mutations may present with expression only within specific tissues. Clinical examples of the effects of mutations are given in the text where appropriate.

Animal models (predominantly rodent) have also provided an enormous insight into endocrine diseases. Some of these mouse and rat strains were the result of naturally occurring mutations. More recently genes have been experimentally inserted (transgenic) or deleted (knockout) in mice and these animal models have provided considerable scientific knowledge. Not all the insights gained from such approaches can be directly extrapolated to the human and it has to be borne in mind that redundancy within endocrine and biochemical systems means that the phenotypic results of such experiments are not always as straightforward as expected.

As the human genome project reaches its target, it is to be hoped that the knowledge gained may be used to further knowledge of the causes of the polygenic disorders so common in endocrinology such as obesity, diabetes mellitus and autoimmune diseases.

# Clinical evaluation of endocrine disorders

It is important to emphasize the oxymoron that patients are bioassays of their circulating hormone concentrations. This is seen repeatedly in the clinical cases that form the springboards for the scientific knowledge throughout this book. Generally, in endocrinology patients come to attention for only two reasons – because of excess hormone action or through its lack. Each has a number of possible causes.

Excessive amounts of a hormone may be secreted by tumors. The normal feedback loop may be reset so that the amount of hormone secreted is abnormal only in the context of the concentration of the variable that it controls. In some cases, the relevant hormone may, in fact, be absent but its receptor may be constitutively activated. On the other hand, there may be a non-physiological stimulator of the receptor such as an antibody. The post-receptor signal transduction pathway may contain an abnormal protein that signals continued receptor occupancy. Finally, excess hormone may be ingested accidentally, deliberately or, indeed, therapeutically.

A lack of hormone effect may result from a lack of the hormone however caused (e.g. genetic deletion, damage to the endocrine gland, lack of a synthetic enzyme) or from the production of a biologically inactive hormone. The hormone receptor (or the down-stream signalling pathways) may be structurally abnormal and inactive leading to hormone resistance.

The pace of progress in endocrinology has always been dictated by the development of assays to measure the hormones. By and large, clinical endocrinology is limited to the measurement of hormone concentrations in venous serum or body fluids such as urine or saliva. Interpretation of the results of these assays should always take into account three factors – the clinical features of the patient, the concentration of the variable regulated by the hormone, and the concentration of other hormones in the feedback loop. For example, a serum insulin concentration can only be interpreted in light of the simultaneous glucose concentration and correct interpretation of thyroid, adrenal or gonadal hormone concentrations requires in many cases the results of the appropriate pituitary hormone concentrations. Tests of the feedback loops may be used; in general, in situations in which hormone concentrations are expected to be high, suppression tests are used and in those in which low concentrations are expected stimulation tests are used.

The practice of clinical endocrinology, like all branches of medicine, has been greatly facilitated by the technological progress in imaging techniques, for example MR and CT scanning. It has also been aided by the exquisite specificity of the biochemistry of individual tissues. Thus, radioactive iodine has been used for over 50 years to image the thyroid gland whilst recent techniques allow the use of radiolabeled agents such as metaiodobenzylguanidine (MIBG) or radio-labeled somatostatin analogs to visualize biologically active endocrine tissues. Examples of these and other techniques are given in appropriate clinical settings.

## CHAPTER 2

# The endocrine pancreas

## Chapter objectives

*Knowledge of*

1. Regulation of blood glucose concentrations
2. Physiological roles of insulin and glucagon
3. Definition, classification and causes of diabetes mellitus and its complications
4. Treatment of diabetes mellitus and its complications
5. Causes of hypoglycemia, their investigation and treatment

*"There was an old person of Dean,*
*Who dined on one pea and a bean;*
*For he said, 'More than that,*
*Would make me too fat,'*
*That curious old person of Dean."*
*One Hundred Nonsense Pictures and Rhymes.*
*Edward Lear.*

Glucose is a small, polar and, thus, water-soluble monosaccharide. Its physiological importance greatly outweighs its size for two reasons. The first is that it has multiple metabolic paths (*Box 2.1*). The second is that neurons have an absolute nutritional requirement for a continuous supply of it; in its absence they die. Thus, homoeostatic regulation of the concentration of extracellular fluid glucose is vital. It is achieved primarily by the actions of the hormones secreted by the pancreas, insulin and glucagon, although other hormones are also involved. Loss of insulin secretion or resistance to its actions (termed insulin resistance) causes an increase in circulating glucose concentrations and the disease diabetes mellitus (DM). As would be expected from the multiple metabolic pathways involving glucose, DM is a multifaceted metabolic disease although it is defined solely in terms of an elevated blood glucose concentration. *Clinical Case 2.1* illustrates many of the clinical features of DM due to a marked reduction in insulin secretion.

## Clinical Case 2.1:

A 23-year-old Caucasian woman presented to the Emergency Room with polyuria, polydipsia and 6 kg weight loss. She had not seen her primary care physician and her only question to the medical staff was to ask whether she had developed diabetes. Biochemical analysis of a blood sample showed that her serum glucose concentration was 15 mmol/l (normal fasting 3–6 mmol/l), urea 6.2 mmol/l (NR 2.5–8.0 mmol/l), potassium 4.2 mmol/l (NR 3.5–4.7 mmol/l), sodium 131 mmol/l (NR 135–145 mmol/l) and bicarbonate 24 mmol/l (NR 22–28 mmol/l). Analysis of urine showed mild ketonuria.

An understanding of the symptoms and biochemical results in *Clinical Case 2.1* requires discussion of the homoeostatic mechanisms regulating blood glucose concentration, that, at any instant, is determined by the amounts entering and leaving. Glucose concentration is increased by the intake of food and by glucose production in the liver and

**Box 2.1:**
**Metabolic paths of glucose**

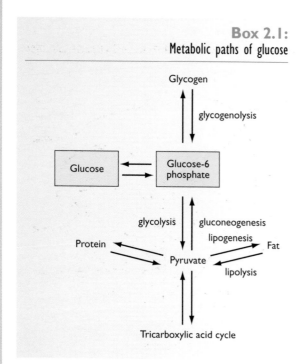

decreased by the uptake of glucose into cells (including those of the liver). The liver is, thus, the most important organ buffering changes in blood glucose concentration. Sitting at the head of the hepatic portal vein (*Box 2.2*), it directly receives digested nutrients and the two major hormones of the endocrine pancreas, insulin that decreases blood glucose concentration and glucagon that increases it.

## Glucose turnover

Carbohydrates exist as polysaccharides (such as starch), disaccharides (such as sucrose, maltose and lactose) and monosaccharides (such as galactose, glucose and fructose). Glucose absorbed from the gut is mainly derived from starch that, in Western societies, constitutes about 60% of the daily carbohydrate intake. The rest is in the form of sucrose (30%) and lactose (10%). In starch, straight chains of glucose molecules are held in amylose (approximately 20% of the total starch) whilst branched chains of glucose molecules are held in amylopectin (80% of the total starch). In the gut, these

large molecules are broken down by digestion but the polarity of the hexoses requires that absorption across the hydrophobic cell membrane of the gut involves specialized transport proteins (*Box 2.3*). Such is the importance of glucose, there are five of these glucose transporters (GLUTs) for the absorption and uptake of glucose into cells. These have distinct tissue distributions and features (*Box 2.4*).

After a meal, some glucose absorbed from the gut is used immediately by cells as a source of energy. Most is either stored in muscle and liver as glycogen or converted to triglyceride in adipocytes. An overview of the uses of glucose is shown in *Box 2.5*.

In skeletal muscle, absorbed glucose is directly converted to glycogen via glucose 6-phosphate. Whilst the same direct process occurs in the liver, approximately two thirds of the liver glycogen is formed from an indirect pathway. Glucose absorbed in the diet is first converted to lactate (a process termed glycolysis) in non-hepatic tissue (for example, the gut) and, in the liver, is converted to glucose 6-phosphate (via pyruvate), a process known as gluconeogenesis. In the liver, this may also occur from some amino acids (*Box 2.5*).

The breakdown of glycogen to glucose is known as glycogenolysis (*Box 2.5*). In the liver pyruvate can be converted to acetyl co-enzyme A (acetyl-CoA) that is not only important in the tricarboxylic acid (TCA) cycle but can also be used to form ketones or fatty acids. In addition, pyruvate can be transaminated to form the amino acid, alanine.

Circulating concentrations of lactate are usually about 1 mmol/l. In conditions such as extreme exercise or when cardiac output is low, glucose is metabolized to lactate. Lactic acid has a $pK_a$ of 3.86 (i.e. in aqueous solution 50% of lactate is ionized at pH 3.86). At a physiological pH of about 7.4, it is completely dissociated leading to the generation of $H^+$ ions and to acidosis if large amounts of lactate are produced and the blood buffering capacity is exceeded (resulting in lactic acidosis).

## Anabolic and catabolic phases of glucose metabolism

The metabolic use of glucose depends on the nutritional situation existing at any time. Before break-

Surface and gross anatomical relationships between the pancreas, small intestine and liver

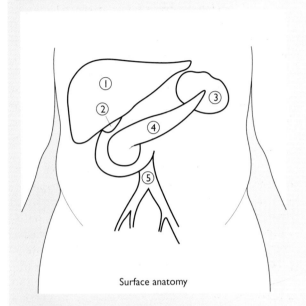

Surface anatomy

① Liver
② Gall bladder
③ Spleen
④ Pancreas
⑤ Aortic bifurcation

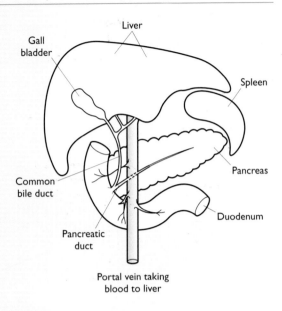

Diagrammatic representation of the pancreas and associated structures: pancreatic secretions and nutrients are transported directly to the liver by the hepatic portal vein.

fast after a 10 h fast (termed the post-absorptive state), the metabolic situation is fairly stable. Depending on prior nutritional state, the glucose stores (glycogen) in the liver may have been partly used and glucose production comes from a combination of hepatic gluconeogenesis and glycogenolysis. Glucose production and utilization are approximately equal at about 12 µmol/kg body weight/min. After breakfast, the blood glucose concentration rises. The magnitude of the increase depends not only on the type of carbohydrate ingested (i.e. its glycemic index) but also on the rates of digestion and absorption. The portal vein glucose concentration rises from, say, 4 mmol/l to around 10 mmol/l and the liver takes up some of this glucose. A smaller fraction is taken up by mus-

cle. Thus, in the anabolic phase of glucose metabolism, that fraction of glucose not directly utilized by cells is stored in the liver or muscle in the form of glycogen. In the catabolic phase (i.e. post-absorptive state), glucose is first obtained from glycogen stores (glycogenolysis) and then by gluconeogenesis. Insulin has anabolic actions on glucose metabolism, glucagon has catabolic actions (*Box 2.6*).

Knowing the average daily intake of carbohydrates, the volume of extracellular fluid and the mean glucose concentration of 5 mmol/l, it can be calculated that the glucose content of the entire extracellular fluid is replaced 25 times daily, i.e. approximately once an hour. Since the venous plasma glucose concentration may only rise by a

## Box 2.3:
### Absorption of monosaccharides in the small intestine

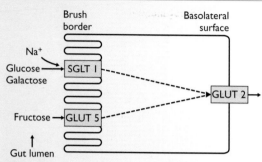

Glucose and galactose are actively taken up by the sodium ($Na^+$)/glucose transport protein I (SGLT I) which is stimulated by the presence of $Na^+$ in the lumen of the gut. Fructose is taken up by GLUT 5 (see Box 2.4). All monosaccharides are transported across the basolateral surface by the GLUT 2 transporter.

few mmol/l (from about 4 mmol/l to, say, 6 mmol/l), even after a large meal, it is clear that blood glucose concentrations are tightly regulated.

The liver is able to buffer changes in blood glucose concentrations after a meal because it sits at the head of the portal vein and has a large capacity to take up glucose. There are four reasons for this. Firstly, hepatic cells express the high affinity GLUT 2 transporter protein (Box 2.4). GLUT 2 transporters are not insulin-responsive and they are present at high density. Secondly, glucokinase, which phosphorylates imported glucose, has a high $K_m$ for glucose and does not undergo product inhibition i.e. glucokinase is not inhibited by its product glucose-6-phosphate that can be converted to glycogen. Thirdly, glucose itself can increase glycogen formation by modulating phosphorylation. Lastly, insulin promotes glycogen synthesis by increasing the activity of two key enzymes (see below).

## Box 2.4:
### The family of glucose transporters (GLUTs 1–5)

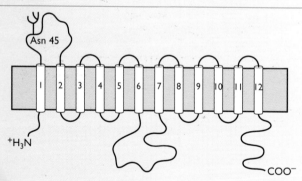

Model of a mammalian glucose transporter (approximately 500 amino acids long) showing the 12 transmembrane α helices. Members of this family of proteins, named GLUT 1–5, have distinctive tissue distribution and features

| Name | Tissue distribution | Important features |
|---|---|---|
| GLUT 1 | Brain, erythrocytes, placenta, fetal tissue | Low $K_m$* (~ 1 mM). Allows relatively constant uptake of glucose independent of the normal extracellular concentration (4–6 mM). |
| GLUT 2 | Liver, kidney, intestine, pancreatic β-cell. | High $K_m$ (15–20 mM). Allows intracellular and extracellular glucose to equilibrate across membrane. |
| GLUT 3 | Brain | Low $K_m$ (<1 mM) compared with GLUT2. Allows preferential uptake in hypoglycemia. |
| GLUT 4 | Muscle and adipose tissue | Medium $K_m$ (2.5–5 mM). Insulin recruits transporters from intracellular stores increasing glucose uptake. |
| GLUT 5 | Jejunum | Medium $K_m$ (~ 6 mM). Responsible for fructose uptake. |

*$K_m$ – the concentration of glucose at which there is a half maximal rate of transport. $K_m$ is inversely proportional to the affinity of glucose for the transport proteins.

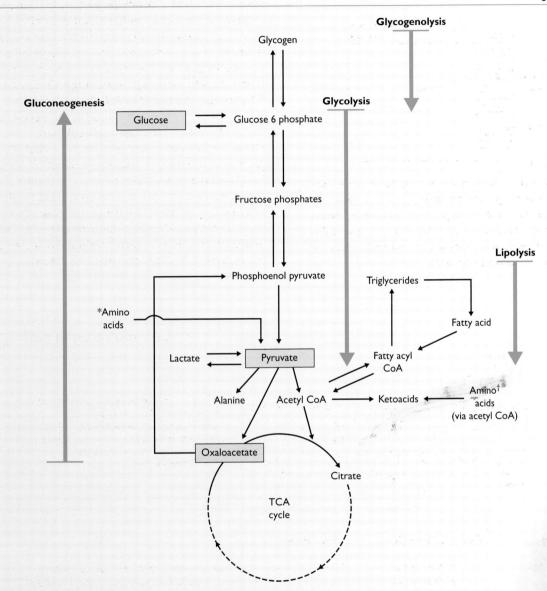

A highly simplified diagram showing an overview of glucose metabolism. Absorbed glucose can be stored in the liver and muscle in the form of glycogen. Alternatively it is converted to pyruvate by a process known as glycolysis and then to acetyl CoA from which it can be converted to triglycerides which are stored in adipose tissue. By a process of lipolysis, triglycerides can be converted back to acetyl CoA to enter the TCA cycle or form ketoacids, as can certain amino acids. Glucose can also be generated from some amino acids. This involves their initial metabolism to pyruvate. Since, however, there is no reverse reaction of pyruvate to phosphenolpyruvate, the pyruvate must be converted to oxaloacetate to overcome this 'block'. Oxaloacetate can then be converted to glucose by a process known as gluconeogenesis.

*Alanine, cysteine, glycine, serine, threonine, tyrosine
†Leucine, phenylalanine, tyrosine, tryptophan, lysine

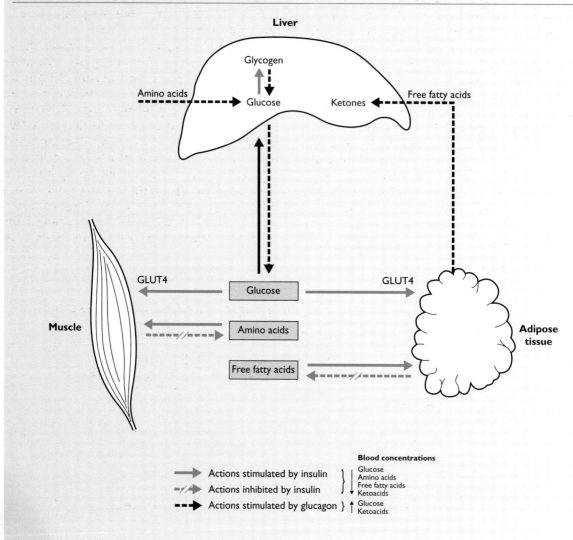

**Box 2.6:**
The actions of insulin and glucagon in liver, muscle and adipose tissue on the overall flow of fuels

Whilst the liver has a high capacity to store and synthesize glucose, nerve cells can neither synthesize, concentrate nor store more than a trivial amount. Glial cells, however, may have a small store of glycogen. Thus, cells of the nervous system have an absolute requirement for a continuous supply of glucose that is usually oxidized fully to carbon dioxide and water. In the post-absorptive state, the brain uses about 60% of hepatic glucose production, although with time, i.e. during prolonged starvation, the brain can adapt metabolically to use ketones. This reduces but does not abolish the glucose need.

## Actions of insulin and glucagon

The major targets for the anabolic actions of insulin are the liver, adipose tissue and muscle. At the cellular level, such target cells possess specific insulin receptors. The actions of insulin and glucagon controlling the overall flow of fuels are summarized in *Boxes 2.6* and *2.7*. In the liver, insulin promotes glycogen synthesis by stimulating glycogen synthetase and inhibiting glycogen phosphorylase although it has no direct effect on the GLUT 2 transporters and, hence, the uptake of glucose into hepatocytes. In contrast, insulin induces a rapid uptake of glucose in muscle and fat tissue by recruiting intracellular GLUT 4 transporters and, thus, increasing their cell-surface expression. As a consequence, muscle converts glucose to glycogen. In adipose tissue, glucose is converted to fatty acids for storage as triglyceride. Insulin also stimulates the uptake of amino acids into muscle. At the same time, insulin suppresses mobilization of fuels by inhibiting the breakdown of glycogen in the liver,

the release of amino acids from muscle and the release of free fatty acids from adipose tissue. This explains, in part, why patients with DM such as *Clinical Case 2.1* lose weight despite normal or increased appetite.

Glucagon has opposing actions (termed 'counter regulatory') to those of insulin, promoting mobilization of fuels, particularly glucose. Its primary action is on the liver where it binds to a seven-transmembrane G-protein-linked glycoprotein receptor and stimulates the production of cAMP. It may also activate the phosphatidylinositol signaling pathway. Through a subsequent cascade of intracellular events, glucagon ultimately stimulates the breakdown of glycogen to glucose and the production of glucose from amino acids (gluconeogenesis). In addition, it stimulates the release of free fatty acids from adipose tissue and, when these

**Box 2.7:**

Major effects of metabolic hormones controlling the overall flow of fuels

| | Liver | Muscle | Adipose tissue |
|---|---|---|---|
| Insulin | + glycogen synthesis<br>+ glycolysis<br>– glycogenolysis<br>– gluconeogenesis<br>– ketogenesis | + glucose uptake<br>+ amino acid uptake<br>– proteolysis | + glucose uptake<br>+ free fatty acid uptake<br>– lipolysis |
| Glucagon | + glycogenolysis<br>+ gluconeogenesis<br>+ ketogenesis | minimal action | minimal action |
| Cortisol | + glycogenolysis<br>+ gluconeogenesis | – amino acid uptake<br>+ proteolysis<br>– insulin action | + lipolysis<br>– insulin action |
| Growth hormone | + gluconeogenesis<br>+ IGFs/IGFBP | + amino acid uptake<br>– glucose uptake | + lipolysis<br>– glucose uptake |
| Epinephrine | + glycogenolysis<br>+ gluconeogenesis<br>+ ketogenesis | + glycogenolysis<br>– insulin action | + lipolysis<br>– insulin action |
| Thyroid hormones | + gluconeogenesis | + proteolysis | + lipolysis |

+stimulates
–inhibits
Abbreviations: IGFs, insulin like growth factors; IGFBP, IGF binding protein

enter the liver, glucagon directs their metabolic fate. Rather than being used for the synthesis of triglycerides, they are shunted towards β-oxidation and the formation of ketoacids (see below). Thus, glucagon is both a hyperglycemic and a ketogenic hormone.

By and large, it is the molar ratio of insulin to glucagon in the portal blood that governs the metabolic state of the liver. As insulin concentrations fall during the post-absorptive state, its inhibitory effect on glycogenolysis is removed whilst the increasing concentration of serum glucagon reduces glycogen synthesis by inactivating (by phosphorylation) glycogen synthetase. In the same way that glycogen synthesis and breakdown is controlled by the molar ratio of insulin to glucagon, so too is gluconeogenesis. Thus, in the post-absorptive state, glycolysis is reduced and gluconeogenesis increases. In the early post-absorptive state, glycogenolysis and gluconeogenesis occur simultaneously but, as the glycogen stores become exhausted, gluconeogenesis becomes the sole source of glucose.

Other hormones that also play major roles in the regulation of blood glucose concentrations include cortisol, adrenaline and growth hormone, all of which act to raise blood glucose concentrations (*Box 2.7*) and are, thus, considered to be counter-regulatory and, in excess, diabetogenic.

## Lipid metabolism – insulinopenia and diabetic ketosis

Lipids are stored as triglycerides (three fatty acids attached to a glycerol molecule) and transported around the body associated with proteins as lipoproteins. *Clinical Case 2.1* had mild ketonuria as a result of disordered lipid metabolism, and these changes that occur in diabetes mellitus cannot be over-emphasized. Indeed, it has been said that, had it been as easy to measure fatty acids and triglycerides as glucose, diabetes would have been better known as a disorder of lipid metabolism rather than that of glucose.

The overall action of insulin on the adipocyte is to stimulate fat storage and inhibit mobilization.

The remarkable effects of locally injected insulin on the accumulation of triglyceride into adipocytes are graphically illustrated in *Box 2.8*. Whilst this was likely to have been caused by *de novo* lipogenesis from glucose, it is generally believed that on a Western diet, triglycerides are usually accumulated in adipocytes by uptake from plasma (*Box 2.9*). This process is also stimulated by insulin-mediated activation of key enzymes inducing hydrolysis of very-low-density lipoproteins (VLDL) and chylomicron triglycerides into non-esterified or 'free' fatty acids (FFAs), thus making them available for uptake into adipocytes.

Insulin reduces fat mobilization from adipocytes by inhibiting hormone-sensitive tissue lipase and stimulating re-esterification of FFAs (*Box 2.8*). As insulin concentrations fall, FFAs are released from adipocytes into the circulation. Taken up by the liver, they can be esterified to form triacylglycerol stored in the liver and used either for hepatic energy needs or as the basis of VLDL formation. Alternatively, the FFAs may undergo β-oxidation that also produces energy for hepatic metabolism together with acetoacetate and 3β-hydroxybutyrate. These ketones are exported into the blood. The relative concentrations of insulin and glucagon regulate the rates of esterification and β-oxidation.

The uptake of FFAs into mitochondria, where β-oxidation occurs, is facilitated by the enzyme carnitine O-palmitoyltransferase-1. The activity of this enzyme is inhibited by malonyl-coenzyme A and when insulin concentrations are high so too are the concentrations of malonyl-CoA. Thus, β-oxidation is inhibited and ketone body formation is low. The reverse occurs when the insulin:glucagon ratio is reduced and ketone body formation increases. This, together with a reduction in insulin's suppressive actions on the release of fatty acids from adipocytes and increased gluconeogenesis, fuels ketone body formation (*Box 2.10*). The presence and degree of ketosis is a sensitive indicator of circulating insulin concentrations, a very important fact for clinical practice.

Ketone bodies are formed as acids (acetoacetic and hydroxybutyric). In cases of mild ketonuria, as seen in *Clinical Case 2.1*, the blood buffers these acids. When, however, ketone bodies are formed in

## Box 2.8:
### Action of insulin on the adipocyte

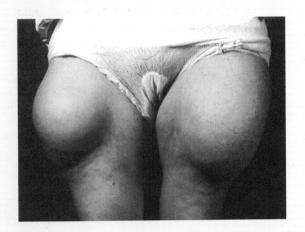

The effects of insulin on adipose tissue.

The patient developed type I diabetes mellitus in 1941 at the age of 17 years. She injected herself daily over a period of some 47 years with approximately 60 Units bovine soluble insulin using only two injection sites on her thighs.

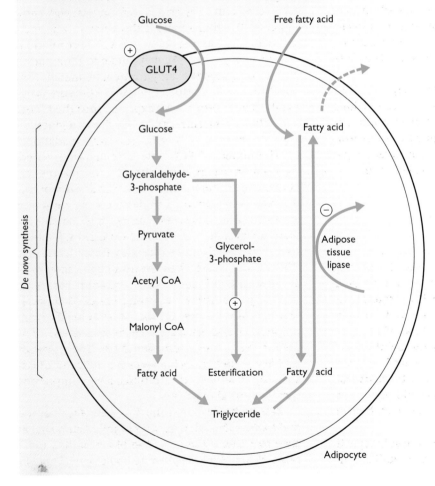

Biochemical reactions for the storage of triglycerides in adipose tissue.

Triglycerides may be formed by *de novo* synthesis from glucose which is stimulated ⊕ by the action of insulin on the GLUT4 transporter and induction of the dehydrogenase which converts glyceraldehyde-3-phosphate to glycerol-3-phosphate. This is required for esterification of fatty acids. Most fat stores, however, are generated from the triglycerides held in chylomicrons and VLDL complexes (see *Box 2.9*). Insulin stimulates lipoprotein lipase which releases the fatty acids from these complexes and at the same time inhibits ⊖ adipose tissue lipase which breaks down triglycerides.

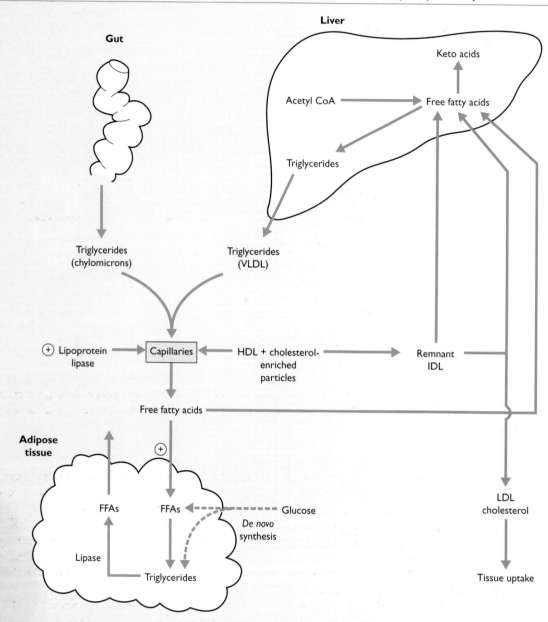

Triglycerides are absorbed from the diet in the form of chylomicrons and are only found circulating after a meal. In the post-absorptive state triglycerides are derived from very-low-density lipoprotein (VLDL) synthesized in the liver. Facilitated by high-density lipoprotein (HDL) and catalyzed by lipoprotein lipase in the capillary endothelium, free fatty acids (FFAs) are released for uptake into tissues. The triglyceride-depleted and cholesterol-enriched particles, together with the HDL, form intermediate-density lipoprotein (IDL) and remnants. The remnant particles and some of the IDL are taken up by the liver while the remainder of the IDL is converted to cholesterol-rich low-density lipoprotein (LDL) which is taken up by virtually all cells by LDL receptors. ⊕, effects stimulated by insulin.

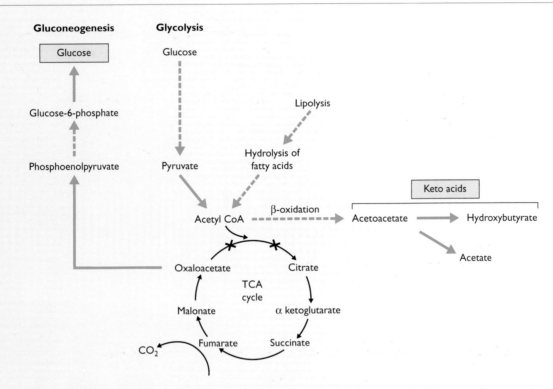

Acetyl CoA, formed from pyruvate and fatty oxidation hydrolysis, enters the TCA cycle. In diabetes or fasting, oxaloacetate is consumed by the gluconeogenic pathway. There is reduced incorporation of acetyl CoA into citrate (**x**) and hence acetyl CoA is converted to form ketone bodies.

large quantities, e.g. 7 mmol/min, the buffering capacity of blood (and the ability of the kidney to excrete protons) may be overwhelmed. This leads to a falling serum bicarbonate concentration, falling blood pH and a rising serum potassium concentration (due to the renal $K^+/H^+$ exchange) even though total body potassium is reduced as a result of the diabetic-induced polyuria. The effects of the acidosis on the chemoreceptor control of respiration lead to the characteristic deep, sighing (Kussmaul) respiration said to be characteristic of diabetic ketoacidosis but also seen in other forms of severe metabolic acidosis.

The interactions between glucose metabolism and the fatty acid cycle were noted more than 30 years ago. Elevated concentrations of free or non-esterified fatty acids (NEFA) increase lipid oxidation and decrease the activity of pyruvate dehydrogenase and phosphofructokinase, enzymes involved in glycolysis. The resulting increase in glucose 6-phosphate (*Box 2.5*) leads to a decrease in glucose uptake and oxidation. There is also evidence that increased concentrations of FFAs decrease non-oxidative glucose metabolism, i.e. glucose to lactate.

The changes in the concentrations of FFAs are translated into changes in the expression of genes by a family of nuclear transcription factors, the peroxisome proliferator-activated receptors (PPAR). After binding FFAs, these heterodimerize with the retinoid X receptor and interact with specific response elements in DNA. There are three PPARs ($\alpha$, $\beta$, $\gamma$) in the family and they share strong structural similarities with other nuclear receptors such as those for steroids and tri-iodothyronine. PPARγ plays an important role in the adipocyte (*Box 2.11*).

## Protein metabolism and the anabolic actions of insulin

The importance of proteins (or, more correctly, their constituent amino acids) in the control of blood glucose concentrations is that they can be converted to glucose by gluconeogensis or form ketoacids by ketogenesis. Alternatively they can be degraded and the released ammonium incorporated into urea in the liver via a biochemical pathway known as the urea cycle. In turn, this cycle is linked to the energy-producing citric acid cycle. Thus, whatever the catabolic fate of proteins, they are all energy-producing pathways.

Insulin promotes the uptake of amino acids (especially the essential amino acids leucine, valine, isoleucine, tyrosine and phenylalanine) into muscle and stimulates protein synthesis. Simultaneously, it prevents protein breakdown and the release of certain amino acids from muscle. Glucagon, acting predominantly on the liver, stimulates the extraction of amino acids from the circulation and increases the activity of the gluconeogenic enzymes whilst decreasing the activity of the glycolytic enzymes (*Box 2.6*).

It may be concluded that *Clinical Case 2.1* had symptoms resulting from the osmotic effects of hyperglycemia and weight loss and ketonuria as a result of a loss of the metabolic effects of insulin on adipocytes, skeletal muscle and the liver (*Box 2.12*).

---

### Box 2.11:
#### Peroxisome proliferator-activated receptors (PPARs)

- The 3 PPARs (α, β, γ) are all activated by naturally occurring fatty acids or fatty acid derivatives.

- PPARs belong to the superfamily of nuclear transcription factors.

- They heterodimerize with retinoid X receptors, bind to specific response elements (interacting in a complex way with protein coactivators or corepressors) and alter the transcription of genes involved in regulating nutritional and metabolic pathways.

- PPARs are also the target of newly developed pharmacological agents, the thiazolidinediones (e.g. rosiglitazone). Some non-steroidal anti-inflammatory drugs also bind to PPARs.

- PPARγ has three isoforms γ1, γ2 and γ3 resulting from alternative transcription start sites and splicing. PPARγ1 is the predominant form.

- PPARγ is involved in the regulation of:

    Adipocyte differentiation

    Adipocyte apoptosis

    Insulin sensitivity

    Extracellular lipid metabolism (e.g. increasing triglyceride clearance)

    Macrophage differentiation

- PPARγ is not expressed in skeletal muscle but PPARγ agonists may reduce insulin resistance in skeletal muscle via an indirect mechanism involving adipocytes.

- Mutations leading to ligand-independent activation of PPARγ have been reported in morbidly obese patients. Certain polymorphisms have been reported to have higher incidence in populations with higher body mass indexes.

- **Polyuria.** The maximal rate ($T_{max}$) at which the kidneys can reabsorb glucose from the glomerular filtrate is ~ 2.0 mmol/min. This is reached when plasma glucose concentrations are between 10–15 mmol/l. Glucose remaining in the tubule causes osmotic retention of water and a consequent diuresis with concomitant loss of sodium and potassium.

- **Polydipsia.** Mechanisms that control plasma volume and osmolality also stimulate thirst (see *Chapter 7*) to match the volume of urine lost.

- **Weight loss.** Insulin has anabolic effects on muscle and fat (*Box 2.6*). Loss of these effects is the main cause of weight reduction although calories are also lost in the urine.

- **Thrush.** The fungus, *Candida albicans*, thrives in conditions of high glucose. The glucose inhibits the functions of leucocytes and, hence, fungal infections of the mouth and vagina are common in diabetics.

- **Blurred vision.** High circulating glucose concentrations cause osmotic swelling of the lens of the eye.

- **Fatigue.** The mechanism for such fatigue is poorly understood but seen in all types of diabetes when circulating concentrations of glucose are high.

# Definition and diagnosis of diabetes mellitus

Diabetes mellitus is defined solely in terms of elevated blood glucose concentrations (*Box 2.13*) and because of the vital role of insulin in regulating glucose metabolism a reduction in insulin secretion and/or insulin resistance is a common cause of DM. The lability of blood glucose concentrations in the post-prandial state makes it important that diabetes is defined in terms that reflect the timing of the last meal. In most human populations, fasting blood glucose concentrations are unimodally (or normally) distributed. Thus, diabetes mellitus must be diagnosed in a way that encompasses as many 'true' diabetics as possible, avoids the inclusion of 'normal' people and, yet, remains clinically relevant. The current WHO and the more recent American Diabetes Association criteria are given in *Box 2.13*.

For many years, the administration of a large oral liquid glucose load (75 g) combined with measurements of the subsequent changes in blood glucose concentration has been used to test pancreatic islet cell function. But a number of factors, apart from loss of insulin secretion, affect the ability of the body to deal with such an unphysiological meal (termed 'glucose tolerance'). These include increasing age, physical inactivity, reduced carbohydrate intake and intercurrent illness, all of which reduce glucose tolerance. Asymptomatic people with decreased glucose tolerance and not meeting the criteria for DM are said to have impaired glucose tolerance (IGT). About 5–10% of people with IGT progress to DM each year.

*Clinical Case 2.1* is used to illustrate the presentation of DM but also because of her very unusual reaction to the diagnosis. She raised questions concerning the etiology of type 1 DM. The biochemical measurements in the presence of classical symptoms confirmed the diagnosis of DM. In response to being told this, she became alternately sullen and monosyllabic and truculently voluble. She refused to give herself insulin and the medical team was forced to admit her to facilitate any treatment, even though physically she was virtually unaffected by her disease.

She demanded antibiotics to treat the newly diagnosed disease and clearly considered that her DM had an infective cause. It became apparent that she thought her diabetes mellitus had been sexually transmitted. Some months prior to the diagnosis, she had returned home early from work to find her husband *in flagrante delicto* with her younger sister (whom she knew had diabetes). Whilst being aware of a genetic tendency for the disease, she was con-

**Box 2.13:**
Definition of DM and diagnostic criteria

**Definition**: DM is a group of metabolic diseases characterized by hyperglycemia resulting from defects in insulin secretion, insulin action or both.

**Diagnostic criteria**

A. *American Diabetes Association (1998)*

1. Symptoms of diabetes plus a plasma glucose concentration >11.1mmol/l obtained at any time of day and without regard to meals, OR

2. Fasting* plasma glucose >7 mmol/l, OR

3. A plasma glucose concentration >11.1 mmol/l 2 h after 75 g of oral glucose[†]

Impaired glucose tolerance is defined by a fasting venous plasma glucose concentration <7 mmol/l, and a value between 7.8 and 11.0 mmol/l 2 h after 75 g of oral glucose.

In the absence of unequivocal hyperglycemia and metabolic decompensation, these criteria should be confirmed by repeat testing on a different day.

B. *World Health Organization (1980)*

1. Symptoms of diabetes plus a plasma glucose concentration >11.1 mmol/l obtained at any time of day and without regard to meals, OR

2. Fasting plasma glucose >7.8 mmol/l, OR

3. A plasma glucose concentration >11.1mmol/l 2 h after 75 g of oral glucose[†].

[†]Impaired glucose tolerance is defined by a fasting venous plasma glucose concentration <7.8 mmol/l and a value between 7.8 and 11.0 mmol/l 2 h after 75 g of oral glucose.
*Fasting is defined as no caloric intake for >8 h.

vinced that her husband had passed the infective agent to her. This proved to be a source of enormous clinical difficulty (not to mention the strain it put on the marriage) but it highlights the possible interaction between genetic and environmental factors.

## Etiology of type 1 DM

Type 1 DM is considered to be a T-lymphocyte-dependent autoimmune disease characterized by infiltration and destruction of the islets of Langerhans, the endocrine unit of the pancreas. The initiation and promulgation of the destructive processes remain poorly understood and genetic associations, environmental factors and immune reaction are all considered as causative agents.

Studies in twins have clearly established a major genetic element to type 1 DM, seen in *Clinical Case 2.1* whose sister had DM. However, less than half of identical twins both develop the disease. Thus, it is considered that genetic elements form approximately 40% of disease susceptibility. Genetic associations with type 1 DM include those on the short arm of chromosome 6 (in the region of human leukocyte antigen (HLA) molecules, termed *IDDM1*), and regions of chromosome 11 upstream of the insulin gene itself (*IDDM2*). Together these putative genes have been numbered *IDDM1–IDDM17*, though some have only been documented in single families or small studies. Some of the genetic regions identified exert only a small influence and the precise genes remain unknown. More detailed studies have been possible in rodent models of type 1 DM and a number of genes have been implicated in the causation.

Type 1 DM is predominantly a disease of Caucasians living away from the equator and, whilst all ethnic groups may be affected, there are isolated areas of high incidence e.g. Sardinia. It tends to occur in patients <20 years of age; prevalence is approximately 0.2% of 20 year olds. Age of onset is no longer essential to its definition that requires both an insulin deficiency of such degree that ketosis occurs and usually the presence of markers of autoimmunity (*Box 2.14*). The geographical observations, together with the secular changes in some areas of the world where the incidence of type 1 DM is increasing, support the involvement of environmental factor(s) (*Box 2.14*). Overall, it occurs with equal frequency in males and females and there are increases in incidence around puberty and before starting school.

Whilst there is a body of experimental work in animal models and circumstantial evidence for infective causes in humans, direct evidence for infective agents as etiological agents of type 1 DM is sparse. Three mechanisms have been proposed by which infective agents may trigger autoimmunity. Damage of the islets and initiation of the 'innocent bystander' effect is thought to occur in congenital rubella, the best-known infective precipitant in the human. 'Molecular mimicry' (for example, structural similarity between the Coxsackie virus protein p2-C and the islet cell protein glutamic acid decarboxylase, GAD) is also postulated.

---

**Box 2.14:**
**Genetic, environmental and immune factors in the etiology of type 1 DM**

**Genetic associations**

- The clearest association is with class II human leucocyte antigens (HLA) coded on the short arm of chromosome 6. This locus has been termed *IDDM1*.

- The region around the gene coding for insulin is termed *IDDM2* and there are associations with loci on chromosomes 15q (*IDDM3*), 11q (*IDDM4*) and 6q (*IDDM5*).

- The number of mutations at other putative sites continues to increase but the exact nature of these associations is not known.

- Studies in twins indicate that approximately 40% of the risk of type 1 DM is genetic.

- Parental 'imprinting' occurs such that the risk of a child of diabetic parents developing type 1 DM is less if the affected parent is the mother rather than the father.

**Environmental factors**

- Viruses. Evidence for a viral etiology of DM in humans is circumstantial though in animal studies the evidence is good. Viruses implicated include rubella (congenital), mumps, cytomegalovirus and Coxsackie B.

- Dietary agents. Controversially, those implicated include cow's milk (containing bovine serum albumin), preserved meats (containing nitrosamines) and coffee.

**Immune markers**

- Type 1 DM is characterized by the presence of T lymphocytes within the pancreatic islets that may play a key role in islet destruction.

- Patients with type 1 DM have circulating antibodies against the islets. Antibodies against the insulin molecule insulin, the enzyme gamma-amino butyric acid decarboxylase (GAD) or the tyrosine kinase IA-2 have been well characterized, others are just termed anti-islet cell antibodies.

- Type 1 DM patients have an increased risk of other diseases that are considered to be autoimmune e.g. hypothyroidism, Graves' disease, pernicious anemia, vitiligo, Addison's disease.

Finally, production of microbial superantigens (proteins that facilitate the interaction of MHC class II molecules and polyclonal T-cells) as the result of activation of a human endogenous retrovirus has been suggested for some forms of adult-onset type 1 DM.

*Clinical Case 2.1* was repeatedly assured that there was no *known* direct sexually transmitted causative agent but, despite being given considerable emotional support, she remained unconvinced. However, she eventually accepted dietary advice and started treatment with subcutaneous insulin.

## Prevention of type I DM

It is generally accepted that the autoimmune destruction of the islet β-cells, once initiated, takes many months or years. The availability of genetic markers of predisposition together with serological markers of on-going autoimmunity such as antibodies to islet cells or insulin has led to trials of treatments to prevent type 1 DM in first-degree relatives of patients. None has proved very successful to date and studies continue.

## Structure, synthesis and metabolism of insulin and glucagon

Human insulin contains 51 amino acids (molecular weight 5700) and is structurally homologous to insulin-like growth factors 1 and 2 (IGF-1 and -2) and also to the ovarian hormone, relaxin. It is synthesized in the β-cells of the pancreatic islets. The gene for insulin codes for pre-proinsulin which is made up of a signal sequence (approximately 23 amino acids that are rapidly cleaved after hormone synthesis has been directed to the endoplasmic reticulum), and the B chain, connecting (or C) peptide and A chain (*Box 2.15*). A and B are joined together by two disulfide bonds between common cysteine amino-acid residues. The C peptide is essential to the formation of these disulfide bonds and is cleaved in the Golgi apparatus leaving the joined A and B chains which form the active insulin molecule. It is to be noted that the cleaved

C peptide is co-secreted with insulin, a point of great clinical importance (see below). Previously considered to have no physiological role, C peptide is now recognized to have G-protein-coupled cellular receptors and is likely to have some function in regulating blood flow and renal function.

Insulin is secreted in pulses every 10 min or so and has a $t_{1/2}$ in the systemic circulation of approximately 3 minutes. About 50% is removed by the liver. This is known as the 'first-pass' effect (i.e. the first time insulin passes through the liver). Insulin that has escaped inactivation by the liver has, of course, important regulatory actions on peripheral tissues. C-peptide is released in a 1:1 ratio with insulin and since it is not significantly removed by the liver and has a $t_{1/2}$ of 30 min its measurement has been used as an index of insulin secretion.

Glucagon contains 29 amino acids (molecular weight 3450) and has no disulfide bonds. The gene for glucagon encodes pre-proglucagon in the α-cells of the pancreas and this gene is a member of a superfamily of structurally similar genes coding for vasoactive intestinal peptide (VIP), gastrointestinal inhibitory peptide (GIP), secretin and growth hormone-releasing hormone (GHRH). After cleavage of the signal peptide, pro-glucagon is cleaved into active glucagon, glycentin-related pancreatic peptide (GRPP) and the major proglucagon fragment (*Box 2.16*). The same glucagon gene is also expressed in the gut where, after translation, it yields a different set of hormones from that of the pancreas (*Box 2.16*). The first-pass clearance of glucagon is also approximately 50% and its $t_{1/2}$ in the systemic circulation is approximately 3 min.

## Anatomical features of pancreatic islets in relation to hormone secretion and its control

The tight coupling between insulin and glucagon secretion in relation to blood nutrients is possible because of the anatomical arrangement of cells in the islets and the direction of the blood flow in each islet. Surrounded by the exocrine pancreas, there are approximately 1 million islets that consti-

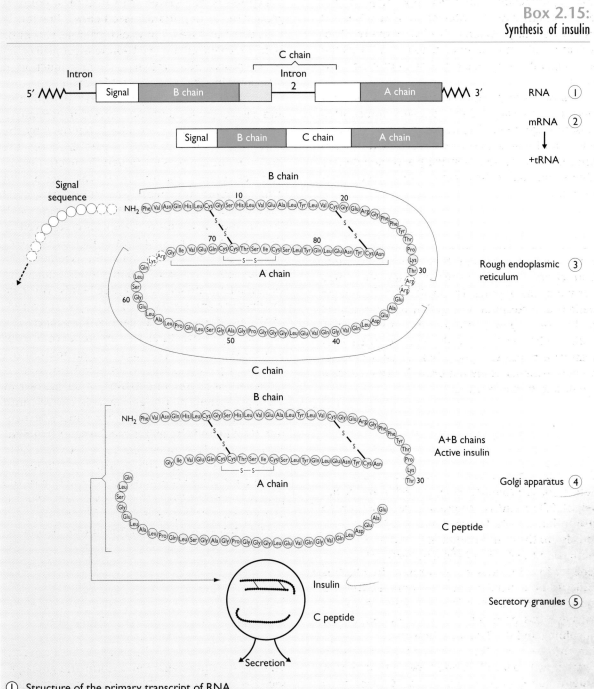

**Box 2.15:**
**Synthesis of insulin**

① Structure of the primary transcript of RNA
② Mature messenger (m) RNA after excision of the introns
③ Structure of proinsulin after cleavage of the signal sequence from pre-proinsulin
④ Cleavage of the C peptide leaving biologically active insulin
⑤ Packaging of insulin and C-peptide in secretory granules for storage and release

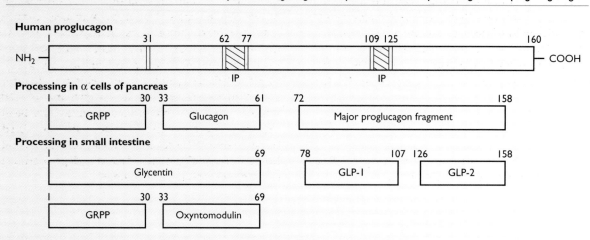

**Human proglucagon**

**Processing in α cells of pancreas**

**Processing in small intestine**

Schematic representation of the major products of proglucagon in the human pancreas and intestine. The processing of glucagon in the gut produces two important peptides – glucagon-like peptide 1 (GLP-1) and oxyntomodulin – which are known as incretins as they increase the insulin response to glucose. GRPP, glucagon related pancreatic peptide; IP, intervening peptide.

tute 1–1.5% of the total human pancreatic mass (*Box 2.17*). Each islet contains a central core of insulin-secreting β-cells and a mantle of glucagon-secreting α- and/or somatostatin-releasing δ-cells (*Box 2.18* Ⓐ) or a mantle of δ- and PP cells, so called because they release pancreatic polypeptide. The δ-cells are dendritic in shape (i.e. they have many branches) and send processes into the core of the islet.

Each islet is highly vascularized with small arterioles entering its core. These break up into a network of capillaries that form venules carrying blood to the mantle. Such an arrangement of blood flow allows high concentrations of insulin to bathe the α-, δ- and PP cells (*Box 2.18* Ⓑ). Additionally, the capillaries within the islets are fenestrated, facilitating peptide entry into the blood stream.

Insulin is secreted in response to increases in glucose concentration in extracellular fluid. This metabolic signal requires metabolism of glucose to pyruvate and appears to be detected by the activity of the enzyme glucokinase that catalyzes production of glucose-6-phosphate. This initiates an insulin-releasing signal involving a rise in ATP, clo-

sure of a $K^+$ channel, depolarization and opening of a $Ca^{2+}$ channel. This process is very rapid and secretion of insulin occurs within one minute of exposure to glucose (*Box 2.19*). Detection of changes in

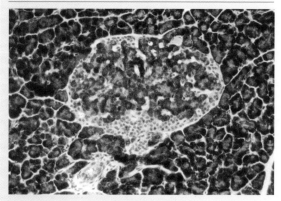

Histology of the pancreas showing a single islet surrounded by exocrine acini.

glucose concentration is facilitated by the presence of canaliculi containing interstitial fluid along the lateral surfaces of neighboring β-cells between the arterioles and venules (*Box 2.18*©). Concentrated in the microvilli of these canaliculi are the specific GLUT2 glucose transporters enabling the intracellular concentration of glucose in the β-cells to be essentially the same as that of the interstitial fluid.

## Control of insulin and glucagon secretion

The control of insulin secretion is complex (*Box 2.20*). The most potent metabolic stimuli to insulin secretion are glucose and amino acids that act synergistically. Triglycerides and fatty acids have only a small stimulatory effect on insulin release. In animals, ketoacids may also induce insulin release but this is insignificant in the human. In response to an oral glucose load, insulin secretion occurs in two phases (*Box 2.19*). The first phase represents the release of insulin stored in secretory granules. Approximately 10 minutes later when pre-formed granules have been depleted, there is a more gradual and sustained increase in insulin release that can last for several hours in normal individuals and is dependent on *de novo* synthesis of the hormone.

**Box 2.18:**
**Arrangement of cells and blood supply in a single islet of Langerhans**

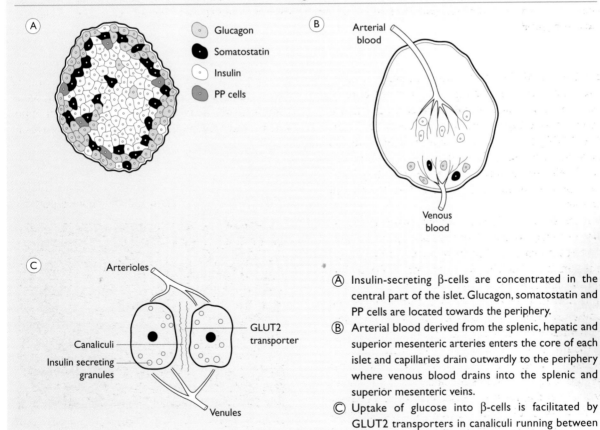

Ⓐ Insulin-secreting β-cells are concentrated in the central part of the islet. Glucagon, somatostatin and PP cells are located towards the periphery.

Ⓑ Arterial blood derived from the splenic, hepatic and superior mesenteric arteries enters the core of each islet and capillaries drain outwardly to the periphery where venous blood drains into the splenic and superior mesenteric veins.

Ⓒ Uptake of glucose into β-cells is facilitated by GLUT2 transporters in canaliculi running between the cells.

41

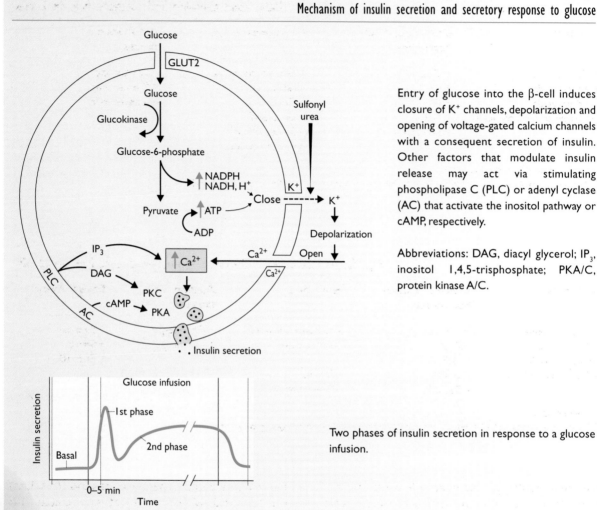

Entry of glucose into the β-cell induces closure of K⁺ channels, depolarization and opening of voltage-gated calcium channels with a consequent secretion of insulin. Other factors that modulate insulin release may act via stimulating phospholipase C (PLC) or adenyl cyclase (AC) that activate the inositol pathway or cAMP, respectively.

Abbreviations: DAG, diacyl glycerol; $IP_3$, inositol 1,4,5-trisphosphate; PKA/C, protein kinase A/C.

Two phases of insulin secretion in response to a glucose infusion.

The secretion of glucagon is stimulated by a reduction in blood glucose concentration. It is also stimulated by a protein meal, particularly by the amino acids, alanine and arginine (*Box 2.21*). These secretory responses are suppressed by the presence of insulin and glucose respectively (reducing transcription of the glucagon gene). Thus, ingestion of an ordinary meal produces much less variation in glucagon secretion than in that of insulin because of insulin's suppressive effect on glucagon release.

The secretion of both insulin and glucagon is potentiated by gastrointestinal hormones (termed incretins) that are released in response to orally ingested nutrients. Thus, an oral glucose load stimulates a greater insulin response than intravenous administration because one or more gastrointestinal hormones are released.

In addition to metabolic stimuli and hormones from the gut, insulin and glucagon secretion are also controlled by neural and paracrine mechanisms (*Boxes 2.20* and *2.21*). Sympathetic, parasympathetic and peptidergic nerves innervate the islets. Sympathetic nerves stimulate insulin release via β-adrenergic receptors (and inhibit via α-adrenergic

**Major factors controlling insulin secretion from the β-cells**

| Nutrients | Gastrointestinal hormones | Hormones | Autonomic nerves |
|---|---|---|---|
| + Glucose | + Gastrin | + Growth hormone | + Cholinergic |
| + Amino acids | + CCK | − Adrenaline | + β adrenergic |
| (+) Keto acids | + GIP | − Cortisol | − α adrenergic |
| (+) Triglycerides/fatty acids | + GLP-1 | + Glucagon* | |
| | + Secretin | − Somatostatin* | |
| | | − Other peptides*† | |

*Paracrine signals; † neurocrine signals
CCK = cholecystokinin; GIP = gastrointestinal inhibitory peptide; GLP-1 = glucagon-like peptide-1

**Major factors contributing to the control of glucagon secretion from the α cells**

| Nutrients | Gastrointestinal hormones | Hormones | Autonomic nerves | Environment |
|---|---|---|---|---|
| + Hypoglycemia | + Gastrin | + Growth hormone | + Cholinergic | + Exercise |
| + Amino acids | + CCK | + Adrenaline | + Adrenergic | + Stress |
| (Arginine/alanine) | + GIP | | | + Starvation |
| − Free fatty acids | − GLP-1 | − Insulin* | | |
| | − Secretin | − Somatostatin* | | |

*Paracrine signals
CCK = cholecystokinin; GIP = gastrointestinal inhibitory peptide; GLP-1 = glucagon-like peptide-1

receptors) whilst parasympathetic vagal nerves stimulate both insulin and glucagon release. This innervation accounts for the increase in insulin secretion that may occur before the entry of food into the gastrointestinal tract. Finally, somatostatin from the δ-cells inhibits the release of both hormones through a paracrine action (this has importance for clinical practice and is discussed in the context of *Clinical Case 2.5*).

## Type 2 DM

It is clear from the foregoing that the complexity of the regulation of carbohydrate metabolism in general, and insulin and glucagon secretion and their actions in particular, means that there are numer-ous ways in which hyperglycemia (and thus, DM) can be caused. Whilst type 1 DM is associated with loss of insulin production, type 2 is classically associated with insulin resistance. However, in many populations it is characterized not only by insulin resistance but also by insulinopenia (loss of β-cell function) and the relative roles of each in the etiology of type 2 DM may vary in different populations and remain contentious (*Box 2.22*). It is noteworthy in rodent models of type 2 DM that even severe insulin resistance is not associated with the development of DM. This suggests that DM does not occur unless there is a failure of β-cell compensatory hypertrophy or hyperplasia.

Elevated circulating concentrations of glucose have an autoregulatory effect in enhancing glu-

---

**Box 2.22:**
**The etiology of type 2 diabetes mellitus**

**Genetic associations**

- Studies in twins indicate that approximately 30–90% of the risk of type 2 diabetes is genetic.

- Prevalence of type 2 DM is very high in certain ethnic groups including Pima Indians in Arizona, Naruans in Polynesia, and Indian sub-continent Asians in the UK.

- These ethnic groups have a high prevalence of obesity. The 'thrifty gene' hypothesis proposes that during evolution of such groups the ability to accumulate triglyceride in fat tissue was a selection advantage for periods of famine.

**Environmental factors**

- Obesity (especially central), aging, physical inactivity. These increase insulin resistance.

- Poor fetal development. This (the 'thrifty phenotype' hypothesis) is thought to lead to metabolic sequelae predisposing to type 2 diabetes, as well as hypertension, lipoprotein abnormalities and coronary disease in later life.

---

cose uptake, decreasing hepatic glucose production and increasing insulin production. However, in DM the prolonged stimulation of the β-cells depletes the insulin granule stores. β-cells are thus unable to secrete 'pulses' of insulin and become 'blind' to changes in glucose concentration. Hyperglycemia may also cause peripheral insulin resistance as a result of a down-regulation (i.e. decreased numbers) of GLUTs in peripheral tissues.

These effects have been termed, rather loosely, 'glucotoxicity' although studies using animal islets of Langerhans suggest that the cells are not actually injured by high glucose concentrations (at least in short-term culture). Histologically, loss of β-cell function in type 2 DM is associated with amyloid deposition within the islets of Langerhans. It is also seen in insulin-secreting tumors of the islets (insulinomas) and the peptide has been termed amylin or islet amyloid polypeptide (IAPP). It is structurally related to calcitonin-gene-related peptide and may act to reduce gastric emptying.

Type 2 DM is a heterogeneous polygenic disorder which is much more common (in the UK) in Afro-Caribbean and Asian populations. It has to be distinguished from type 1 DM presenting in adulthood and rarer forms of inherited DM (see below). The next two clinical cases illustrate acute and chronic presentations respectively of type 2 DM.

## Clinical Case 2.2:

A 63-year-old Jamaican man was admitted from the Emergency Room to which he had been brought by ambulance. A medical history was obtained from his wife who had returned from work and found him unrousable. Until 4 days previously, the patient had been well, apart from treatment for high blood pressure. He was not known to have had DM but both his parents had had the disease in later years of life. He had developed a chest infection and, despite taking time off work, his health had gradually deteriorated. On admission, the medical team noted his height (1.65 m) and weight (81 kg) and estimated that he was about 20 kg overweight. They could find no signs of illness apart from physical signs of fluid depletion and the chest infection. He was barely conscious and responded only to painful stimuli by moving all limbs. The blood results were markedly abnormal. The venous serum $Na^+$ was 121 mmol/l (NR 135–145 mmol/l), $K^+$ 4.0 mmol/l (NR 3.5–4.7 mmol/l), $Cl^-$ 98 mmol/l (NR 98–109 mmol/l), $HCO_3^-$ 24 mmol/l (NR 22–28 mmol/l), urea 38 mmol/l (NR 2.5–8.0 mmol/l), creatinine 250 μmol/l (NR 60–110 μmol/l), glucose was 84 mmol/l (NR fasting 3.0–6.0 mmol/l). Analysis of urine when it was obtained by catheterization of the bladder was negative for ketones.

*Clinical Case 2.2* illustrates a number of issues. The first important clinical observation is that type 2 DM is an insidious disease and patients with type 2 DM do not necessarily know that they have the disease. Metabolically, it is important to note that despite the very high blood glucose there was no ketosis indicating that there was sufficient circulating insulin to suppress the drive to ketone body formation. The extreme hyperglycemia lowered the serum sodium concentration by its osmotic action causing cellular dehydration (attracting water out of cells). The renal failure (evidenced by the marked elevation of serum urea and creatinine) was caused by the osmotic diuresis producing polyuria exacerbated by the fever and general prostration (reducing fluid intake) of the pneumonia. Such severe episodes in which conscious level is affected (due to dehydration of brain cells) are termed hyperosmolar non-ketotic coma (HONK).

Type 2 DM has an inherited component, though the strength of its effect continues to be debated. Twin studies have been variously interpreted as showing that as much as 90% or as little as 30% of disease susceptibility is inherited. In populations such as that of the Pima native Americans or the Pacific island of Narua, as many as 60% of the population may be diabetic or have impaired glucose tolerance. In the UK, the Caucasian population has an overall prevalence of the disease of 4% whilst the Asian and Afro-Caribbean population prevalence is four times higher. Type 2 DM is a complex heterogeneous disease and much work remains to be done to clarify the precise genes involved in its etiology.

*Clinical Case 2.2* illustrates the two main environmental or acquired factors increasing the incidence of type 2 DM, age and obesity. The effect of age was reflected in the previous name for type 2 DM, maturity onset DM. Obesity markedly increases insulin resistance and also the likelihood of developing DM in a predisposed population. Other factors include a high-fat diet and 'Western' lifestyle. 'Lipotoxicity', the effect of increased concentrations of FFAs may also be involved. It was suggested nearly 40 years ago that relative skeletal muscle insulin resistance leading to increased deposition of triglyceride in adipose tissue was an evolutionary adaptation 'thrifty gene' allowing survival during periods of famine in hunter-gatherer populations. It is argued that exposure of such populations to cheap, easily available and plentiful high-fat foods in the twentieth century has led to epidemic obesity and type 2 DM.

Insulin resistance can arise as a result of mutations in the receptor itself. These are uncommon and many have unusual phenotypes (e.g. Leprechaunism or Rabson-Mendenhall syndrome) presenting in infancy. Insulin receptors are tetramers made up of two extracellular α-subunits, joined by disulfide bonds, and two transmembrane β-subunits each of which is joined to an α-subunit by disulfide bonds (*Box 2.23*). The binding of insulin to its receptor activates the intracellular tyrosine kinase on the β-subunits causing autophosphorylation of the receptor. In turn, the fully active tyrosine kinase phosphorylates a number of insulin receptor substrates (numbered IRS-1–5) and these can initiate a cascade of further events which ultimately alter enzyme activity, translocate glucose transporters to the cell membrane and stimulate or inhibit transcription in the nucleus. More than 70 mutations have been described and these have been classified according to the defect caused. Some decrease the rate of receptor synthesis whilst others impair transport of the receptor to the membrane or accelerate its degradation. Some decrease receptor affinity for the hormone and others impair tyrosine kinase signaling.

The vast majority of insulin resistance is, however, manifest by changes in the signalling pathways distal to the receptor. Studies on mice models (such as the IRS knock-outs) have thrown light on the mechanisms of insulin signalling. To date, the only defined defects in type 2 DM have been reductions in insulin receptor kinase or IRS protein tyrosine phosphorylation or PI3 kinase activation.

Epidemiological studies have suggested that people born with low birthweights are more likely to develop type 2 DM, hypertension and heart disease in later life. It has been suggested that poor early nutrition damages islet cell development and in the presence of a 'Western' lifestyle leads to impaired glucose tolerance and DM, the 'thrifty phenotype' hypothesis. It is to be noted that insulin is the major intrauterine growth factor and that inherited insulin resistance would be predicted to produce impaired intrauterine growth and later

## Box 2.23:
### Signaling at the insulin receptor

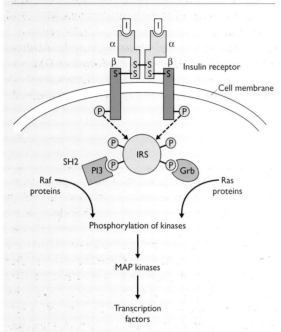

Insulin (I) binds to the two extracellular α domains of the insulin receptor that are linked by a disulfide bond (S–S). This induces phosphorylation (P) of the intracellular tyrosine kinase region of the two β-subunits which are connected to their α-units by a disulfide bond. Activated tyrosine kinase phosphorylates an insulin receptor substrate (IRS) and subsequent binding of proteins with SH2 domains. These include phosphatidylinositol 3-kinase (PI3) and Grb. Subsequent signal transduction linkages may involve Ras and Raf proteins with activation of MAP kinases and activation of nuclear transcription factors (see Box 1.10).

## Box 2.24:
### Etiological classification of diabetes mellitus

**Type 1 DM** – β-cell destruction, usually leading to absolute insulin deficiency
a) immune mediated
b) idiopathic

**Type 2 DM** – a combination of insulin resistance and insulin deficiency

**Other specific types**
- Genetic defects of β-cell function
  Glucokinase
  Hepatic nuclear factor 1α
  Hepatic nuclear factor 4α
  Mitochondrial DNA
  Others

- Genetic defects in insulin action e.g. type A insulin resistance, leprechaunism, Rabson-Mendenhall syndrome, lipoatrophic DM

- Diseases of the exocrine pancreas e.g. pancreatitis, hemochromatosis, cystic fibrosis

- Endocrinopathies e.g. acromegaly, Cushing's syndrome, pheochromocytoma

- Drug- or chemical-induced

- Infections e.g. congenital rubella, cytomegalovirus

- Uncommon forms of immune-mediated DM e.g. stiff-man syndrome

- Other genetic syndromes associated with DM e.g. Down's syndrome, Prader Willi syndrome or Wolfram syndrome

**Gestational DM**

type 2 DM. Indeed, the IRS-1 knockout mouse has this phenotype. Thus, the low birthweight may just be an early reflection of insulin resistance rather than an etiological factor *per se*.

## Causes of DM

A complete list of the causes of DM is dauntingly long. It is, however, possible to abbreviate it sub-

stantially whilst maintaining pathophysiological relevance and clinical utility (*Box 2.24*). It is obvious that all processes that damage islets cells are likely to lead to insulin deficiency whether they be trauma, pancreatitis, cystic fibrosis or the deposition of iron (hemochromatosis); these may, therefore, all be lumped together. Note that they do not give rise to type 1 DM since this is by definition autoimmune in origin (and idiopathic when markers of autoimmunity are absent). Note also that processes that damage *all* the islet cells and not just the β-cells lead to marked decrease in *both* insulin and glucagon. Such patients are likely, therefore, to need substantially less insulin and be less prone to ketosis.

Similarly, it makes little sense endocrinologically to maintain an inclusive list of all drugs that damage the β-cell unless the mechanism by which the damage is done is informative of the biochemistry of the cells themselves. Equally, long lists of excessively rare syndromes associated with DM serve only to test the memory unless the mechanism(s) (often due to single gene defects) underlying the DM add to our knowledge of β-cell function. This is exemplified in the following group of diseases.

## Genetic disorders of β-cell function

As discussed previously, type 2 DM was previously termed maturity-onset DM. It was also termed non-insulin-dependent DM since treatment with insulin was not required to prevent ketosis. Some forms of non-insulin-dependent DM may present at an early age, typically between 15 and 30 years. This has been termed maturity-onset diabetes of youth (MODY), a term used to define a relatively small percentage of diabetic patients who have a strongly familial form of diabetes mellitus (autosomal dominant inheritance). Patients with MODY do not have ketosis or markers of autoimmunity. Genetic studies have defined a number of subtypes of MODY. These include mutations in the glucokinase gene that lead to abnormalities in sensing the circulating concentrations of glucose (MODY2). Mutations in the transcription factor hepatic nuclear factor HNF-1α (MODY3), -4α (MODY1) or HNF-1β (MODY5) could lead to abnormal gene regulation in the liver or pancreas whilst those in insulin promoter factor-1 (IPF-1, MODY4) have been associated with pancreas agenesis in homozygous form (*Box 2.24*).

Mitochondrial (mt) DNA is double-stranded, circular, highly polymorphic and only inherited from the mother. Because there are potentially many mitochondria in cells, the mutational burden (or percentage of mutant mt DNA) may vary in different tissues. There is a tendency for mutant mt DNA to accumulate in slowly or non-dividing cells (such as neurons). Mutations at np3243 are believed to account for 1–2% of all non-insulin-dependent DM patients and may be found in MELAS syndrome (Mitochondrial Encephalopathy, Lactic Acidosis and Stroke-like episodes). Such forms of DM may be misdiagnosed unless the link of maternal inheritance and associated neurological features is noted.

## Counter-regulatory hormones and DM

Whilst most DM is caused by a loss of β-cell function and/or insulin resistance, it may also result from an excess secretion of the hyperglycemic (counter-regulatory) hormones – cortisol (see *Clinical Case 4.1*), catecholamines (see *Clinical Case 4.7*) and somatotrophin (see *Clinical Case 7.4*). The clinical features of these cases are discussed elsewhere but the effects of such hormone excess on carbohydrate tolerance have not been emphasized. Patients with these diseases frequently develop secondary diabetes or impaired glucose tolerance because the excess hormone-induced hyperglycemia may lead to insulinopenia and/or peripheral resistance to insulin. The mechanisms by which these hormones induce hyperglycemia are summarized in *Box 2.25*.

Although DM is compatible with a normal life span, on average it shortens life expectancy by about 30%. It causes damaging complications, the treatment of which absorbs approximately 10% of the NHS budget.

## Complications of DM

Diabetes is the most common cause of blindness in adults of working age, the most common cause of end-stage renal failure requiring dialysis or transplantation and the most common cause of non-traumatic amputation. It is an important factor in the etiology of heart attack and stroke. *Clinical Cases 2.3* and *2.4* illustrate the range and scope of complications and discussion will focus on the mechanisms of their generation.

**Box 2.25:**
Endocrine causes of secondary diabetes mellitus

| Disease | Excess hormone | Mechanism of disease |
|---|---|---|
| Cushing's | Cortisol | Peripheral insulin resistance<br>Increased hepatic glucose production as a result of peripheral catabolic effects |
| Acromegaly | Growth hormone (somatotrophin) | Peripheral insulin resistance |
| Pheochromocytoma | Epinephrine/ Norepinephrine | $\alpha2$ adrenergic inhibition of insulin secretion<br>$\alpha2$ adrenergic increase in glycogenolysis in liver and muscle and lipolysis in fat<br>$\beta$ receptor mediated increase in peripheral insulin resistance |

## Clinical Case 2.3:

In October, a 22-year-old woman was diagnosed as having type I DM. For just 3 days she had symptoms of polyuria, polydipsia and fatigue, and blood tests showed her 3 h post-prandial serum glucose was 19 mmol/l with a trace of ketonuria. She was started on a dietary regimen and twice-daily subcutaneous insulin but had only moderate diabetic control. One Saturday in December she noticed that she lost the sight in the left eye and then in the right eye on Sunday. Returning to the clinic on Monday with the help of her mother, her visual acuity was so reduced that she was only able to perceive hand movements up to I meter distance. Examination showed that she had lost the 'red reflex' (the red appearance of the eye seen, most commonly, in color photographs taken with a flash), indicating that she had developed acute cataracts. The Ophthalmology department confirmed acute diabetic cataracts. After a period of much improved diabetic control in hospital without benefit, she underwent bilateral cataract removal in two stages. One year later, she became pregnant during which her diabetes control was also poor. The fetus was large for the documented duration of the pregnancy ('large for dates') and delivery by Cesarean section was performed 3 weeks early at 37 weeks of pregnancy. The baby (*Box 2.26*) was very large at birth (4.8 kg) and developed neonatal hypoglycemia (serum glucose 0.6 mmol/l at 2 h of age).

## Clinical Case 2.4:

A 56-year-old Indian unemployed accountant was referred to the Emergency Room of the hospital by his primary care physician because of problems with his right foot. He had never attended a specialist diabetes clinic although he had had DM for an unspecified period of years. Physically, he was lean with a blood pressure of 160/80. His ankle reflexes were absent and he had, indeed, serious problems with his right foot (*Box 2.31*). After attempting to leave the department barefoot, it became apparent that he thought that God talked to him via the birds and that the universe was controlled by a dinosaur that had bitten his foot. He initially refused all treatment and was convinced that God would heal his foot through the further personal intervention of the dinosaur. Later discussion with his family revealed that he had been psychotic for 20 years but that he had always refused medical help. He had a strong family history of type 2 DM and had been known to have the disease for at least 15 years. Clinical examination demonstrated markedly reduced visual acuity and bilateral diabetic retinopathy (*Box 2.29*). He was in renal failure with a serum urea of 14 mmol/l (NR 2.5–8.0 mmol/l) and a creatinine of 199 μmol/l (NR 60–110 μmol/l). A 24 h urine collection showed that there was 1.5 g/d of proteinuria (NR <0.1 g/d).

---

*Clinical Case 2.3* like *Case 2.1* illustrates the rapid onset of the clinical features in type 1 DM once more than about 80% of islet β-cell function has been lost. It is reasonably certain that she only had diabetic symptoms for a few days or weeks before she was diagnosed in the autumn (the most common time of the year in the UK for type 1 DM to present). In less than 3 months, her diabetes had made her virtually blind. Such acute diabetic cataracts are rare. More usual are the chronic cataracts that typically develop over the age of 40 years and are more common in diabetics. Acute cataractogenesis may arise from an increased production of sorbitol through the polyol pathway

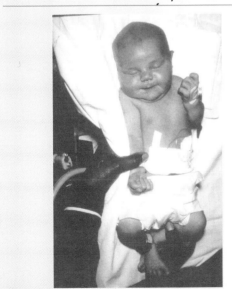

**Box 2.26:**
### Macrosomic baby of Clinical Case 2.3

Note the large size of the newborn baby and also the plentiful deposits of adipose tissue.

(*Box 2.28*) that may cause osmotic swelling and damage to the lens.

The underlying diagnosis of schizophrenia made it more difficult to be certain of the duration of type 2 DM in *Clinical Case 2.4*, but the complications have clearly taken some years to become apparent.

## Macrovascular circulatory changes

Most diabetic complications arise from damage to blood vessels. Those arising from accelerated atherosclerosis particularly affect the coronary, carotid and femoral arteries (and are termed macrovascular, *Box 2.27*). Those more specific to diabetes affecting the retina, kidney and nervous system (and termed microvascular) give rise to retinopathy, nephropathy and neuropathies respectively (see below).

The atheromatous plaques in diabetic macrovascular disease are no different from those in non-diabetics though they tend to be more common and more extensive. The processes through which diabetes is thought to induce atherosclerosis are, in part, due to the hyperglycemic effects on endothelial cell structure, platelet adhesion and stimulatory factors in plaque formation (*Box 2.27*). DM also has a prothrombotic effect.

## Microvascular changes – diabetic retinopathy, nephropathy and neuropathy

A number of hypotheses (that are not mutually exclusive) have been proposed to account for the etiology of microvascular complications (*Box 2.28*). An increase in the polyol pathway that reduces glucose to fructose increases the NADH/NAD+ ratio and decreases the intracellular concentration of myo-inositol, a precursor of phosphatidylinositols, has been suggested. The increased NADH:NAD+ ratio (reflecting 'oxidative stress') leads to increased protein kinase C activation and increased intracellular glyceraldehyde concentration. Non-enzymic glycation of proteins occurs (the same chemical reaction that causes the browning of a peeled apple). Such protein glycation may affect protein

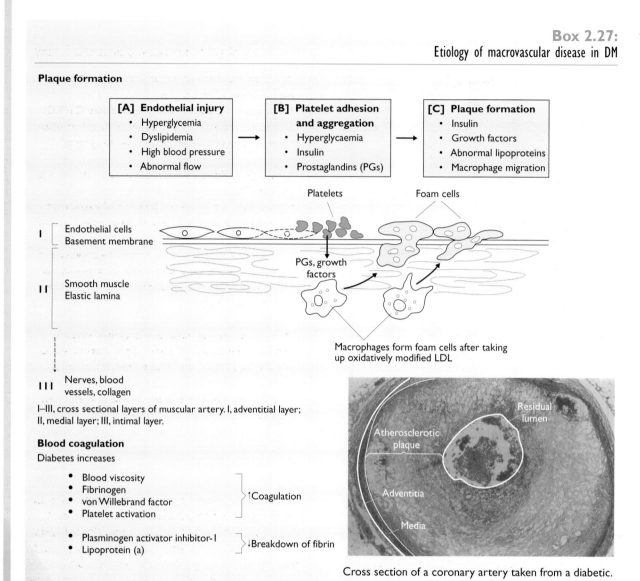

**Plaque formation**

| [A] Endothelial injury | [B] Platelet adhesion and aggregation | [C] Plaque formation |
|---|---|---|
| • Hyperglycemia | • Hyperglycaemia | • Insulin |
| • Dyslipidemia | • Insulin | • Growth factors |
| • High blood pressure | • Prostaglandins (PGs) | • Abnormal lipoproteins |
| • Abnormal flow | | • Macrophage migration |

Platelets

Foam cells

PGs, growth factors

I   Endothelial cells
    Basement membrane

II  Smooth muscle
    Elastic lamina

III Nerves, blood
    vessels, collagen

Macrophages form foam cells after taking up oxidatively modified LDL

I–III, cross sectional layers of muscular artery. I, adventitial layer; II, medial layer; III, intimal layer.

**Blood coagulation**

Diabetes increases

- Blood viscosity
- Fibrinogen
- von Willebrand factor
- Platelet activation

  }↑Coagulation

- Plasminogen activator inhibitor-1
- Lipoprotein (a)

  }↓Breakdown of fibrin

Residual lumen

Atherosclerotic plaque

Adventitia

Media

Cross section of a coronary artery taken from a diabetic.

function and, thus, alter the structure and function of the microvasculature or lens of the eye. Glycation of proteins such as hemoglobin (hemoglobin $A_{1c}$) may be used as an index of diabetic control.

The structural changes in the microvasculature include thickening of the basement membrane of capillaries, affecting both their permeability and structural integrity, probably via increased synthesis and reduced catabolism of glycoproteins. *Clinical*

*Case 2.4* had retinopathy and renal failure as a result of his DM. Whilst microvascular changes can be seen in almost all tissues of the body, the poorly supported capillaries of the retina and kidney are very vulnerable in DM. Examination of the microcirculation of the retina with an ophthalmoscope provides a valuable way of assessing the degree of structural and functional microangiopathy.

Retinopathy is usually graded into background and proliferative retinopathy (*Box 2.29*). Tiny hem-

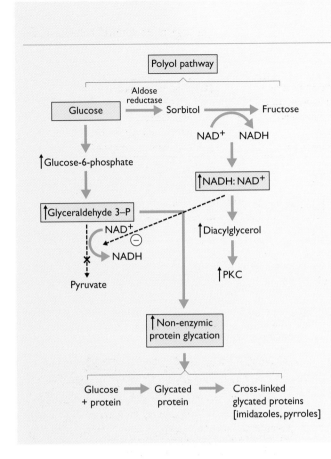

**Box 2.28:**
Etiology of microvascular diabetic complications

Increased activation of the polyol pathway increases the $NADH:NAD^+$ ratio. This:

- increases the activation of protein kinase C (PKC)
- reduces activity of 3-phosphate dehydrogenase which converts glyceraldehyde 3-P to pyruvate

Excess glyceraldehyde induces non-enzymic protein glycation. This:

- alters the structure and function of extracellular matrix proteins e.g. basement membrane of blood vessels
- induces interactions with intracellular receptors which stimulates prothrombic changes in the endothelial surface through release of cytokines and growth factors

In some tissues sorbitol accumulation leads to a decrease in intracellular myoinositol, a precursor of phosphoinositides, and additional deleterious effects.

Note: Aldose reductase is only found in nerve, lens, retina, glomerulus and blood vessel wall.

orrhages and areas of capillary exudate are characteristic of background retinopathies. They do not cause visual impairments, unless they encroach on the macula. When they do aggregate on the macula, visual acuity is reduced and the retinopathy is classified as a maculopathy. Background retinopathy may progress to proliferative retinopathy because the ischemia, resulting from the damaged capillaries, induces growth of new capillaries (angiogenesis). These new vessels are fragile and bleed readily into the vitreous humor and, if the proliferation is left untreated, will lead to total blindness within 5 years. Proliferative retinopathy is prevented by laser photocoagulation of the retina. This is believed to remove the source of growth factors released from the leukocytes that accumulate in the venule end of the capillaries as a result of their structural changes.

The first clinical sign of nephropathy in a diabetic patient is the presence of small amounts of protein in the urine (termed microalbuminuria). Once established, it leads, over a period of years, to larger amounts of proteinuria and chronic renal failure. Hypertension develops at about the same time in type 1 DM but may already be established in type 2 DM. Uncontrolled hypertension is a major factor in the progression of DM complications, particularly nephropathy.

Diabetes has many effects on the nervous system (*Box 2.30*) and whilst the majority of these are thought to arise from metabolic effects, some such as the cranial neuropathies or the mononeuropathies may arise as a result of microvascular occlusion which removes the blood supply to individual nerve bundles. Several studies have shown that careful glycemic control may reduce

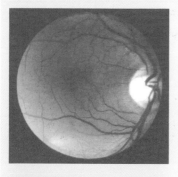

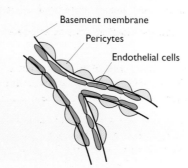

Basement membrane

Pericytes

Endothelial cells

(A) Normal eye and intact blood supply. The retina is part of the brain and the tight junctions between the endothelial cells maintain the blood–retinal barrier.

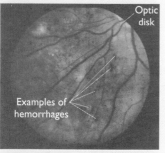

Optic disk

Examples of hemorrhages

Increased blood flow

Thickening of basal lamina

Loss of pericytes

Hemorrhage

(B) Early features of retinopathy include thickening of basement membrane and loss of pericytes that normally wrap themselves around the capillaries and may control blood flow. Capillary permeability and blood flow is increased causing tiny hemorrhages and accumulation of serum as hard exudates.

(C) Maculopathy where exudates occur on the macula and reduce visual acuity.

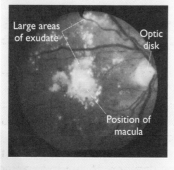

Large areas of exudate

Optic disk

Position of macula

Activated leukocytes

Growth factors

Ruptured basement membrane

Growth of endothelial cells

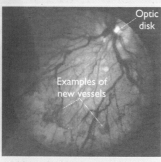

Optic disk

Examples of new vessels

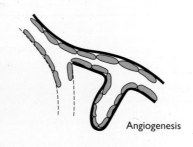

Angiogenesis

(D) Structural changes in the capillary and prothrombic serum changes cause capillary closure and ischemia. Leukocytes accumulate in the venule end of the capillary and their production of growth factors induces angiogenesis. The new blood vessels are fragile and rupture easily. Hemorrhages into the vitreous humor lead to loss of vision.

These clinical photographs are available in color on the website.

**Progressive neuropathies**: gradual in onset, progressive and associated with other diabetic complications.

- Distal neuropathy, predominantly sensory ('glove and stocking'); may be associated with numbness or with altered or reduced sensation.

- Autonomic neuropathy; may be associated with other forms of neuropathy and be asymptomatic or give rise to most disagreeable symptoms including sweating after eating (gustatory sweating), postural hypotension, diarrhea, vomiting from delayed stomach emptying (termed gastroparesis), and impotence. Gustatory sweating is the most common.

- Diffuse small-fiber neuropathy; commonly associated with symptomatic autonomic neuropathy, ulceration of the feet and disruption of the bones of the feet (termed Charcot arthropathy). It may have a different etiology from other forms of neuropathy and some have suggested an autoimmune cause. This is fortunately a less common neuropathy that affects young type I DM patients in their 20s and 30s, particularly women.

**Reversible neuropathies**: sudden onset; not necessarily associated with other diabetic complications nor related to the duration of DM.

- Mononeuropathies: cause symptoms related to the nerve or nerve root involved and sudden onset is often attributed to vascular occlusion of blood supply to the nerve. The most common nerves to be affected are the femoral nerve leading to pain, and sometimes muscle wasting, in the anterior thigh. Most commonly seen in middle-aged patients and normally recovers, though slowly. Cranial neuropathies usually affect the 3rd and 6th nerves.

- Compression neuropathies: diabetic nerves are more readily damaged by compression. Median (carpal tunnel syndrome), ulnar and lateral popliteal neuropathies may occur more frequently than in non-diabetic people.

the prevalence and severity of diabetic complications.

The insidious nature of the onset of type 2 DM means that about 20% of patients have microvascular changes at the time of diagnosis indicating that they had elevated blood glucose concentrations for a considerable period prior to presentation. This has implications for the screening for type 2 DM in predisposed populations.

## Diabetes and the neuropathic foot

It is clear from the attempt by *Clinical Case 2.4* to leave the Emergency Room barefoot that his right foot must have been painless, despite its appearance (*Box 2.31*). This patient had a neuropathic foot, one of the most common neurological sequelae of the disease; it is usually bilateral and symmetrical. The problem in this man's right foot arose because of a progressive distal sensory neuropathy (*Box 2.30*) resulting from the metabolic effects of

DM on the nervous system. This predisposed the foot to unnoticed injury. His poor footwear led to an ulcer that was secondarily infected.

Angiography confirmed that macrovascular disease, which causes arterial ischemia and makes tissues vulnerable, played no role in the pathology of this man's foot problems (*Box 2.31*). He was treated with bed rest, local chiropodial surgery to the ulcer, intravenous antibiotics and improved control of blood glucose concentrations. He refused major surgery on his leg because his belief in the dinosaur remained unwavering, despite medication for his schizophrenia. He needed many months in hospital and his mental state raised medicolegal issues regarding his ability to give consent (see Website).

## Diabetes and insulin resistance of pregnancy

One of the dominant metabolic effects of normal pregnancy is an increase in insulin resistance, probably induced by placental hormones including

## Box 2.31: Angiograms and feet of two diabetic patients

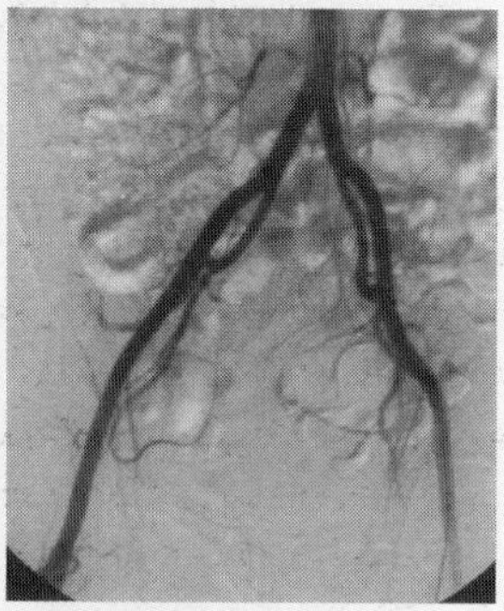

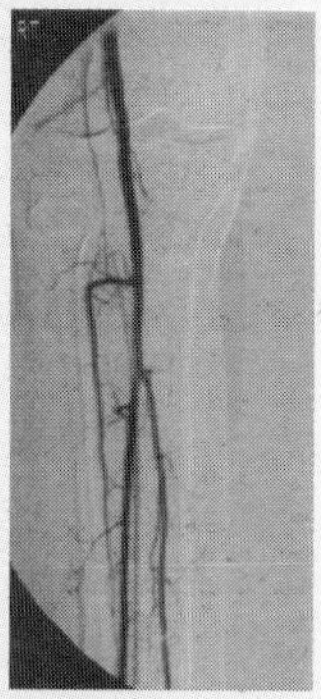

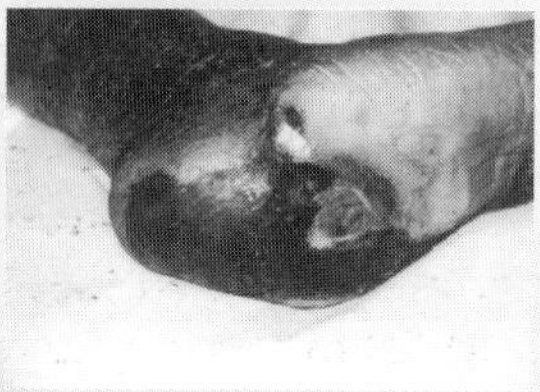

Neuropathic ulcers tend to be at points of pressure or wear

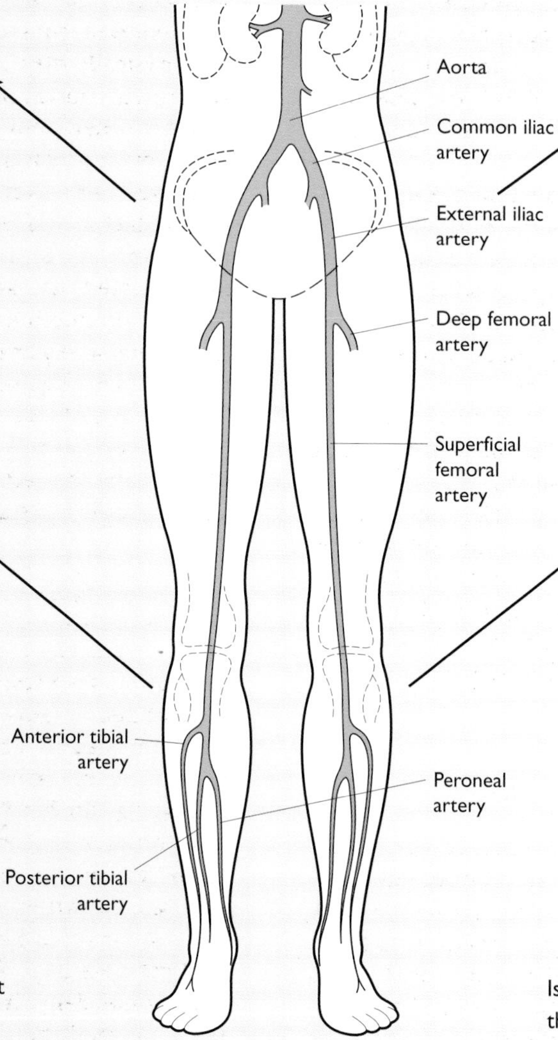
Aorta
Common iliac artery
External iliac artery
Deep femoral artery
Superficial femoral artery
Anterior tibial artery
Peroneal artery
Posterior tibial artery

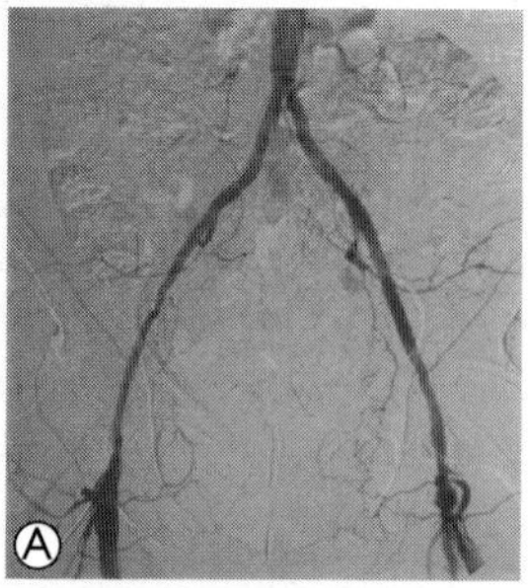
A

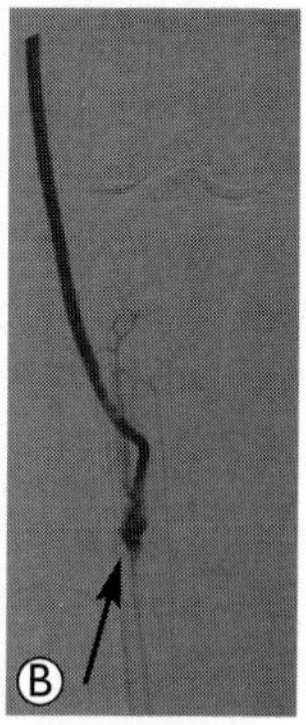
B

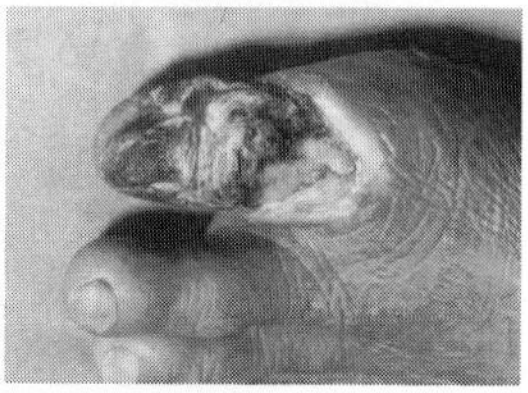

Ischemic lesions tend to occur at the ends of toes

Angiogram: A fine tube is inserted in the femoral artery in the groin and passed into the lower aorta. After a radiopaque dye is rapidly injected, a series of X-rays is taken. The background bone and muscle are removed from the pictures digitally so only appear as 'ghosts'.

Left: The angiogram and foot of *Clinical Case 2.4*. Angiogram was normal showing absence of macrovascular disease. The 'dinosaur bite' (ulcer), towards the heel, was the result of a neuropathic foot.

Right: The angiogram and foot of a 65-year-old diabetic smoker. Angiogram was abnormal showing macrovascular disease. Very little dye entered the profunda femoris arteries and at point Ⓐ her femoral artery had been surgically replaced by a vein that runs to the popliteal artery Ⓑ. Blood flow to the toe was minimal causing a typical diabetic ischemic toe.

These images are available on the website.

progesterone and placental lactogen. This leads to higher postprandial glucose concentrations that are considered to improve fetal growth; it is termed 'facilitated anabolism'. Fasting glucose concentrations decrease as a result of placental glucose transfer and in the later stages of pregnancy, there is also enhanced maternal lipolysis. This is considered to spare glucose for the fetus and is termed 'accelerated starvation'.

In genetically predisposed women, the normal insulin resistance of pregnancy may lead to the diagnosis of DM for the first time, termed 'gestational diabetes'. This may disappear within hours of giving birth depending on individual factors such as islet β-cell function and predisposing factors such as obesity. Women with pre-existing DM require higher doses of insulin during pregnancy and patients who are usually controlled using oral hypoglycemic agents are transferred to insulin at this time.

The effects of pregnancy-induced insulin resistance in women with DM lead to poorer control of blood glucose and also an increased likelihood of ketoacidosis. The hyperglycemia in early pregnancy has considerable effects on the development of the fetal pancreas. Maternal ketoacidosis leads to fetal loss.

## Development of the pancreas: effects of DM on organogenesis

The pancreas develops from two buds of gut endoderm termed the ventral and dorsal initially though they are affected by gut rotation (*Box 2.32*). The islets arise from specialized buds of the cells that give rise to the pancreatic ducts and exocrine cells. Insulin is present within the fetal pancreas by 9 weeks gestation. Islet development in both animal models and in humans is affected by the metabolic environment. Poor maternal diabetic control in early pregnancy leads to an increase in fetal islet β-cell mass. This programming may continue during later pregnancy so that the increase in β-cell mass may continue to have fetal effects even though maternal DM control has improved.

Poor DM control at the time of fetal organogenesis is teratogenic, producing malformations of the heart, nervous system and skeleton in particular. The terato-

genicity is related to the degree of diabetic control and has been termed 'fuel-mediated teratogenesis'.

The patient in *Clinical Case 2.4*, who became pregnant a year after her diabetic cataracts had been removed, subsequently delivered a very large and physically disproportionate baby due to fetal overgrowth (macrosomia – *Box 2.26*). This was caused by her poorly controlled hyperglycemia which, by transplacental transfer, caused increased fetal insulin secretion. Insulin, like IGF-1 and -2 is a growth factor and is the major factor for fetal growth *in utero*. In addition, diabetic pregnancies are associated with an increased incidence of miscarriage, intrauterine death, pre-eclamptic toxemia and neonatal respiratory distress syndrome. Tight control of blood glucose during pregnancy can prevent many of these problems but the high incidence of congenital malformations (approximately 10%) means that efforts to achieve good glucose control should be established prior to conception.

## Treatment of DM – rationale and practical considerations

It is important to emphasize basic principles.

Treatment targets should be clinically relevant. Thus, the degree of glycemic control set for a 20-year-old pregnant woman will not be the same as that, say, for her 80-year-old grandmother. The monitoring of glucose control should be practical and reflect these clinical targets. Thus, measuring glucose concentrations in urine may be all that is required for some patients whilst others may need to check capillary blood glucose concentrations several times daily. Within these limitations, it is to be emphasized that DM complications are less in those with better DM control.

Insulinopenia of such a degree as to cause ketosis requires immediate insulin therapy. A corollary of this is that keto(acido)sis is *always* a medical emergency. The degree of ketosis and acidosis should be carefully documented and monitored during therapy. In an established diabetic, the cause of the ketoacidosis should always be sought and particular attention should be paid to the possibility of poor DM management, infection and vascular events (such as myocardial infarct or stroke)

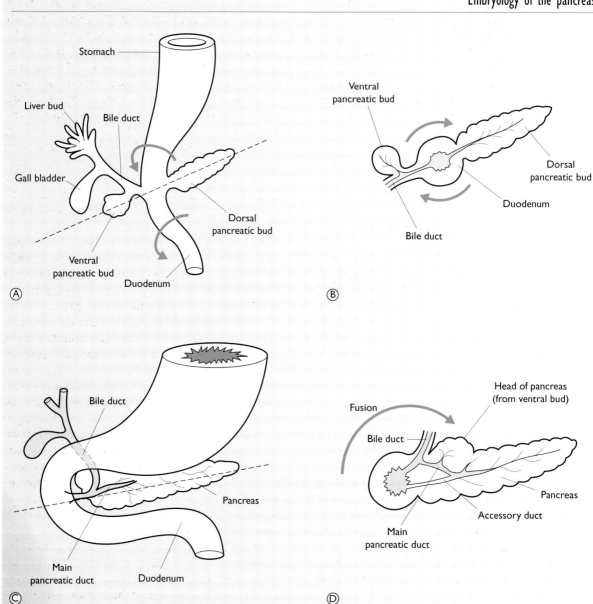

Schematic drawings of the development of the human pancreas at 6 weeks Ⓐ and Ⓑ and 8 weeks Ⓒ and Ⓓ gestation. Growth and rotation of the duodenum (indicated by arrows in Ⓐ and Ⓑ cause movement of the ventral pancreatic bud towards the dorsal bud and their eventual fusion Ⓓ. Union of the distal part of the dorsal pancreatic duct and the entire ventral pancreatic duct forms the main pancreatic duct. The proximal part of the dorsal pancreatic duct usually disappears but it may persist as an accessory duct Ⓓ. Dotted lines indicate the level of the corresponding diagrammatic transverse sections shown on the right.

The genetic implications of the diagnosis for the rest of the family should also be given consideration. Relatives of diabetic probands should be screened on a regular basis. Prevention of DM will receive greater attention as the worldwide epidemic threatens. For type 2 DM, prevention or reduction of obesity and the use of exercise programs has been shown to prevent or delay disease onset. Large-scale (and expensive) public health measures to reduce obesity have not proved successful to date. In type 1 DM, a variety of preventative measures are under consideration or trial.

Dietary modification is fundamental to the long-term treatment of *all* forms of DM. The generally recommended diet, the so-called 'healthy-eating diet', contains >55% carbohydrate, 10–15% protein and <30% fat (<10% saturates) and, in general, needs no modification other than to add an injunction to reduce sources of simple sugars (<25 g per day added sucrose) and to replace them with complex carbohydrates. In the case of type 1 DM there is a requirement to balance the amount of carbohydrate with the insulin dose at any meal, with the proviso that this may be altered by the amount of exercise to be done. The need for between meal or bedtime carbohydrate snacks is dependent on the time course of action of the insulin used. Alcohol should be taken in moderation and smoking should be scrupulously avoided.

Treatable causes of insulin resistance should be removed or minimized. The main one is obesity. There is good evidence that even modest weight loss (say 5–10 kg in an adult) results in improved diabetic control and, long-term, in a decrease in cardiovascular events and deaths. Regular exercise (that improves insulin sensitivity) should be encouraged. Generally, this succeeds best if it is incorporated into normal life; examples include cycling or walking to work and using the stairs rather than the elevator. It is important to emphasize that significant weight loss cannot easily be achieved by increased exercise *alone*. Calculating the exercise required to consume 1 kg fat (based on the assumption that this contains 7000 kcal/ 30 000 kJ energy) one would need to jog for about 14.5 h, play football for 12.7 h or cycle 175 km.

Drug therapies (*Boxes 2.33–2.35*) should be kept to the minimum that is effective. They should not be used as an alternative to changes in eating patterns, but as adjuncts. Glucosidase inhibitors, such as acarbose, may help reduce post-prandial peaks of serum glucose, but have major gastrointestinal side effects. The effects of the soluble form of amylin pramlintide on gastric emptying (and, thus, slowing glucose absorption) in type 1 DM have been studied. Agents such as the pancreatic lipase inhibitor orlistat may aid the reduction in obesity. For the obese, metformin or the recently introduced PPARγ agonists thiazolidinediones e.g. rosiglitazone may aid the improvement in insulin resistance. It is to be emphasized that adjunctive therapies may be needed for additional metabolic problems such as hyperlipidemia or for the treatment of systemic hypertension that is so often an accompaniment to type 2 DM.

Specific treatments are being developed to prevent the complications of DM. These include orally active inhibitors of aldose reductase, inhibitors of non-enzymatic glycation such as aminoguanidine or the protein kinase C inhibitor LY333531.

Insulin and sulfonylureas should be used with due circumspection. In Western countries, the majority of insulins now available are human. However, it will be immediately clear that there is virtually nothing else physiological about current insulin replacement therapy. Physiologically, insulin is secreted from β-cell granules (probably as hexamers and dimers) and enters the circulation through specialized fenestrations in the capillary endothelium that increase permeability 5–10 fold. The insulin is carried directly to the liver in the portal vein. Its short-lived pulses ($t_{1/2}$ approximately 3 min) are exquisitely related to the metabolic milieu that is regulated within fine limits.

In contrast, replacement insulin is injected subcutaneously into the systemic circulation. Absorption is slow, extremely variable and dependent on multiple factors including the site in the body, capillary density, temperature, blood flow and, not least, the method used to slow its absorption. The vast majority of modifications of insulin have, to date, involved the use of materials such as zinc or proteins such as protamine to slow absorption (*Box 2.33*). As a result, after a meal *all* patients taking insulin are inadequately replaced early and over-replaced some hours after. Recently, molecular

## A Medical

### Human insulins

| Type | Synonym | Timing of effect (h) | | |
|------|---------|------|------|----------|
| | | Onset | Peak | Duration |
| Insulin lispro[†] | LysB-28, ProB-29 | 0.25 | 1 | 4 |
| Insulin aspart[†] | B-28Asp | 0.25 | 1 | 3.5 |
| Unmodified | Soluble, Regular | 0.5–1 | 2–4 | 5–9 |
| NPH[*] | Isophane | 1–2 | 3–6 | 8–14 |
| Lente | Insulin-zinc suspension (mixed) | 1–2 | 5–10 | 8–16 |
| Ultralente | Insulin-zinc suspension (crystalline) | 2–3 | 4–8 | 8–16 |
| Insulin glargine[**] | HOE901 | 2–3 | No peak | 24 |

[*]NPH=Neutral Protamine Hagedorn

[†]These insulins were developed by site directed mutation of the insulin gene to give insulin molecules with less tendency to form multimers. They have the advantage of being very rapidly absorbed but the disadvantage that patients with no endogenous secretion of insulin rapidly run out of insulin unless another type with a longer duration of action is used in addition.

[**]Similar molecular biological techniques were used to alter the isoelectric point of insulin (and, thus, its solubility) to generate molecules with much slower absorption. Extended duration insulins have also been obtained by fatty acid acylation of LysB29 that results in the insulin binding to albumin.

Note that a large number of mixtures of insulins are available commercially many using proprietary administration systems. By and large they offer convenience but no greater efficacy.

## B Surgical

| Procedure | Advantages/indications | Side-effects/disadvantages |
|-----------|------------------------|-----------------------------|
| Islet cell transplantation | Offers option of 'cure' of type I DM | Shortage of donor islets<br>Not routinely available<br>Often only performed when complications have occurred (e.g. in patients requiring renal transplantation)<br>Requires immunosuppression |

techniques have been used to alter the structure of human insulin. Site-directed mutagenesis has been used to create novel human insulins (e.g. human insulin lispro) with structures that have a decreased tendency to form dimers and hexamers. The absorption of these is much more rapid, less variable and as a result improves post-prandial control of glucose.

A wide variety of sulfonylureas is available (*Box 2.34*). These act on the sulfonylurea receptor of the K[+]-ATPase channel (*Box 2.19*) to increase insulin secretion. They all bind strongly to albumin. They vary in cost and duration of action and are best used in those in whom insulin resistance due to obesity has been addressed. They have the serious side-effect of weight gain and the potentially fatal one of hypoglycemia (*see Clinical Case 2.6*). A recent development has been a non-sulfonylurea agonist repaglinide that has a shorter duration of action and may improve post-prandial glucose

**Box 2.34:**
Therapies for DM – 2 Insulin secretagogues*+ and sensitizers

**Secretagogues**

| **Drug** | **Duration of action** | **Advantages** | **Disadvantages/side effects** |
|---|---|---|---|
| Sulfonylureas† | | | |
| Tolbutamide | Short | Short-lasting and cheap | Large tablet size |
| Glibenclamide | Long | Cheap | Long action |
| Glimepiride | Long | Once daily | |
| Meglitinides | | | |
| Repaglinide | Short | Rapid action and short duration | Hepatic metabolism. Use with care in hepatic or renal impairment |
| Amino acid derivative | | | |
| Neleglinide | Short | Rapid action and short duration | Too early to determine side effects |

*Note that these are ineffective in the absence of adequate β-cell function.

†This is a large group of agents, including gliclazide, glipizide, gliquidone, tolazamide. All increase the likelihood of hypoglycemia particularly when availability of the drug is increased e.g. as a result of decreased excretion.

**C Incretins (potentiators of insulin secretion)***

| **Drug** | **Advantages** | **Disadvantages/side effects** |
|---|---|---|
| e.g. GLP-1 7-36 amide, exendin 4 | Increases insulin secretion<br>Inhibits glucagon secretion<br>Delays gastric emptying<br>Promotes satiety | Currently research only<br>Given by injection<br>Expensive |

*None currently licensed in the UK.

**D Insulin sensitizers**

| **Drug** | **Advantages** | **Disadvantages/side effects** |
|---|---|---|
| Biguanide | | |
| Metformin | First choice in obese patient<br>Increases glucose utilization<br>Decreases hepatic glucose production<br>No hepatic metabolism<br>No hypoglycemia | Gastrointestinal upset<br>Lactic acidosis especially in renal impairment |
| Thiazolidinediones | | |
| e.g. Rosiglitazone or pioglitazone | PPAR-γ agonist<br>No stimulation of insulin secretion<br>May be used with metformin or sulfonylurea<br>Reduces circulating FFAs | Expands plasma volume; avoid in heart failure<br>Anemia<br>Weight gain |

**Effects on carbohydrate absorption**

| Drug | Advantages | Disadvantages/side effects |
|------|-----------|----------------------------|
| α-glucosidase inhibitor e.g. Acarbose | Slows starch and sucrose absorption and, thus, reduces post-prandial hyperglycemia | Gastrointestinal upset |

**Prevention (or treatment) of complications**

| Drug | Advantages | Disadvantages/side effects |
|------|-----------|----------------------------|
| Inhibitor of glycosylation e.g. Aminoguanidine | Inhibits glycation in experimental studies Also thought to reduce NO synthase (and, thus, oxidative stress) Beneficial effects on nerve conduction in animal studies | Outcome of clinical trials awaited |
| Aldose reductase inhibitor[*] e.g. Tolrestat | Beneficial effects on nerve conduction in animal and clinical studies Reduces cataractogenesis in animal models | Little or no clinical improvements. Note that many of the trials have been criticized methodologically |
| Protein kinase-C inhibitor e.g. LY333531 | Beneficial effects on renal and peripheral nerve function in animal models | Awaiting clinical trial data |
| Growth factors | | |
| e.g. Platelet derived growth factor (PDGF, Becaplermin) | Improves rate of healing of neuropathic diabetic foot ulcers | Relatively expensive adjunctive therapy |
| Nerve growth factor (NGF) | Improvement in parameters of nerve function in animal studies | Clinical studies underway |

[*]None currently licensed in the UK.

**Treatment of obesity**

| Drug | Advantages | Disadvantages/side effects |
|------|-----------|----------------------------|
| (i) Appetite suppressants e.g. Sibutramine | Serotonin and noradrenaline reuptake inhibitor Approx 5 kg weight loss in clinical trials Fewer side effects than previous agents e.g. dexfenfluramine | Currently not licensed in UK |
| (ii) Pancreatic lipase inhibitors e.g. Orlistat | Approx 10 kg weight loss in clinical trials Not absorbed Side effects encourage maintenance of low fat diet | Side effects of fat malabsorption Potential for malabsorption of fat soluble vitamins |

contd

**Prevention of DM**

| Drug | Advantages | Disadvantages/side effects |
| --- | --- | --- |
| Nicotinamide | Cheap. Some evidence for efficacy in rodent models of DM | Little evidence of efficacy in published clinical trials |
| Insulin | Cheap and given orally | Little evidence of efficacy in published clinical trials |

Adjunctive therapies. These include all the treatments used in the treatment of conditions associated with DM (including hypertension and hyperlipidemia) and all those associated with attempts to improve the condition of those living with its complications (including those for neuropathic pain, gastroparesis, postural hypotension etc.).

excursions. Newer sulfonylureas have greater potency (i.e. effect per milligram) but there is little evidence that they have any greater maximal effect on insulin secretion and improved clinical benefit. Older drugs are often cheaper and available from generic manufacturers.

The treatment of DM is bedeviled by the problem of hypoglycemia, the sword of Damocles that hangs over every patient attempting to normalize his or her blood glucose. Were it not for hypoglycemia, the treatment of DM would be child's play.

## Hypoglycemia

Most cases of hypoglycemia seen in clinical practice are diabetics over-treated with insulin or sulfonylureas.

### Clinical Case 2.5:

A 56-year-old woman, a known diabetic taking sulfonylurea tablets (but with no other known medical problems) was brought to the Emergency Room by ambulance with her husband. The night before he had left his wife watching television and drinking a can of beer, but when he returned in the morning from his night-shift he had found her unconscious on the bedroom floor jerking her limbs continuously. She was still in her day clothes and the remains of a four-pack (4 × 500 ml) of strong lager (9% ethanol) were on the sitting room carpet. The television had been switched off but there were no signs of washing up. In the Emergency Room, her fits were treated with an intravenous glucose infusion and intravenous diazepam, a benzodiazepine. Her conscious level was poor (she responded with groans to painful stimuli) and she later required ventilatory support and transfer to the Intensive Care Unit. Her pretreatment venous serum glucose was extremely low at 0.6 mmol/l.

The brain with its absolute dependency on a continuous supply of glucose is central to discussions on hypoglycemia and on how hypoglycemia is defined. Glucose crosses the blood–brain barrier by facilitated diffusion via endothelial GLUT 1 receptors (*Box 2.4*) and this is the major rate-limiting step. At normal blood glucose concentrations, the rate of supply is approximately twice that of neuronal glucose utilization. As the arterial plasma glucose concentration falls below approximately 3.6 mmol/l, this transfer becomes rate limiting to neuronal glucose metabolism. Clearly what matters, therefore, in determining hypoglycemia is cerebral capillary glucose concentration. However, in ordinary clinical practice the only available measure is venous serum glucose concentration and there has been long discussion as to what this value should be in order to define hypoglycemia. A commonly used value is 2.2 mmol/l but this value can only be used to diagnose hypoglycemia when two other criteria have also been established viz. the symptoms experienced should be compatible with hypoglycemia and they should be improved when the hypoglycemia is corrected. These three criteria form Whipple's triad. However, the rigid use of a single value of glucose concentration in the definition of hypoglycemia is difficult to justify both physiologically and clinically.

The symptoms and signs of hypoglycemia have been divided into those due to lack of glucose to the brain (neuroglycopenia) and those due to increased activity of the sympathetic nervous system (*Box 2.36*). The causes of hypoglycemia are given in *Box 2.37*. Mechanistically, it is clear that the causes can be divided into those that increase its removal from the blood (i.e. hormones and drugs) and those that reduce its entry into the blood (i.e liver failure, hormone deficiencies). The hypoglycemia seen in *Clinical Case 2.5* was caused by both of these.

She was taking regular glibenclamide, the long-acting second-generation sulfonylurea responsible for most cases of hypoglycemia reported in the medical literature. On the night she became ill she also drank the best part of 180 g ethanol. If taken over, say, a 2 h period, (assuming total body water to be 39 l with a clearance rate of alcohol at 8 g/h) her serum ethanol concentration would have been approximately 400 mg/d – approximately 5 times the current U.K. legal drink-drive limit. Ethanol is not taken up by tissues and stored. It, thus, forces its metabolism by hepatic alcohol dehydrogenase. This changes the hepatic $NAD^+/NADH$ ratio that reduces hepatic gluconeogenesis, particularly from lactate.

Ethanol is an important dietary component in a significant proportion of the population and discussion continues as to whether it is a macronutrient or a poison. It can cause either hyper- or hypoglycemia. This depends on the nutritional state of the imbiber and the carbohydrate intake with the ethanol. The original descriptions of ethanol-induced hypoglycemia were in patients in poor nutritional state (with poor hepatic glycogen

stores) who were fasted. In the well-nourished, non-fasting subject ethanol may well cause hyperglycemia by a peripheral action to increase insulin resistance. *Clinical Case 2.5* was not in a poor nutritional state and it is unlikely that ethanol alone would have caused her hypoglycemic presentation

---

**Box 2.36:**
**Symptoms of hypoglycemia**

Autonomic
- Hunger
- Shakiness/tremor
- Palpitations
- Sweatiness
- Nervousness

Neuroglycopenic
- Tiredness or drowsiness
- Blurred vision
- Confusion
- Difficulty speaking
- Weakness
- Seizures
- Coma
- Death

---

**Box 2.37:**
**Causes of hypoglycemia**

Fasting hypoglycemia
- Drugs – especially insulin, sulfonylureas, alcohol, rarely salicylates, sulfonamides
- Hormone deficiencies – cortisol, somatotrophin, glucagon, epinephrine
- Liver failure
- Critical illness – heart failure, renal failure, extreme starvation e.g. anorexia
- Endogenous hyperinsulinism – β-cell disorder – insulinoma
  autoimmune – e.g. insulin or insulin receptor antibodies
- Hypoglycemias of infancy and childhood

Postprandial hypoglycemia
- Congenital deficiency of enzyme of carbohydrate metabolism e.g. galactosemia, fructose intolerance
- Gastrointestinal

with continuous generalized fits. What is more likely is that she took her glibenclamide in the evening and did not eat her usual meal; ethanol would have reduced awareness of the resultant hypoglycemia. The absence of oral carbohydrate intake and the alcohol-induced inhibition of gluconeogenesis meant that the drug-induced hyperinsulinemic hypoglycemic state was not correctable. Prolonged hypoglycemia, particularly when followed by epileptic activity, leads to neuronal death (through mechanisms that remain ill-understood). Indeed, this patient never recovered and remained dependent on full nursing care.

Whilst alcohol was pivotal to this patient's demise, the question sometimes arises as to whether episodes of hypoglycemia are accidental or deliberately induced by the patient (suicide) or by someone else (murder). To understand these important medicolegal possibilities it is important to reconsider the synthesis and secretion of insulin (*Box 2.15*). Cleaved C-peptide is co-secreted with insulin but is not cleared by the liver and has a longer $t_{1/2}$ in the systemic circulation. Commercially available human insulin contains no C-peptide, so in the case of exogenous hyperinsulinemia circulating concentrations of insulin would be high but the C-peptide low or absent. If the hyperinsulinemia were induced by sulfonylurea stimulated β-cell function, then the concentrations of both immunoreactive insulin and C-peptide would be high.

## Physiological responses to hypoglycemia and its treatment

As arterial blood glucose falls below about 4.5 mmol/l, serum insulin concentrations fall. With a continued lowering of blood glucose to below about 3.8 mmol/l there is secretion of the counter-regulatory hormones, glucagon, catecholamines, cortisol and somatotrophin (of which the most important in the acute situtuation are glucagon and epinephrine). With further reductions of blood glucose (at about 3.0 mmol/l) there is symptomatic awareness and at around 2.6 mmol/l cognitive dysfunction is apparent. However, it is clear that recent episodes of hypoglycemia can alter

(increase) these thresholds so that greater reductions in serum glucose concentrations are required before hormonal responses and symptoms are manifest. This is true both for normal volunteers and diabetics. The reverse occurs (decreased thresholds) in diabetics who have had a period of high serum glucose concentrations. Thus, depending on preceding blood glucose concentrations, a diabetic may be symptomatically hypoglycemic at a 'normal' serum glucose concentration or asymptomatic with a serum glucose of, say, 2.5 mmol/l.

The immediate treatment of a hypoglycemic emergency is to restore circulating glucose concentrations using a glucose infusion if necessary (*Box 2.38*). Additional therapy is used to reduce circulating insulin concentrations. *Clinical Case 2.5* was additionally given an octapeptide analog of somatostatin, octreotide, to try to reduce the glibenclamide-induced insulin secretion. In this case it had little demonstrable effect, probably because of the delay in the patient's clinical presentation. Glucagon may be given to stimulate hepatic gluconeogenesis, but in sulfonylurea-induced hypoglycemia it may cause additional insulin release. Other drugs used in this situation include diazoxide (*Box 2.38*) this drug opens the K+-ATPase channel in the β-cell and this inhibits insulin secretion (see *Box 2.19*).

## Hypoglycemia and insulinoma

The next case, though rare, illustrates the fact that not all cases of hypoglycemia are caused by diabetic drugs.

### Clinical Case 2.6:

A 66-year-old obese woman regularly attended the clinic for control of her hypertension. She was referred back to the clinic by her primary care physician with a history of being unwell over several months. The blood pressure control was reasonable but her husband had found her difficult to rouse in the mornings and seeming quite confused. This wore off as the morning progressed. Her weight had been increasing and she had been treated with a number of therapies including antidepressants. On one occasion her right arm twitched. She was thought to have epilepsy and an EEG was reported to show a focal abnormality. She was referred to the neurologists and a CT brain scan was normal. She was admitted and noted by the nurses to have a capillary blood glucose of 1.9 mmol/l during a morning 'attack'. The formal venous serum glucose was 1.0 mmol/l and she was referred to the endocrine unit. The time from the onset of symptoms to the establishment of the diagnosis was in excess of 1 year.

This patient has severe symptomatic spontaneous hypoglycemia with low venous serum glucose (1.0 mmol/l). The serum insulin (78 pmol/1) and C-peptide (916 pmol/1) concentrations were high at the time of hypoglycemia. From the foregoing, it is clear that this patient has an endogenous source of hyperinsulinism and an insulinoma was top of the diagnostic list.

These are rare tumors (0.5 per 100 000 per annum) occurring most frequently between the ages of 30 and 60 years and with equal incidence in both sexes. The vast majority (>99%) occur in

**Box 2.38:**
Treatment of hypoglycemia

**Medical**

| Drug | Advantages | Disadvantages/side effects |
|------|-----------|---------------------------|
| Glucose (oral liquid/gel or intravenous infusion according to conscious state) | Cheap, rapidly effective<br>Oral can be given by relatives | Intravenous infusion requires medical intervention |
| Glucagon | Stimulation of gluconeogenesis<br>Can be given by relatives subcutaneously or intra-muscularly | Nausea/vomiting<br>May cause insulin secretion<br>Effect may be transient |
| Diazoxide | Inhibition of insulin secretion<br>Some peripheral actions | Hypotension, hair growth<br>Retention of $Na^+$ and water<br>Nausea/vomiting<br>Long $t_{1/2}$ (48 h) |
| Somatostatin analog e.g. octreotide or lanreotide | Inhibition of insulin secretion<br>Some peripheral actions | Expensive, gallstones<br>Gut upset |

**Surgical**

| Procedure | Advantages/indications | Disadvantages/side effects |
|-----------|-----------------------|---------------------------|
| 95% distal pancreatectomy | Offers surgical 'cure' in PHHI | Operative morbidity ~30%[*]<br>Operative mortality ~2%<br>DM later in life ~95% |
| Adenomectomy or Distal pancreatectomy | Cure for insulinoma[†] | Operative morbidity ~30%[*]<br>Operative mortality ~2% |

[*]This includes fistula in approximately 10%, pancreatitis in approximately 5%, abscess in approximately 3%, wound infection in approximately 3% and hemorrhage or peritonitis in approximately 2%.
[†]95% success in first operations.
Abbreviation: PHHI, persistent hyperinsulinemic hypoglycemia of infancy.

the pancreas and about 10% are malignant. Thirty per cent are less than 1 cm diameter at diagnosis. The diagnosis of insulinoma may well be achieved late in the course of the disease. Once diagnosed, the problem is to localize it within the pancreas (*Box 2.39*) and to remove it

**Box 2.39:**
Localization of insulinoma[*]

| Technique | Advantages | Disadvantages |
|---|---|---|
| CT scan | Non-invasive<br>Sensitivity 50–70%<br>Widely available | Ionizing radiation |
| MR scan | Non-invasive<br>Sensitivity 50–70%<br>No ionizing radiation exposure | Less widely available than CT |
| Ultrasound<br>    Cutaneous | No ionizing radiation exposure<br>Cheap, widely available<br>Non-invasive | |
|     Endoscopic | Improved resolution and sensitivity | Invasive |
|     Peroperative | Improved resolution and sensitivity | Invasive and restricted to surgery |
| Angiogram | Quoted as 'gold standard' | Invasive |
| [111]In-octreotide | Non-invasive<br>Sensitivity 50%<br>May detect metastases | Less good for insulinomas than for other pancreatic tumors e.g. gastrinoma |

[*]Note that techniques are constantly improving and are subject to major differences in local expertise. As a result, for example, sensitivities quoted for CT scans may not apply to spiral CT or multi-slice techniques.

[111]In-octreotide scan of *Clinical case 2.6.*

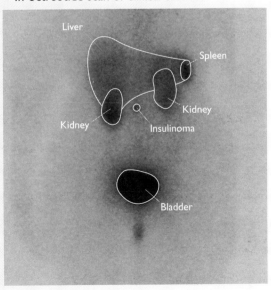

65

surgically. In *Clinical Case 2.6*, a CT scan of the pancreas and the liver was normal. However, a [III]In-labeled octreotide (somatostatin analog) scan showed a clear, but small, midline area of increased uptake (binding) of this somatostatin analog (*Box 2.39*). After initial medical treatment with diazoxide, the small benign adenoma of β-cells causing the insulinoma was removed with resolution of the symptoms.

## Hypoglycemia in infancy

There are some causes of hypoglycemia that come to light early in childhood. These include transient hypoglycemia in the neonatal period (more common in pre-term or small-for-gestational-age infants), hyperinsulinism and congenital enzyme defects. Some of these such as hereditary fructose intolerance and galactosemia present with post-prandial hypoglycemia. Such hypoglycemia has been termed 'reactive hypoglycemia'. This diagnosis was overused in the 1960s and 1970s and fell into disrepute. It is probably preferable to use the term post-prandial hypoglycemia, to remember to enquire as to the types of food that precipitate symptoms and to insist on the criteria in Whipple's triad being met.

The causes of hypoglycemia in infancy and childhood form another rather daunting list (*Box 2.40*). However, it is possible to clarify the subject somewhat and make some generalizations. The first is that all infants are prone to hypoglycemia, probably as a result of greater brain mass relative to body size. In addition, there may be some immaturity of gluconeogenic pathways in the pre-term and small-for-gestational-age infants. Second, the most common cause of hyperinsulinism is maternal DM (as seen in the child of *Clinical Case 2.3*). Fetal hormonal adjustments to maternal pathology may cause problems neonatally. In the case of fetal hyperglycemia, this leads to hyperinsulinism and hypoglycemia in the early neonatal period. Third, the majority of enzyme defects leading to hypoglycemia will be those disrupting glycogenolysis and gluconeogenesis, fatty acid oxidation or amino acid supply for gluconeogenesis. Examples of each of these are given in *Box 2.40*.

---

**Box 2.40:**
**Causes of hypoglycemia with onset in infancy and childhood**

**Transient intolerance of fasting**
- Preterm or small for gestational age infants
- Endocrine deficiency, e.g. cortisol deficiency

**Hyperinsulinism**
- Infant of diabetic mother
- Maternal drugs, e.g. sulphonylurea
- Persistant hyperinsulinemic hypoglycemia of infancy
- Miscellaneous, e.g. Beckwith–Wiedeman syndrome

**Enzyme defects**
- Carbohydrate metabolism, e.g. glycogen storage diseases types I, III, VI, fructose 1,6 bisphosphatase deficiency
- Protein metabolism, e.g. branched chain α-ketoacid dehydrogenase complex deficiency
- Fat metabolism, e.g. fatty acid oxidation defects

---

Mutations in the $K^+$-ATP channel in β-cells may lead to inactivation of the channel and membrane depolarization and insulin release. These may be inherited in autosomal dominant or recessive forms and give rise to persistant hyperinsulinemic hypoglycemia of infancy (PHHI) previously termed nesidioblastosis.

## Disorders of the α, γ and PP cells of the islets

Both insulin deficiency and its excess have been discussed. Functional glucagon deficiency may be seen in diabetics, increasing with the duration of the disease and being virtually universal after about 20 years of DM. Though α-cells are present within the islets they become functionally insensitive to hypoglycemia through mechanisms that are unknown. As would be predicted from the actions of glucagon, this results in markedly slower recovery from hypoglycemia.

Clearly, a state of clinical glucagon excess might be expected to result in DM. Glucagon excess may be seen in rare tumors (glucagonomas) of the α-cells. These are seen in the middle aged and older and the catabolic effects on muscle result in weight loss and wasting. The increased uptake of amino acids leads to a reduction in circulating concentrations. The DM is usually mild (resulting from increased hepatic gluconeogenesis) and is not associated with ketosis. For reasons that are not understood glucagonomas produce a necrolytic rash that migrates to different areas of skin and to thrombosis in blood vessels.

An excess of somatostatin (seen with extremely rare somatostatinomas of the γ-cells of the islet) also causes mild DM and circulating concentrations of both glucagon and insulin are low. The gut effects are noteworthy with malabsorption of fat (termed steatorrhea) and the formation of gallstones. Treatment of patients with octreotide or lanreotide results in similar gut effects that can limit their use. Tumors of the islet PP cells secreting pancreatic polypeptide occur but seem not to be associated with clinical sequelae. The principles of treatment of these tumors of the islets are the same as those in insulinoma.

# CLINICAL CASE QUESTIONS

The following are examples of applied pathophysiology and these clinically based questions can be answered with the information provided in this chapter. Answers and additional material are available on the website.

---

**Clinical Case Study Q2.1:**

A 26-year-old woman was transferred to the Intensive Care Unit from another hospital. She had been diagnosed as having DM for some 8 years. She had a strong family history of DM. Her grandfather, father, paternal uncle, cousin and younger brother all had early onset DM and one received insulin therapy. When initially diagnosed at another hospital she had been treated with insulin but was later treated with diet and the oral hypoglycemic agent metformin. Three weeks prior to hospital transfer she had been taking these drugs and had been seen in the Emergency Room of another hospital with an infection of her right foot. When seen, she had gangrene of her lateral three toes with cellulitis of her lower leg. She was 1.61 m tall and weighed 140 kg. Her blood pressure was 70 mmHg systolic and she was pyrexial (39°C). She was noted to have an acidosis (arterial pH 7.18, NR 7.35–7.45) and moderate ketonuria on urinalysis. The serum $Na^+$ was 130 mmol/l (NR 135–145 mmol/l), the $K^+$ 4.9 mmol/l (NR 3.5–4.7 mmol/l), $HCO_3^-$ 8 mmol/l, urea 8.6 mmol/l (NR 2.5–8.0 mmol/l), creatinine 130 μmol/l (NR 60–110 μmol/l). A diagnosis of diabetic ketoacidosis was made. She was admitted to the hospital and treated with intravenous antibiotics and soluble insulin. During the admission she developed anuria with renal failure and was transferred to the Intensive Care Unit for dialysis.

---

**Question 1:** The patient was diagnosed at the age of 16 years as having type 1 DM. Was this diagnosis correct? If not, why not?

**Question 2:** What was the cause of the acidosis?

**Question 3:** How would you confirm this?

## Clinical Case Study Q2.2:

A 30-year-old Caucasian woman booked into the Antenatal clinic at 17 weeks gestation. She was 1.65 m tall and weighed 55.8 kg. Uterine ultrasound confirmed the gestational age and was otherwise unremarkable. She complained of vaginal thrush and on routine testing had 2+ glycosuria. There was no polydipsia or polyuria. She had a past medical history of an operation for hiatus hernia at the age of 9 months. At the age of 25 years, she had undergone a partial esophagectomy (with continuity restored using a piece of colon) for a benign tumor. There was no relevant family history. The thrush was treated.

At 28 weeks gestation, she presented to Ob-Gyn again with pre-term labor. She was noted to have marked polyhydramnios (an excess of amniotic fluid). Ob-Gyn considered the polyhydramnios to be due to gestational DM and performed a 75 g glucose tolerance test:

| Time (min) | Serum glucose concentration (mmol/l) |
| --- | --- |
| 0 | 3.6 |
| 30 | 14.0 |
| 60 | 15.4 |
| 90 | 8.1 |
| 120 | 3.7 |

Question 1: Were Ob-Gyn correct in diagnosing gestational diabetes mellitus?

Question 2: If not, how may the glucose tolerance test be interpreted?

Question 3: How would you have treated the patient at the time of the presentation at 28 weeks gestation?

## Clinical Case Q2.3:

A 27-year-old Caucasian woman presented to the out-patient department with a cough productive of white sputum, fatigue and general malaise of several months standing. She had a complicated past medical history that included neurosurgery and radiotherapy to treat an optic nerve glioma at the age of 9 years. Following this she was registered blind and had epilepsy and hypopituitarism. She was treated with phenytoin for the epilepsy and thyroxine and somatotrophin for her hypopituitarism. Examination showed her to have poor sight with a visual field defect and to be thin and apyrexial. Physical signs in the chest suggested infection in the left lung which was confirmed by the chest X-ray (Box Q2.3). She declined to undergo a bronchoscopy. Three sputum samples were obtained for culture and she was started on treatment for presumed pulmonary tuberculosis. After 2 days treatment with rifampicin, pyrazinamide, isoniazid and pyridoxine, she was admitted after a collapse at home. She had a systolic blood pressure of 80 mmHg and responded only to painful stimuli. She was jaundiced with no palpable liver. Her serum glucose was 0.6 mmol/l. Biochemical tests of her liver showed the serum bilirubin was 129 μmol/l (NR 0–17 μmol/l), the albumin 35 g/l (NR 35–48 g/l), the alanine transaminase 580 (NR 0–40 IU/l). Ultrasound of her liver showed non-specific changes only. The admitting medical team attributed the hypoglycemic coma to isoniazid-induced liver failure (with resultant loss of hepatic gluconeogenesis).

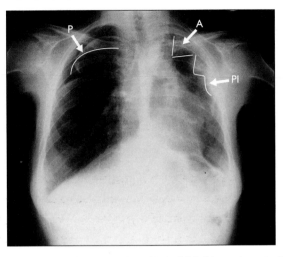

Chest X-ray of *Clinical Case Study Q2.3*. Note the apical shadowing (A) on the left. The elevation of the left hilum indicates volume loss in this area. There is also involvement of the pleura on the left (Pl) and a pneumothorax on the right (P).

Question 1: Which investigations would you perform?

Question 2: In the light of these results, was the admitting team correct? If not, what other possibilities should be considered?

## CHAPTER 3

# The thyroid gland

## Chapter objectives

*Knowledge of*

1. Importance of iodine in thyroid metabolism
2. Mechanisms of iodination of tyrosine and their regulation
3. Physiological roles of thyroxine and tri-iodothyronine, their transport and metabolism
4. Physiological control of thyroid growth and hormone secretion
5. Causes and clinical effects of insufficient and excessive thyroid hormone secretion
6. Investigation and treatment of thyroid disease

*'See, see! what showers arise,*
*Blown with the windy tempest of my heart.'*
*King Henry VI Part III, William Shakespeare.*

Thyroid hormones are extremely important and have diverse actions. They act on virtually every cell in the body to alter gene transcription: under- or over-production of these hormones has potent effects. Disorders associated with altered thyroid hormone secretion are common and affect about 5% women and 0.5% men.

Like the catecholamines epinephrine and norepinephrine, thyroid hormones are synthesized from the amino acid tyrosine. The synthesis of thyroid hormones requires the iodination of tyrosine molecules and the combination of two iodinated tyrosine residues (*Box 3.1*). Whilst tyrosine is relatively easily iodinated, iodine is rare, ranking 61st in the list of most common elements and forming just 0.000006% of the Earth's mantle. The thyroid gland has evolved not only to trap this element avidly from dietary sources but also to maintain a large store of the iodinated tyrosines to maintain the secretion of thyroid hormones during periods of relative iodine deficiency. *Clinical Case 3.1* illustrates the importance of iodine in thyroid function and, whilst it is relatively unusual, it demonstrates the problems of excess iodine intake and a consequent increase in thyroid hormone synthesis and release.

## Clinical Case 3.1:

A 25-year-old city high-flyer was in an interview for a position with a merchant bank. During the interview she suddenly found herself unable to speak and left the room unsteadily and in tears under the gaze of her disbelieving interviewers. The sympathetic secretary in the outer office ordered her a taxi to the hospital. She was found to have an irregular pulse rate of 180 beats per minute and remained unable to find her words (termed an expressive dysphasia). By writing, she was able to inform the medical team that she was taking the drug amiodarone for a heart condition that runs in her father's family. She had attributed recent anxiety, poor sleeping patterns, intolerance of summer weather and a 3 kg weight loss to the worry over the job interview. An electrocardiogram confirmed the irregular tachycardia and a diagnosis of a left cerebral hemisphere stroke (causing the expressive dysphasia), secondary to atrial fibrillation, was made. The atrial fibrillation was treated. Clinical examination revealed a diffusely enlarged thyroid gland (Box 3.4) and blood tests later confirmed that she was hyperthyroid.

**Box 3.1:**
Structures of hormones derived from tyrosine

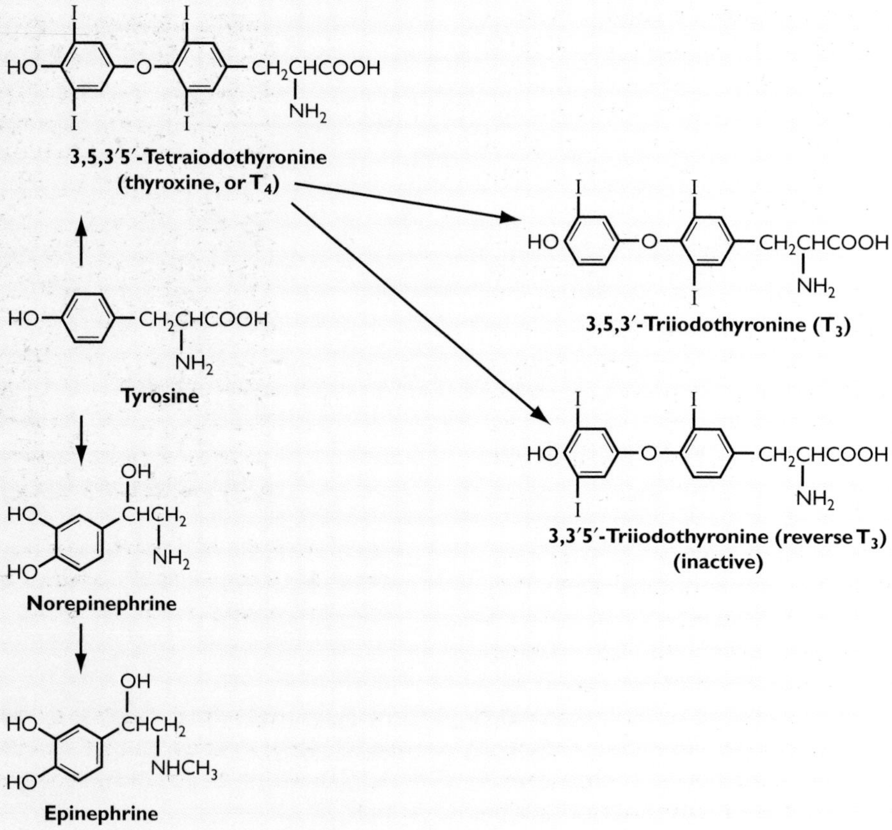
HO
O
$CH_2CHCOOH$
$NH_2$
I
3,5,3′5′-Tetraiodothyronine
(thyroxine, or $T_4$)
Tyrosine
OH
$CHCH_2$
Norepinephrine
$NHCH_3$
Epinephrine
3,5,3′-Triiodothyronine ($T_3$)
3,3′5′-Triiodothyronine (reverse $T_3$)
(inactive)

The important clue to *Clinical Case 3.1*, which led to her diagnosis, was the drug she had been prescribed to treat her inherited cardiac condition. Amiodarone (*Box 3.2*) contains 30% by weight of iodine and, at the dose prescribed (one 200 mg tablet daily), she was ingesting approximately 70 mg iodine per day.

**Box 3.2:**
Structure of amiodarone

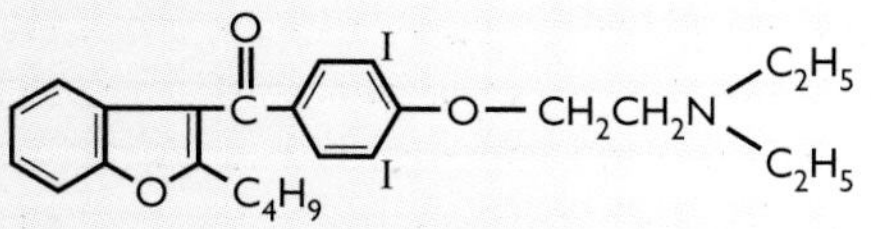
O
C
I
O
$CH_2CH_2N$
$C_2H_5$
$C_4H_9$
Amiodarone

## Iodine intake

The normal European daily dietary intake of iodine is about 150 μg, of which approximately 125 μg is taken up by the thyroid gland and used for hormone synthesis. The patient in *Clinical Case 3.1* was, thus, taking over 500 times the normal intake (released upon the breakdown of amiodarone) resulting in an excess production and release of thyroid hormones and symptoms of hyperthyroidism. In contrast, lack of iodine in the diet leads to hypothyroidism.

Iodine (as the iodide, I⁻) is relatively abundant in seawater and seafood is a rich dietary source. Fruit and vegetables also contain significant concentrations of iodine, although the amount depends on the soil and growing region. Areas of iodine deficiency tend to be inland, at high altitude and isolated and daily iodine intake may be as low as 25 μg. The term cretinism, used to define the severe impairment of physical and neurological development resulting from iodine deficiency during fetal and post-natal development, derived from 'cretein', a term first used in the Swiss Alps. The word cretin entered the vernacular as a term of abuse indicating severe mental retardation. In 1994, nearly 30% of the world population was at risk of iodine deficiency. The commitment from the World Health Organization in 1990 to eliminate iodine deficiency disorders by the year 2000 (with a policy of iodide supplementation of salt) had reduced the population at risk to less than 15% by 1997.

Increased iodine intake or a deficiency of dietary iodine can both induce goiter formation (*Box 3.4*). The former results from increased thyroid hormone synthesis and storage as seen in *Clinical Case 3.1*. Goiter formation in regions of dietary deficiency (the most common cause of goiter), is graphically illustrated in *Box 3.3*. It is due to reduced thyroid hormone synthesis and the compensatory increased secretion of the pituitary hormone thyrotrophin as a result of the loss of negative feedback (see below).

## Anatomical features of the thyroid gland

The thyroid gland consists of two lobes lying on either side of the ventral aspect of the trachea. Each lobe is about 4 cm in length and 2 cm thickness connected together by a thin band of connective tissue called the isthmus (*Box 3.4*). Weighing approximately 20 g, it is one of the largest classical endocrine glands in the body and receives a high blood flow from the superior thyroid arteries (arising from the external carotids) and the inferior thyroid arteries (arising from the subclavian arteries). The gland is so important that it takes more blood

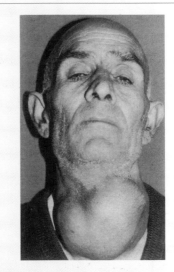

In the mountains of Kashmir patients such as this are said to find it easy going up mountains, but much more difficult negotiating an accurate descent.

per unit weight than the kidney and sometimes, when there is a goiter, blood flow in the gland may be heard with a stethoscope. The sound is termed a bruit.

The functional unit of the thyroid gland is the follicle, a roughly spherical group of cells arranged around a protein-rich storage material called colloid. The follicular cells are orientated with their bases near the capillary blood supply and the apices abutting the colloid.

## Iodine trapping and thyroid function

The active uptake of iodide (I⁻) by the follicular cells involves an energy-requiring (ATPase-dependent) transport mechanism which allows I⁻ to be taken up from capillary blood against both a concentration and an electrical gradient with Na⁺ (*Box 3.5*). This enables the thyroid gland to concentrate iodide 30–50 times that of the circulating con-

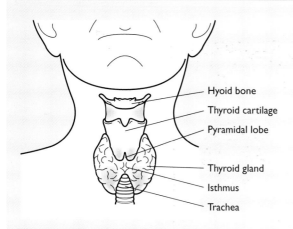

Hyoid bone
Thyroid cartilage
Pyramidal lobe
Thyroid gland
Isthmus
Trachea

Gross anatomy

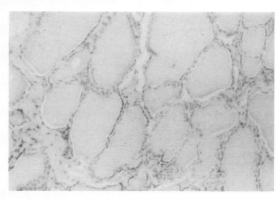

Histological appearance of normal thyroid follicles

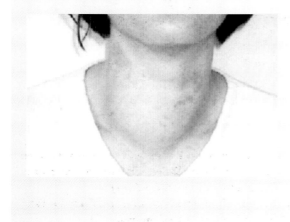

**WHO classification of goiter.**
This classification is useful for epidemiological studies but not for routine clinical practice.

| Grade | Definition |
|---|---|
| 0 | No palpable or visible goiter |
| I | Palpable goiter |
| | A  Only palpable |
| | B  Palpable and visible with the neck extended |
| 2 | Goiter visible with neck in normal position |
| 3 | Very large goiter visible from distance |

centration and allows radioactive isotopes to be used to investigate patients with thyroid disease (*Box 3.6*). Other ions such as bromide, chlorate or pertechnetate (though not fluoride) may also compete with I⁻ for this uptake process and this has important clinical uses (see *Box 3.19*). On a normal daily iodide intake the thyroid gland clears approximately 20 ml of plasma iodide per minute.

The active uptake of iodide appears to be the main control point for hormone synthesis and is stimulated by the pituitary hormone thyrotrophin (thyroid stimulating hormone, TSH). Iodide itself, however, plays an important role in regulating the activity of the thyroid gland (termed autoregulation). Excess iodine given to a person with normal thyroid gland activity leads to an initial reduction in organification and hormone synthesis and secretion, the Wolff–Chaikoff effect. 'Escape' from this inhibition (as was seen in *Clinical Case 3.1*) generally occurs after several days. The exact

Box 3.5:
Uptake and organification of iodine by the thyroid gland

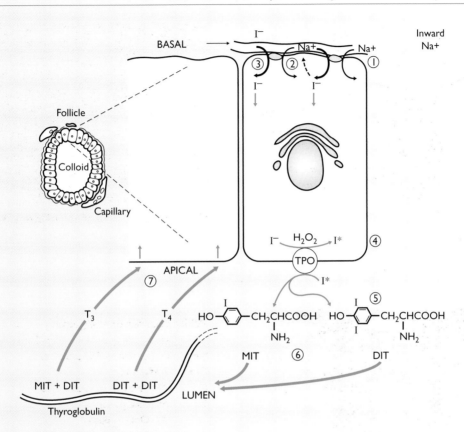

① Active uptake of iodide (I⁻) with Na⁺.

② Iodide may be discharged from the follicular cell by administration of competing ions such as perchlorate, bromide or chlorate.

③ Iodide uptake, the main control point for hormone synthesis, is stimulated by TSH.

④ Oxidation of iodide by hydrogen peroxide ($H_2O_2$) to form active iodine. The reaction is catalyzed by thyroid peroxidase (TPO).

⑤ Incorporation of active iodine into the tyrosine residues of thyroglobulin molecules to form mono- and di-iodotyrosines (MIT and DIT).

⑥ Linking of iodinated tyrosine residues to form triiodothyronine ($T_3$) and thyroxine ($T_4$).

⑦ About 1% of stored colloid is removed each day. When the gland is very active this may rise to nearly 100% and colloid stores are depleted.

mechanism(s) of such autoregulation is unknown but the Wolff–Chaikoff effect is useful clinically because pharmacological doses of iodine may be used to reduce acutely the activity of the thyroid gland (see *Box 3.19*). When dietary intake of iodine is insufficient, overactivity of the thyroid gland is a more common initial response to excess iodine.

Uptake of a radioactive isotope by the thyroid gland is used to determine:

- localization of the gland
- approximate size
- overall or regional function of the gland.

**Isotopes.** $^{125}I$ has a radioactive half-life ($t_{1/2}$) of 60 days, $^{131}I$ a $t_{1/2}$ of 8 days and $^{123}I$ a $t_{1/2}$ of 13 hours. A radioisotope of technetium ($^{99m}$pertechnetate) is often used because it has a usefully short radioactive $t_{1/2}$ (approximately 6-h) and, unlike radioactive iodine, is not organified in the thyroid gland. Radiation dose to the thyroid is thus low.

- **Localization and size.** Uptake of isotope in a normal gland ① and in a patient whose left lobe was surgically removed ②. Arrow indicates uptake of iodine in the salivary glands.
- **Overall function.** More rapid and increased uptake of the isotope in primary hyperthyroidism ③ compared with normal thyroid activity ① and slower, reduced uptake in hypothyroidism ④.
- **Regional function.** 'Hot' nodule in upper left lobe of the thyroid gland (arrow) showing increased isotope uptake and suppression of uptake in surrounding tissue ⑤. 'Cold' nodule in lower left lobe (arrow) showing reduced isotope uptake ⑥.

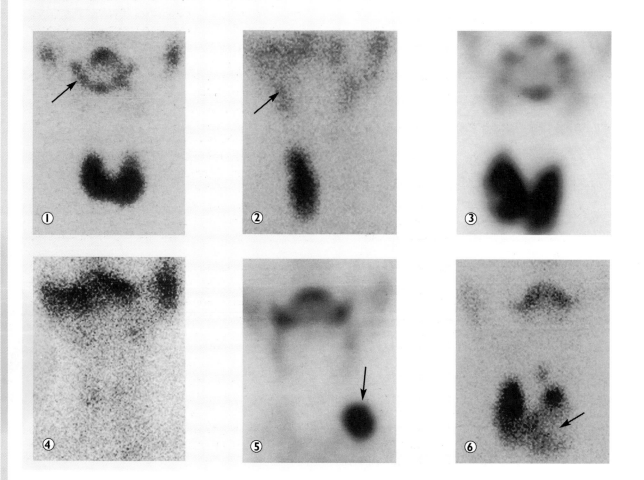

# Synthesis of thyroid hormones

The synthesis and storage of thyroid hormones occurs between the follicular cells and the colloid (*Box 3.5*). Different follicles may be in different states of activity. Less active follicles contain cells with a more cuboidal appearance, whilst the active follicles contain columnar cells.

The process of thyroid hormone synthesis is complex. Once inside the follicular cell, iodide is oxidized to active iodine by hydrogen peroxide. This reaction is catalyzed by the heme-containing enzyme thyroid peroxidase (TPO). Iodine is then actively transported across the apical surface of the follicular cell by the same active process that occurs at the basal surface.

At the apical-colloid interface, iodine is immediately incorporated into the tyrosine residues of the large glycoprotein thyroglobulin molecules. Thyroglobulin is synthesized in the follicular cells and has a molecular weight of around 650 000 with about 140 tyrosine residues, depending on the form of thyroglobulin. Approximately one quarter of these residues can be iodinated. Once iodinated, thyroglobulin is taken up into the colloid of the follicle where, still incorporated in the protein, a coupling reaction between pairs of iodinated tyrosine molecules occurs. The coupling of two tyrosine residues each iodinated at two positions (di-iodotyrosine, DIT) produces tetra-iodothyronine or thyroxine ($T_4$) whilst the combination of DIT with mono-iodotyrosine (MIT) produces tri-iodothyronine ($T_3$). Such coupling can occur within a single molecule of thyroglobulin or between dimerized molecules of the protein. This coupling is catalyzed by TPO.

Thyroid hormones are stored in this state and are only released when the thyroglobulin molecule is taken back up into the follicular cells (*Box 3.7*). Stimulated by TSH, thyroglobulin droplets are captured by the follicular cells by a process of pinocytosis. Fusion of the droplets with lysosomes results in hydrolysis of the thyroglobulin molecules and release of $T_4$ and $T_3$. About 10% of $T_4$ undergoes mono-deiodination to $T_3$ before it is secreted and the released iodine is recycled.

Approximately 100 µg of thyroid hormones are secreted from the gland each day, mostly in the form of $T_4$ with about 10% as $T_3$. Eighty percent of the $T_4$ undergoes peripheral conversion to the more active $T_3$ in the liver and kidney ($T_3$ is ten times more active than $T_4$) or to reverse $T_3$ ($rT_3$) that has little or no biological activity (*Box 3.1*). Very small quantities of other iodinated molecules, such as MIT and DIT as well as thyroglobulin, are also measurable in the circulation. As this thyroglobulin originates from the normal secretory process, its measurement in the serum is used, for example, to detect endogenous thyroid secretion when patients are taking oral $T_4$ replacement (an important clinical use).

# Actions of thyroid hormones

The effects of thyroid hormones on virtually every cell in the body is manifest in the widespread clinical effects of their lack or excess (*Box 3.8*). They are very important in growth and development and their role in these processes will be discussed in relation to *Clinical Case 3.3* (see page 94).

Many of the actions of thyroid hormones are mediated by their binding to nuclear receptors (*Box 3.9*) that have a preferential affinity for $T_3$. $T_3$ receptors are, like all the steroid hormone receptors, members of a family of nuclear transcription factors that, in combination with other transcription factors, regulate gene expression in target cells. Unlike some steroid receptors (i.e. those for sex steroids and glucocorticoids), thyroid hormone receptors exist in the nucleus, not the cytoplasm, and may remain bound to DNA in the absence of hormone binding.

Thyroid hormones are lipid soluble and readily cross cell membranes. Once inside the nucleus, $T_3$ binds to its receptor. This dimerizes with another $T_3$ receptor (to form a homodimer) or with a different receptor, notably the retinoic acid receptor, to form a heterodimer (*Box 3.9*). In this form, the dimers interact with DNA. This occurs between recognition sites in the 'zinc fingers' of the DNA-binding domains of the receptors and particular base sequences in the DNA helix known as hormone response elements (HRE). The location of HREs determines which genes are regulated by $T_3$.

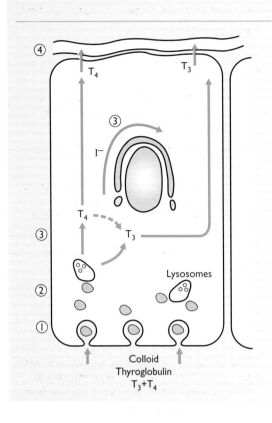

① Under the influence of TSH, colloid droplets consisting of thyroid hormones within the thyroglobulin molecules are taken back up into the follicular cells by pinocytosis.

② Fusion of colloid droplets with lysosomes causes hydrolysis of thyroglobulin and release of $T_3$ and $T_4$.

③ About 10% of $T_4$ undergoes mono-deiodination to $T_3$ before it is secreted. The released iodide is reutilized. Several-fold more iodide is reused than is taken from the blood each day but in states of iodide excess there is loss from the thyroid.

④ On average approximately 100 μg $T_4$ and about 10 μg $T_3$ are secreted per day.

There is also evidence that thyroid hormones can have rapid, non-genomic effects on membrane receptors independent of protein synthesis. These include stimulation of sugar transport, $Ca^{2+}$ATPase activity and increased $Na^+$ transport in muscle. The receptors for these effects have not been identified.

In most tissues (exceptions include brain, spleen and testis), thyroid hormones stimulate the metabolic rate by increasing the number and size of mitochondria, stimulating the synthesis of enzymes in the respiratory chain and increasing membrane $Na^+$-$K^+$ ATPase concentration and membrane $Na^+$ and $K^+$ permeability. Since as much as 15–40% of a cell's resting energy expenditure is used to maintain its electrochemical gradient (pumping $Na^+$ out in exchange for $K^+$), increasing the $Na^+$-$K^+$ ATPase activity, therefore, increases the resting metabolic rate (RMR). RMR may increase by up to 100% in the presence of excess hormones or decrease by as much as 50% in a deficiency.

The clinical signs of intolerance to heat, weight loss and fatigue, as seen in *Clinical Case 3.1*, are typical symptoms of patients presenting with hyperthyroidism (*Box 3.10*) and provide evidence of the metabolic action of thyroid hormones on their target tissues. In contrast, the hypothyroid patient is intolerant to cold, is lethargic, gains weight and has a cool, dry skin.

Whilst these metabolic changes associated with hyperthyroidism increase cardiac output, the increase is disproportionate to the increase in metabolic rate. The reason for this is that thyroid hormones have positive inotropic and chronotropic effects on the heart. The chronotropic effects of thyroid hormone (increases in sinoatrial node firing rate, decreases in atrial excitation threshold, decreased refractory period of conduction tissues)

Clinical manifestations of thyroid hormone deficiency and excess

| Tissue/organ | Deficiency | Excess |
|---|---|---|
| Skin/hair | Pale, dry, puffy skin (myxedema)<br>Dry, brittle hair, brittle nails | Pink, warm, moist skin<br>Onycholysis of nails |
| Cardiovascular | Decreased blood volume and cardiac output; dilated, pale, poorly contractile myocardium; pericardial effusion; sinus bradycardia | Increased cardiac output, decreased peripheral resistance; supraventricular tachycardia/atrial fibrillation |
| Respiratory | Pleural effusions (small), alveolar hypoventilation in severe hypothyroidism, obstructive sleep apnea | Decreased vital capacity (myopathy of respiratory muscles) |
| Gut | Modest weight gain, decreased motility (ileus or constipation), small ascites, associated pernicious anemia and achlorhydria | Increased appetite, weight loss, increased motility (loose motions), nausea and vomiting (especially in pregnancy), associated pernicious anemia and achlorhydria or celiac disease |
| CNS | *In childhood* – poor neuronal development and myelination (cretinism)<br>*In adulthood* – slowed intellectual functions, paranoid or depressive psychiatric disorder, perceptive deafness, night blindness, cerebellar ataxia, slow-relaxing reflexes, carpal tunnel syndrome | Nervousness, emotional lability, hyperkinesia, tremor |
| Muscle | Stiffness and aching (especially in cold), firm, tender muscles, myoclonus, loss of type 1 muscle fibres | Weakness and fatigability; proximal myopathy with loss of type 2 myocytes; may be associated with myasthenia gravis; hypokalemic periodic paralysis may be seen especially in Chinese |
| Skeleton | Poor growth and maturation of bone, decreased urinary excretion of $Ca^{2+}$ | Demineralization of bone; increased urinary excretion of $Ca^{2+}$ and $PO_4^{3-}$; hypercalcemia |
| Kidney | Renal blood flow, glomerular filtration rate and tubular resorption and secretory functions all decreased; decrease in urinary free water excretion | Renal blood flow, glomerular filtration rate and tubular resorption and secretory functions all increased |
| Bone marrow | Decreased red cell mass; normochromic normocytic anemia; associated pernicious anemia and macrocytic anemia | Increased red cell mass; associated pernicious anemia and macrocytic anemia |
| Gonad | *In childhood* – delayed puberty but occasional paradoxical precocious sexual development<br>*In adulthood* – menorrhagia, decreased libido, erectile dysfunction, infertility | *In childhood* – delayed puberty, though physical development is normal<br>*In adulthood* – increased libido, oligomenorrhea, pregnancy loss |
| Metabolic | Low resting metabolic rate (RMR), decreased appetite, weight gain, cold intolerance, reduced body temperature, flat glucose tolerance curve with delayed insulin response; increased insulin sensitivity; decreased synthesis and degradation of lipids | Increased RMR, and appetite; weight loss; decreased glucose tolerance; increased synthesis and degradation of both lipids and proteins |

- There are two genes which code for $T_3$-receptors; one on chromosome 17 coding for the $\alpha$ receptor, the other on chromosome 3 coding for the $\beta$ receptor. There are at least two alternative messenger RNA splice products for each gene and thus four major $T_3$ receptors – $\alpha1, \alpha2, \beta1$ and $\beta2$. Unusually, the $\alpha2$ receptor does not bind $T_3$, but $T_3$ receptors have functions in the absence of the hormone.

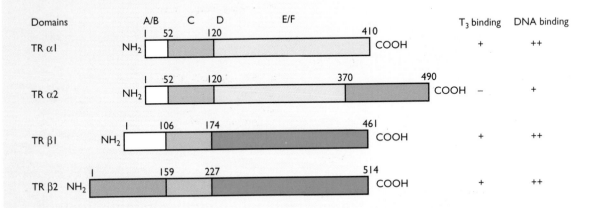

- Binding of T3 to its receptor (TR) causes formation of homo- or heterodimers.

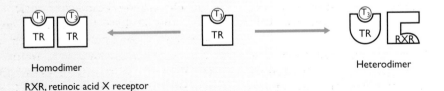

RXR, retinoic acid X receptor

- As dimers, the zinc fingers of the DNA binding domain slot into a hormone response elements (HRE) on the DNA helix. Along with other transcription factors (co-activators/repressors), they regulate gene expression.

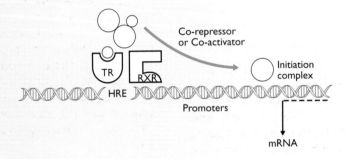

| Symptoms | Signs |
|---|---|
| **Common** | |
| Anxiety and irritability (~ >90%) | Tachycardia (~ 100%) |
| Palpitations (~ 90%) | Tremor (~ 95%) |
| Increased perspiration and heat intolerance (~ 90%) | Goiter (~ 100%) |
| Fatigability (~ 80%) | Warm moist skin (~ 95%) |
| Weakness (~ 70%) | |
| Increased appetite and weight loss (~ 85%) | |
| **Less common** | |
| Dyspnea (~ 65%) | Atrial fibrillation (~ 10%) |
| Increased bowel frequency (~ 30%) | Onycholysis (~ <5%) |
| Anorexia (~ 10%) | 'Liver palms' (~ 5%) |
| Weight gain (~ <5%) | Heart failure (~ 5%) |
| Oligomenorrhea (~ 25%) | |
| **Rare** | |
| Pruritus (~ <1%) | |
| Periodic paralysis (~ <1%) | |

may be due to increases in sarcolemmal $Na^+$ transport and $Ca^{2+}$ influx. The inotropic effects (increase in contractile force) may be mediated by increases in $Ca^{2+}$-ATPase activity in sarcoplasmic reticulum and increases in the expression of the α-myosin heavy chain.

Thus, it is reasonable to assume that it was these effects of excess thyroid hormones on the cardiovascular system that led to the onset of atrial fibrillation in *Clinical Case 3.1*. This led to the disastrous formation of atrial thrombus with subsequent embolization to the left cerebral hemisphere producing a stroke and the consequent temporary loss of speech.

# Control of thyroid hormone synthesis and secretion

Like the adrenal cortex and the gonads, the thyroid gland is controlled by hormone secretions from the hypothalamo-pituitary axis. The synthesis and secretion of TSH from the thyrotrophs is stimulated by the tripeptide, thyrotrophin-releasing hormone

(TRH). This small peptide, cleaved from a larger pro-hormone, is released from neurosecretory cells in the hypothalamus into the hypothalamo-hypophyseal portal capillaries where it is transported to the pituitary thyrotrophs (*Box 3.11*). TSH secretion is inhibited by other hormones (including somatostatin and dopamine) and also cytokines, particularly IL-1β, IL-6 and TNF-α.

TSH is a complex glycoprotein hormone, containing approximately 16% carbohydrate. It contains 211 amino acids in two sub-units and has a molecular weight of about 28 000–30 000. The α unit is identical to that of two other glycoprotein hormones secreted by the human anterior pituitary gland, luteinizing hormone (LH) and follicle stimulating hormone (FSH, see *Box 6.13*). The β unit is unique to TSH and confers biological specificity. The structural homology between TSH, LH and FSH includes 'knots' of three disulfide bonds in both α and β sub-units. The glycosylation of TSH is heterogeneous and this affects both its bioactivity and clearance. TSH has a $t_{1/2}$ in the circulation of about 1 h.

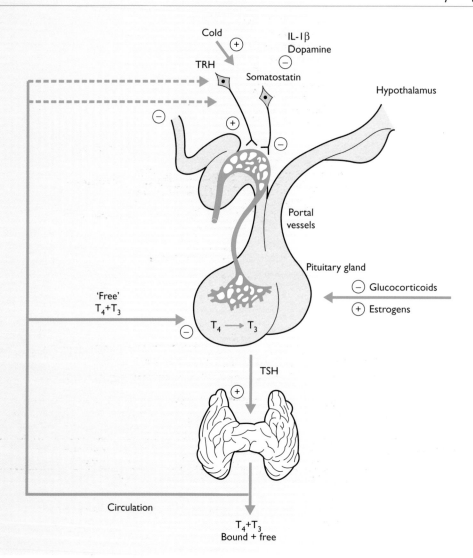

The cell surface receptor for TSH is a typical G-protein linked receptor with 7 helical transmembrane domains, 3 external (E) loops and three internal (I) loops (*Box 3.12*). The hormone binds to the long extracellular amino terminus whilst the carboxyl terminus is intracellular. There are approximately 1 000 TSH receptors on the basal surface of each follicular cell.

The binding of TSH to its receptor activates the G proteins associated with the I loops. This involves the replacement of GDP bound to the $\alpha\beta\gamma$ G-protein heterotrimer with GTP. The $\alpha$ sub-unit then dissociates from the complex and activates intracellular enzymes. The G proteins coupled to the TSH receptor, Gs and Gq, stimulate adenylate cyclase and phospholipase C, respectively. Adenylate cyclase activates protein kinase A whilst phospholipase C stimulates the hydrolysis of phosphoinositides to inositol trisphosphate ($IP_3$) and diacylglycerol. $IP_3$ transiently increases the concentration of intracellu-

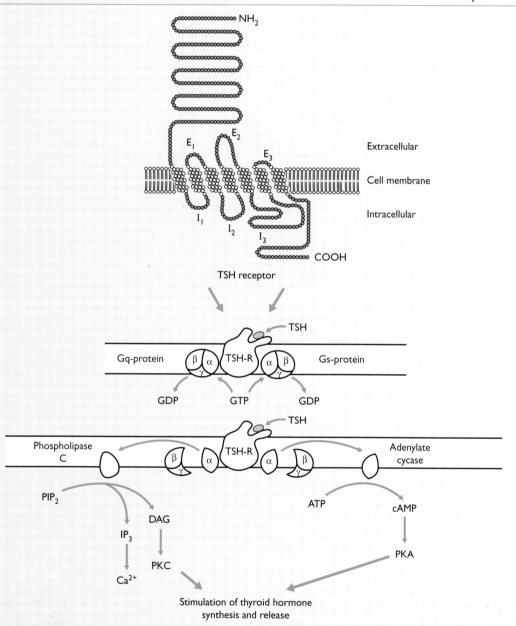

Interaction of TSH with the extracellular amino-terminal domain of its receptor activates its associated G-protein. Bound GDP is replaced by GTP and the α sub-unit of the G protein dissociates. The α sub-unit of a Gs-protein activates adenylate cyclase while that of the Gq-protein phosphorylates and activates phospholipase C. The adenylate cyclase stimulates the conversion of ATP to cAMP which, in turn, phosphorylates and activates protein kinase A (PKA). Phospholipase C stimulates the conversion of phosphatidyl inositol 4,5-bisphosphate ($PIP_2$) to inositol 1, 4, 5-trisphosphate ($IP_3$) and diacylglycerol (DAG). These release $Ca^{2+}$ from intracellular stores and activate protein kinase C respectively. In the human, much higher concentrations of TSH are required to activate the inositol pathway.

lar $Ca^{2+}$ whilst diacylglycerol activates protein kinase C (*Box 3.12*). These kinases activate further signal transduction mechanisms that eventually stimulate several processes involved in thyroid hormone synthesis and release and thyroid growth. These include iodine uptake, production of hydrogen peroxide and TPO and uptake of colloid droplets.

Inactivating mutations in the long extracellular amino-terminal of this receptor have been described and lead to hypothyroidism. In contrast, activating mutations have been described in E1 and E2 and I3 and the 2nd, 3rd, 6th and 7th transmembrane domains, though most are around the 6th and 7th domains. Activating mutations have been reported most frequently in autonomous 'hot' nodules (areas of increased growth and activity) of the gland. If present in the germ line and thus heritable (which is extremely rare), such activating mutations cause familial hyperthyroidism. Mutations of Gs (termed gsp) that result in constitutive activation of the G protein have also been described in 'hot' nodules.

The concentration of thyroid hormones in the circulation is regulated by an homeostatic feedback loop involving the hypothalamo-pituitary axis (*Box 3.11*). The main effect of thyroid hormones is to reduce the response of the pituitary thyrotrophs to TRH rather than altering the secretion rate of TRH from the hypothalamus. The sensitivity of the thyrotrophs to TRH depends on their intracellular concentration of $T_3$, 80% of which is derived from the intrapituitary conversion of $T_4$ to $T_3$ (see *Box 3.29*). When circulating concentrations of $T_4$ are low, there is an increase in the number of TRH receptors and in TSH synthesis resulting in an increased TSH response to TRH. The reverse is true in the presence of high circulating concentrations of thyroid hormones. The TSH response to a bolus injection of TRH has been used to diagnose the exact cause of hypo- and hyper-thyroidism, but measurement of thyroid hormones and TSH, using sensitive modern assays, is usually sufficient for diagnosis. Thus, in *Clinical Case 3.1* concentrations of thyroid hormones in peripheral blood were high and the negative feedback resulted in unmeasurably low serum concentration of TSH.

This regulatory loop is affected by internal and external factors that alter the rate at which TSH is secreted. It is secreted in a pulsatile fashion with a diurnal variation, peaking around midnight. Environmental temperature may stimulate or inhibit the release of TSH by adjusting TRH secretion. Thus, after 24 h exposure to a cold environment, the plasma concentrations of thyroid hormones increase with a consequent rise in basal metabolic rate and an increase in the endogenous production of body heat. This effect is more marked in rats than humans. Pharmacological doses of glucocorticoids, as prescribed in anti-inflammatory therapy, or seen in Cushing's syndrome inhibit thyroid hormone secretions by reducing the TSH secretory response to TRH. In contrast, estrogens have the opposite effect, increasing TSH secretion and, hence, increasing the activity of the thyroid gland.

## Hyperthyroidism – Graves' disease

The importance of the TSH receptor in regulating the activity of the thyroid gland is exemplified by *Clinical Case 3.2*. This patient has Graves' disease, an autoimmune disease resulting in the production of autoantibodies that stimulate the TSH receptor. This highly unusual action of an antibody (most block receptor activation) not only stimulates thyroid hormone synthesis and secretion but also thyroid growth. Autoantibodies to thyroglobulin and TPO may also be present.

### Clinical Case 3.2:

A 35-year-old woman came to the outpatient clinic with her 5-month-old child. She had noted increasing tenseness and irritability with her baby, poor sleep, weight loss and palpitations. Her husband was concerned that she had post-natal depression and had taken time off work to look after the family. She had an unremarkable past medical history and had sailed through pregnancy without any problems; she denied depression but felt exhausted all the time. She recalled that her late mother had an operation on her neck in her twenties and that her younger sister had regular vitamin injections for anemia. She ruefully admitted that the recent strain had led her to restart smoking ten cigarettes daily. On examination, she had a moderate diffuse goiter with an audible bruit, a tremor and a resting tachycardia of 100/min. Her eyes were prominent and puffy (see *Box 3.16*).

Like *Clinical Case 3.1*, this patient with hyperthyroidism is also a young woman with cardiac problems and a diffuse goiter indicating that the pathology was affecting all parts of the gland. The differences between these two cases are that in the second case there was a suggestive family history of thyroid disease, a recent pregnancy, evidence of eye problems and no evidence of an excess intake of iodine.

### Incidence and diagnosis of Graves' disease

Graves' disease is the most common cause of hyperthyroidism and other causes are uncommon or, indeed, rare (*Box 3.13*). For reasons that remain unknown, it is much commoner in women, particularly those aged 30–50. It affects approximately 3% women and 0.3% men. The family history indicates a genetic predisposition to autoimmune disease. In *Clinical Case 3.2*, the patient's mother had had Graves' disease and her sister pernicious anemia (also considered to be autoimmune in nature). The exact nature of this genetic predilection remains uncertain but experimental studies have suggested linkage with a number of other genes. These include a linkage with certain histocompatibility complex genes (on chromosome 6) and associations with other diseases that are characterized by markers of autoimmunity, suggesting a primary genetic defect in immune function. The familial associations include pernicious anemia, Sjogren's syndrome, Addison's disease, type 1 diabetes mellitus and primary biliary cirrhosis.

The relationship of thyroid disease to a recent pregnancy is noteworthy for several reasons. First, pregnancy alters thyroid physiology and, overall, increases circulating concentrations of thyroid hormones (*Box 3.14*). Second, pregnancy is associated with an amelioration of symptoms associated with

---

**Box 3.13:**
*Causes of hyperthyroidism*

**Common**
- Graves' disease (~80%) – autoimmune with stimulating antibodies to the TSH receptor.
- Toxic multinodular goitre (~ 15%).

**Uncommon**
- Toxic adenoma ('hot' nodule, ~ 2%).
- Thyroiditis (~ 1%).

**Rare**
- TSH secreting pituitary tumor (<0.01%) – biochemically this must be distinguished from thyroid hormone resistance when TSH secretion is high due to loss of negative feedback effects.
- Trophoblastic tumors (<0.001%) – high concentrations of the homologous chorionic gonadotrophin hormone interacting with the TSH receptor.
- Thyrotoxicosis factitia (<1%) – excess thyroxine ingestion in patients who perceive weight loss and other benefits.
- Thyroid follicular carcinoma (<0.01%).

---

autoimmune diseases (i.e. immunosuppression) although the causes of this are not understood. Third, the immunological changes that occur post-partum induce a recrudescence of (or, indeed, first appearance of) autoimmune hyperthyroidism or hypothyroidism; it is likely that this caused the hyperthyroidism seen in *Clinical Case 3.2*. It is estimated the 2–15% women become hyperthyroid (often transiently) post-partum.

Graves' disease may be distinguished from other causes of hyperthyroidism because it is associated with abnormalities of the eyes and integument. The diagnosis may be confirmed by the detection of autoantibodies to the TSH receptor (*Box 3.15*). However, the presence of such antibodies is not essential to the diagnosis; indeed, the absence of autoantibodies is usually attributed to the assay.

## Box 3.14:
### Effect of pregnancy on thyroid gland physiology

- Increased renal I⁻ clearance (increasing dietary requirements in deficient areas).
- Increased serum TBG increasing total $T_4$ and $T_3$ concentrations (see *Box 3.28*).
- Increased plasma volume that increases $T_4$ and $T_3$ pool size.
- Increased inner-ring deiodination of $T_4$ and $T_3$ (see *Box 3.29*) by placenta, increasing hormone degradation.
- Increase in free thyroid hormone concentrations and reduction in TSH concentrations. The first trimester increase in human chorionic gonadotrophin (hCG, a glycoprotein hormone with structural similarities to TSH) has been implicated in this effect.

## Ophthalmopathy and dermopathy of Graves' disease

The patient in *Clinical Case 3.2* presented with prominent and puffy eyes and, indeed, eye disease is the most common associated feature of Graves' disease. Since the ophthalmopathy is linked to Graves' disease rather than other autoimmune diseases of the thyroid (such as Hashimoto's disease, see below), it is generally considered that the eye disease results from autoimmune interactions within the orbit involving the TSH receptor. However, attempts to identify the expression of the TSH receptor protein or receptor fragments within the eye have been problematical. In addition, the eye disease may arise before, during or after raised thyroid hormone secretions. Thus, its etiology appears to be independent of thyroid function.

The features of Graves' ophthalmopathy are given in *Box 3.16*. There are three phases to the eye disease; an active period of inflammation is followed by regression and a third inactive or 'burnt out' period. Those elements of the disease that are expressed within the orbit are far more serious than those expressed extraorbitally because they can endanger vision. Within the orbit, antibodies stimulate the production of glycosaminoglycans by the fibroblasts. These attract large amounts of water and, thus, increase retro-orbital pressure causing bulging of the eyes (proptosis). The increased pressure may jeopardize the vascular supply to the eye. Inflammatory activity within the orbit (involving T lymphocytes, macrophages and local production of cytokines) may lead to muscle fibrosis and cause diplopia (double vision). In contrast, the extra-orbital lid retraction and chemosis do not threaten vision though they may be awkward for the patient.

Treatment of the severe symptoms of eye disease (*Box 3.17*) are problematic although minor symptoms such as grittiness or sensitivity can be treated with synthetic tears or darkened and wind protective glasses. An interesting point about *Clinical Case 3.2* is that she was a smoker. Smoking increases the risk of thyroid eye disease some 7-fold, although the relationship to the number (or duration) of cigarettes smoked is poorly defined and the cause unknown.

The effects of Graves' disease on the integument are shown in *Box 3.18*. Graves' dermopathy is the least frequent of all the associated symptoms and even less is known about its etiology. Like the ophthalmopathy it is associated with an increased production of glycosaminoglycans (predominantly hyaluronic acid and chondroitin sulfate) that causes edema, as in the orbit.

## Treatment of hyperthyroidism

There are three methods of treating hyperthyroidism – drugs, surgery and radioisotopes. None is ideal; each has its own advantages and disadvantages (*Box 3.19*). None is exclusive and, not infrequently, a combination of therapies is used.

### Antithyroid drugs

There are three types of drugs used to inhibit thyroid hormone synthesis and release.

### Thiocarbamides

These are the most widely used and were developed after the discovery that feeding certain plants (particularly those of the genus *Brassica*) to animals caused goiter formation. Thiocarbamides reduce thyroid hormone synthesis by inhibiting TPO. The synthetic thiocarbamides now used are carbimazole (or its main metabolite methimazole in the US) and propylthiouacil (abbreviated to PTU) (*Box 3.19*). They have short half-lives, particu-

**Box 3.15:**

## Assay of antibodies to the human TSH receptor – competitive binding assay

Principle:

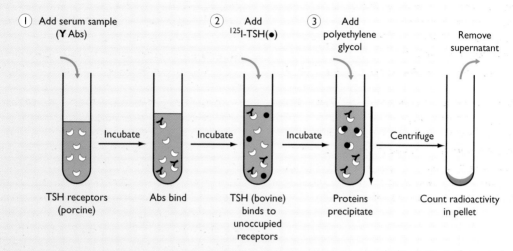

① Add serum sample (**Y** Abs)   ② Add $^{125}$I-TSH(●)   ③ Add polyethylene glycol   Remove supernatant

Incubate → Incubate → Incubate → Centrifuge

TSH receptors (porcine) — Abs bind — TSH (bovine) binds to unoccupied receptors — Proteins precipitate — Count radioactivity in pellet

① Patient's serum containing antibodies (Abs) is incubated with TSH receptors.
② $^{125}$I–bovine TSH is added that competes with Abs for binding to TSH receptors.
③ Receptors precipitated with polyethylene glycol, supernatant removed and radioactivity in pellet counted.

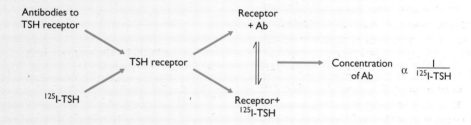

Antibodies to TSH receptor →  ← $^{125}$I-TSH → TSH receptor ⇌ Receptor + Ab / Receptor + $^{125}$I-TSH → Concentration of Ab $\alpha \dfrac{1}{^{125}\text{I-TSH}}$

### NOTE

- It is a heterologous assay and not all human antibodies may react with the porcine receptor or compete with bovine TSH.
- It does not measure function of the Ab, just its ability to bind to the porcine receptors.
- The assay uses TSH rather than a standard human IgG preparation to prepare a standard curve.
- Activating TSH receptor antibodies in serum can be assessed by bioassay e.g. measuring radioactive thymidine uptake by thyroid cells as an index of growth or colloid droplet production by thyroid slices.

larly so in the case of PTU, and for this reason carbimazole is more widely used. However, PTU tends to be prescribed to pregnant and lactating women because it binds to plasma proteins and less crosses the placenta or enters the breast milk. It also has the added advantage of reducing the hepatic conversion of the less active $T_4$ to $T_3$ (*Box 3.29*).

High doses of anti-thyroid drugs are initially prescribed to patients with Graves' disease and the dose gradually reduced whilst aiming to keep the patient euthyroid. Alternatively, some clinicians use the 'block and replace' regimen in which patients are maintained on high doses of anti-thyroid drugs with replacement thyroxine as appropriate.

**Extraorbital features**

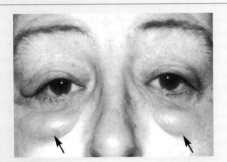

- Periorbital edema — swelling around the eye, the result of accumulation of mucopolysaccharides and associated water.

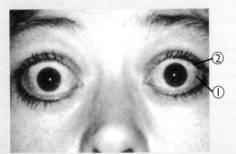

- Chemosis — swelling and redness of the conjunctivae ① Lachrymal glands may show mononuclear cell infiltration.
- Lid retraction — the upper lid is above the junction of the sclera and cornea ② .
- Lid lag — as the eye travels from up-gaze to down-gaze the upper lid lags behind.

**Intraorbital features**

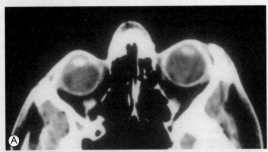

- Proptosis or exophthalmos — the 2 MR scans of the orbits are not technically identically but it can be seen that the globes of the eyes in Ⓑ (lower) are pushed forward compared with those in Ⓐ (upper, normal). There is infiltration of retro-orbital tissues by lymphocytes, macrophages and plasma cells, together with the accumulation of mucopolysaccharides.
- Extraocular muscle involvement — the muscles are affected by the retro-orbital accumulation of cells, inflammatory cytokines and mucopolysaccharides. This can be seen particularly in the inferior rectus in Ⓑ (arrowed).

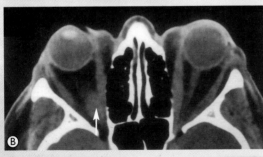

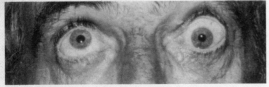

- The resultant fibrosis impairs function (seen here with the patient looking up) leading to diplopia.

These images are available in color on the website.

**Medical**

| Drug | Use | Advantages | Disadvantages/side effects |
|------|-----|-----------|---------------------------|
| Thiocarbamides (e.g. carbimazole) | Maintenance of euthyroid state (see Box 3.19) | Cheap, effective | Rashes, pruritis (~ 4%), neutropenia (~ 0.4%), hepatitis or pneumonitis (~ <0.1%) |
| Glucocorticoid (e.g. prednisolone) | Immunosuppression | Cheap, effective | Cushing's syndrome (see Chapter 4) |
| Azathioprine | Adjunct to glucocorticoids | Cheap, steroid sparing effect | Few in low doses (e.g. 2 mg/kg/d) |
| Somatostatin analog (e.g. octreotide or lanreotide) | Suppression of lymphocytes | Less side effects than glucocorticoids | Expensive; gastrointestinal side effects; gall stones |
| Plasmaphoresis | Reduce circulating autoantibodies | Short term effects | Expensive, invasive |

**Surgical**

| Procedure | Use | Advantages | Disadvantages/side effects |
|-----------|-----|-----------|---------------------------|
| Lid suture | Maintain corneal integrity | Simple | Does not address essential orbital disease |
| Orbital decompression | Decompress the orbit when retro-orbital pressures are high. Relieve proptosis | Effective in reducing pressure and proptosis (by about 6 mm) | Risks of anesthesia and surgery (~ <1% mortality, ~ 10% morbidity). Infection |
| Strabismus (squint) correction | Corrects diplopia | Cosmetic and functional benefits | Only used when the inflammatory process has settled |
| Lowering upper lid | To reduce lid retraction | Cosmetic benefit | |

**Radiotherapy**

| Procedure | Use | Advantages | Disadvantages/side effects |
|-----------|-----|-----------|---------------------------|
| 2000cGy $^{60}$Co photons in 10 fractions | Reduce retro-orbital inflammatory processes | Reduces steroid dependency/dose | Side effects include cataract formation, optic neuropathy and long-term risk of malignancy (~ <1%) |

Anti-thyroid treatment is continued for a somewhat arbitrary length of time (about 18 months) with the hope that the patients will be 'cured' (in remission) after a single course. Unfortunately, many patients relapse after stopping the drug.

*Iodine*

The fastest acting anti-thyroid agent is iodine itself, reducing thyroid hormone synthesis within three days through a presumed autoregulatory mechanism. It may be given as drops of 'Lugol's solution of iodine' or a saturated solution of potassium iodide for 10 days or so. This form of treatment is no longer widely used but is particularly useful in the short term in hyperthyroid 'storm' where the degree of thyrotoxicosis becomes life threatening (with, for example, cardiac failure). It has also been used prior to thyroid surgery to reduce the high blood supply to the gland.

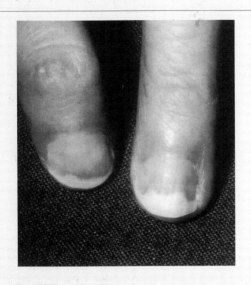

**Onycholysis** – fingernails detached from the nail beds at the free margins.

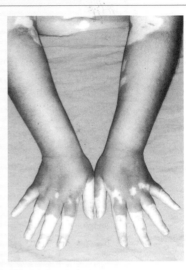

**Vitiligo** – patchy depigmentation of the skin (seen here in an Asian patient), often occuring peripherally and symmetrically. There may also be a streak of leucotrichia – white hair.

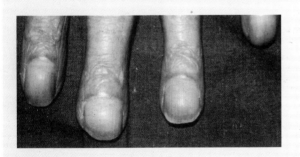

**Acropachy** – a form of finger clubbing.

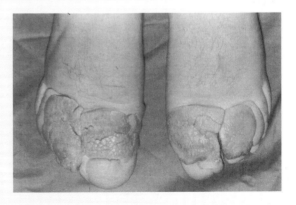

**Infiltrative dermopathy** – localized firm red thickening of skin. There is marked accumulation of glycosaminoglycans and water.

These images are available in color on the website.

### Perchlorate

Perchlorate reduces thyroid hormone synthesis by competing with iodine for uptake into the thyroid gland and discharging iodine from the trapped pool. It is no longer used routinely because it is relatively toxic with adverse effects on bone marrow. However, it is used in cases such as that of *Clinical Case 3.1* in which there has been an excess of iodine.

## Medical

| Drug | Use | Advantages | Disadvantages/side effects |
|---|---|---|---|
| Thiocarbamides e.g. PTU, carbimazole | Patients with mild thyroid disease and small goiter or those with eye disease, cardio-respiratory disease, pregnancy, children | Cheap, effective | Rashes, pruritis (~ 4%), neutropenia (~ 0.4%), hepatitis or pneumonitis (~ <0.1%) |
| β-adrenergic receptor blockers (e.g. propranolol) | Symptomatic relief (especially cardiac), hyperthyroid storm | Propranolol inhibits hepatic conversion of $T_4$ to $T_3$ | Asthma, heart failure |
| Glucocorticoids (e.g. prednisolone) | Hyperthyroid storm | Prednisolone inhibits hepatic conversion of $T_4$ to $T_3$ | Iatrogenic Cushing's syndrome |
| Iodine (e.g. Lugol's solution) | Hyperthyroid storm Prior to surgery to reduce blood flow | Rapid inhibition of thyroid hormone synthesis (Wolff-Chaikoff effect) | 'Escape' occurs with time |
| Perchlorate | Iodine-induced hyper-thyroidism | Discharge iodide excess from thyroid gland | Rash, gastric upset, lymphadenopathy (~ 5%). Agranulocytosis or aplastic anaemia (~ 0.5%) |
| Lithium | Second-line alternative to thiocarbamides | Inhibits $T_4$ and $T_3$ release | Lithium toxicity[*] (tremor, ataxia, coma); polydipsia, polyuria (~10%) |

## Surgical

| Procedure | Use | Advantages | Disadvantages/side effects |
|---|---|---|---|
| Partial thyroidectomy | Patients with large goiter, severe disease, nodular disease, relapsed after medical treatment | 'Definitive' | Expensive and scarring. Recurrent laryngeal nerve palsy (~ 0.5%) hypoparathyroidism (~ 5%), hypothyroidism (~ 5–40%), recurrent hyperthyroidism (~ 5%), carotid/jugular damage and hemorrhage (~ 0.5%). Relative contraindications include previous surgery and pregnancy |

## Radioisotope

| Procedure | Use | Advantages | Disadvantages/side effects |
|---|---|---|---|
| [131]Iodine | Patients with cardio-respiratory disease, severe disease, previous thyroid surgery, toxic nodule | Cheap, effective, shrinks goiter without a scar | Sialadenitis, worsening eye disease, hypothyroidism. Absolute contraindication: pregnancy. Relative contraindication: youth and eye disease – many clinicians do not treat <18 years old and eye disease may be treated with glucocorticoids |

[*]Lithium toxicity is related to the blood concentration of the ion.

The patient in *Clinical Case 3.1* was treated with a combination of perchlorate and carbimazole and her anti-arrhythmic drug was changed to one that did not contain iodine, a β-adrenergic receptor blocker that has additional benefits in hyperthyroidism, particularly on cardiac symptoms.

Destruction of thyroid tissue is the alternative to drug therapy. This can be done using radioactive isotopes of iodine or surgically.

### Radioiodine

Radioactive isotopes of iodine have been in use for over 50 years and today [131]I, with a radioactive half-life of 8 days is the most commonly used for therapy. Since it has proved almost impossible to calculate a dose of the isotope that would result in euthyroidism in individual patients and [131]I treatment is remarkably safe, many clinicians now use a fixed dose of isotope (for example 15mCi or 550MBq) and aim to produce hypothyroidism. Once hypothyroidism is induced, such patients can be treated with oral thyroxine that is cheap, effective and easy to monitor. [131]I is also used to treat euthyroid goiters (so as to avoid surgery) and such treatment usually results in a reduction of about 40% in the volume of the thyroid gland.

### Thyroid surgery

The ancient Egyptians considered that a goiter added grace and beauty to a female neck. Whilst most women in the 20th century might not agree with this view, they are often reluctant to exchange a goiter for a 7 cm scar on the neck. Thus, unless the goiter is malignant, surgery is usually restricted to large and unsightly goiters that are not treatable medically or with radioiodine. It is important to note that, prior to surgery, the patient must be rendered euthyroid with drugs because of the increased risks of anesthesia and surgery in the hyperthyroid patient.

## Surgical anatomy and embryology of the thyroid gland

The surgical anatomy of the thyroid gland is complex and important because of its proximity to the common carotid artery and internal jugular vein, the laryngeal and vagus nerves and its close associa-tion with the parathyroid glands (*Box 3.20*). The thyroid gland is the first endocrine gland to develop in the embryo and begins to form about 24 days after fertilization. Like Rathke's pouch, that develops into the anterior pituitary gland (see *Box 7.2*), the thyroid gland also develops from an outgrowth of the pharyngeal endoderm. As the embryo grows the thyroid gland descends into the neck and for a short time the gland is connected to the developing tongue by a narrow tube, the thyroglossal duct. At around 7 weeks, the gland has assumed its definitive shape and has reached its final destination in the neck. By this time the thyroglossal duct has normally disappeared although its remnants persist as a small pit, the foramen cecum (*Box 3.21C*).

The parathyroid glands that are closely associated with the thyroid gland also develop from the pharyngeal endoderm, in this case the 3rd and 4th pharyngeal pouches (see *Box 3.21B*). The inferior parathyroid glands (sitting at the lower poles of the two lobes of the thyroid gland) migrate with the thymus gland, and the superior parathyroids from the 4th pharyngeal pouch migrate laterally.

The embryology of these glands results in three important clinical sequelae (*Box 3.21D*). First, the thyroglossal duct may not disappear completely and this may result in mid-line thyroglossal cysts. The connection with the tongue means that such cysts move upwards when the tongue is protruded. Second, ectopic thyroid and parathyroid tissue may be found in a number of positions from the tongue to the chest. Third, surgery to the thyroid gland may result in the removal of parathyroid tissue and subsequent hypoparathyroidism.

## Primary hypothyroidism – Hashimoto's disease and myxedema

The most common causes of hypothyroidism are autoimmune in etiology (*Box 3.22*). Like Graves' disease they may have a number of autoimmune markers, including the presence of autoantibodies. However, unlike Graves' disease, T-cell mediated actions result in thyroid gland destruction rather than stimulation. The symptoms of hypothyroidism are vividly demonstrated in the next case.

**Box 3.20:**
Schematic views of the surgical anatomy of the thyroid gland

(A) Anterior view of the blood supply and relationship to other important vessels

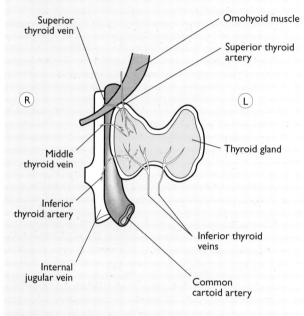

- Superior thyroid vein
- Omohyoid muscle
- Superior thyroid artery
- R
- L
- Thyroid gland
- Middle thyroid vein
- Inferior thyroid artery
- Inferior thyroid veins
- Internal jugular vein
- Common cartoid artery

(B) Left lateral view of the relationship to important nerves

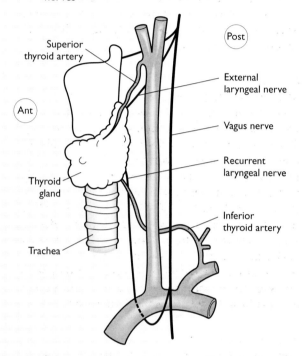

- Superior thyroid artery
- Post
- External laryngeal nerve
- Ant
- Vagus nerve
- Recurrent laryngeal nerve
- Thyroid gland
- Inferior thyroid artery
- Trachea

(C) Transverse view of the relationship to other important structures in the neck

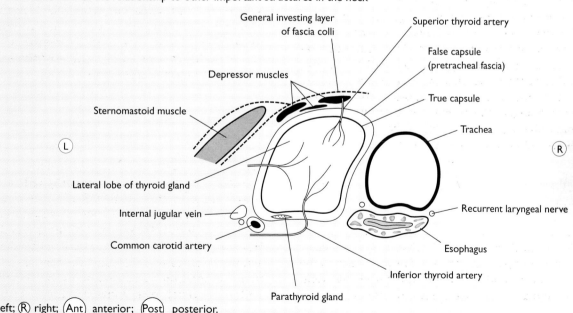

- General investing layer of fascia colli
- Superior thyroid artery
- Depressor muscles
- False capsule (pretracheal fascia)
- Sternomastoid muscle
- True capsule
- L
- Trachea
- R
- Lateral lobe of thyroid gland
- Internal jugular vein
- Recurrent laryngeal nerve
- Common carotid artery
- Esophagus
- Inferior thyroid artery
- Parathyroid gland

(L) left; (R) right; (Ant) anterior; (Post) posterior.

## Clinical Case 3.3:

A 19-year-old young man presented to the Emergency Room with pain in the left hip and knee. X-rays showed that he had a slipped femoral epiphysis Ⓐ. At the age of 19.7 years, he was 1.544 m tall and weighed 57 kg. His mother, who had type 1 diabetes mellitus and hypothyroidism, reported him to be a 'lazy sod … difficult to get out of bed in the morning'. His schoolwork had been poor and he had worn sweaters even during the summer. He looked much younger than his age Ⓒ and, indeed, his bone age (an index of skeletal development) was markedly delayed at 13.4 years. His pubertal development was also delayed by several years (Tanner stage 3) and his serum testosterone concentration was low at 4 nmol/l (NR 9–25 nmol/l). A moderate size goiter was palpable.

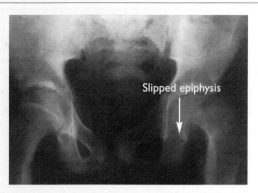

Ⓐ X-ray appearances of the hips at presentation. Comparison of the epiphyses of the right and left femurs shows that the left has 'slipped' sideways at the junction with the diaphysis (arrowed).

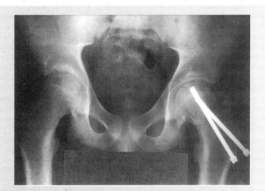

Ⓑ X-ray appearances of the hips after surgical correction.

These images are available on the website.

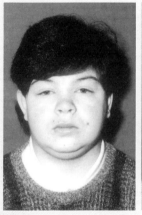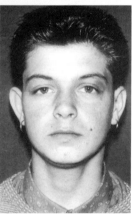

Ⓒ Facial appearance at presentation (left) and after 7 months treatment of T$_4$ (right).

Hashimoto's disease is similar to Graves' disease in that it occurs with about the same incidence and with the same sex bias, peak age of presentation and family history of thyroid disease or related autoimmune diseases. In this regard, *Clinical Case 3.3* was atypical in being male and younger, but serves to illustrate the catastrophic effects of the lack of thyroid hormones.

### Etiology and clinical features of Hashimoto's disease

The cause of the autoimmunity is unknown and since the autoimmune processes in Hashimoto's disease induce destruction of the thyroid gland, it may be surprising to note that it is marked by goiter formation. The goiter is the result of diffuse lymphocytic infiltration (which gives it a number of alternative names such as chronic lymphocytic thyroiditis), together with TSH-stimulated hyperplasia of surviving thyroid tissue due to loss of feedback inhibition from the thyroid hormones. The goiter is usually diffuse with a characteristic – at least to the experienced clinician – 'rubbery' feel to palpation. It is rare for it to be painful or problematic by its size and surgery is infrequently required.

Diagrammatic view of sagittal Ⓐ and transverse Ⓑ views of the pharyngeal regions of a human embryo during the fifth week of gestation, showing the endodermal pharyngeal pouches and mesodermal pharyngeal arches. Diagrams show the embryonic origin of the thyroid gland and parathyroid glands. Migration of the thyroid gland and parathyroid glands (anterior view) is shown in Ⓒ. Diagram Ⓓ illustrates various abnormalities which can occur during embryonic development. Each diagram is not drawn to relative scale.

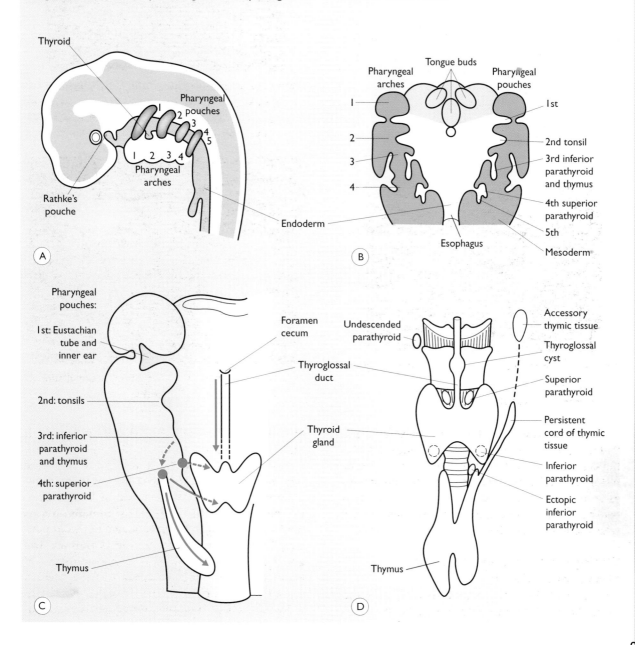

### Causes of hypothyroidism[*]

**Primary disorders**

Common (~ 95%)
- Hashimoto's disease – autoimmune thyroid destruction
- Primary (atrophic) hypothyroidism (Probably endstage Hashimoto's disease)
- Post-radioiodine therapy which destroys thyroid tissue
- Post-surgery of the gland

Uncommon (~ 5%)
- Thyroiditis (non-lymphocytic)
- Impaired $T_4$ synthesis due to genetic defect
- Antithyroid drugs

Rare (<1%)
- Loss of function TSH receptor mutations
- Thyroid hormone resistance

**Secondary** (or pituitary, ~ 1%) disorders
- Hypopituitarism caused by e.g. tumors, surgery, radiotherapy
- Impaired TSH synthesis

**Tertiary** (or hypothalamic, ~ <1%) disorders
- Hypothalamic damage due to tumors, radiotherapy or trauma

[*]In most Western countries iodide deficiency is not a cause of hypothyroidism. It is a major cause in known deficient areas.

Other features of this disease are antibodies against TPO and thyroglobulin (usually in much higher titers than in Graves'). Some patients are affected by a period of hyperthyroidism, in which case it is termed 'Hashitoxicosis', but the degree of hyperthyroidism is usually milder than in Graves' disease.

Hypothyroidism is also associated with primary thyroid atrophy and termed primary myxedema. The relationship between Hashimoto's disease and myxedema has been much discussed but it seems highly likely that non-goitrous myxedema is simply an end-stage of autoimmune destruction leaving only fibrous remnants. A role for antibodies to the TSH receptor that block the actions of TSH (rather than stimulating the receptor as in Graves' disease) has also been proposed.

The symptoms of hypothyroidism are extremely diverse, as might be predicted (*Box 3.23*). *Clinical Case 3.3* showed a number of classic features including those affecting mental processes, gut motility, metabolic rate and the skeleton. He also presented with pubertal delay, though it is to be noted that hypothyroidism can occasionally present in the teenage years with precocious puberty.

## Diagnosis of hypothyroidism

The diagnosis of Hashimoto's disease is usually easy, based on the presence of goiter, circulating thyroid autoantibodies and low circulating concentrations of thyroid hormones with high TSH concentrations. Biochemical investigation in *Clinical Case 3.3* was performed to investigate the cause of his poor growth and pubertal delay that culminated in his presentation to orthopedic surgeons with a slipped femoral epiphysis. These revealed total serum $T_4$ to be unmeasurable at <10 nmol/l (NR 70–150 nmol/l) with a very high serum TSH (>110 mU/l, NR 0.5–4 mU/l). Anti-TPO antibodies were positive in high concentration. Surgical procedures in hypothyroidism are associated with increased risk of morbidity and mortality. He was started on oral thyroxine therapy and subsequently underwent surgery. After some 7 months, he was seen in the outpatient department complaining that his friends did not recognize him (*Clinical Case 3.3*, C). His growth and pubertal development matched the change in his facial appearance.

## Treatment of primary hypothyroidism

Use of the prohormone thyroxine in the treatment of primary hypothyroidism is cheap and easy to monitor. The conversion of $T_4$ to $T_3$ is physiologically regulated and the dose can be altered according to serum TSH concentrations. No attempt is made to treat the underlying immune disorder. Severe hypothyroidism resulting in 'myxedema coma' is not often seen nowadays but may require parenteral $T_4$ or $T_3$ in addition to general supportive measures and hydrocortisone.

It is to be noted that some physiological conditions such as pregnancy may increase $T_4$ require-

Box 3.23:
Clinical features of hypothyroidism

| Symptoms | Signs |
|---|---|
| **Common** ||
| Fatigue (~ 90%) | Dry, scaly skin (~ 90%) |
| Cold intolerance (~ 80%) | Coarse, brittle thinning hair (~ 60%) |
| Depression (~ 70%) | Bradycardia (~ 40%) |
| Poor concentration (~ 65%) | Hair loss or dryness (~ 70%) |
| Musculoskeletal aches and pains (~ 25%) | Anemia |
| Carpal tunnel syndrome (~ 15%) | Puffy eyes (~ 90%) |
| **Less common** ||
| Constipation (~ 50%) | Edema (~ 30%) |
| Hoarse voice (~ 40%) | Cerebellar signs[*] |
| Menorrhagia (~ 30%) | Deafness[*] |
|| Psychiatric[*] |

[*]Note:'Myxedema madness', cerebellar ataxia and deafness are always cited in thyroid texts but are usually only seen in very severe cases, unusual in modern practice

ments whilst gastrointestinal diseases or drugs such as sucralfate may decrease its absorption. Requirements may also be increased by drugs increasing its clearance such as rifampicin whilst some such as amiodarone may decrease $T_4$ to $T_3$ conversion. Diseases such as cirrhosis of the liver or the natural processes of ageing may decrease requirements.

The terms 'compensated hypothyroidism' or 'decreased thyroid reserve' have been used to indicate the situation in which circulating $T_4$ or $T_3$ concentrations are low-normal but serum TSH concentrations are elevated. There has been discussion over when such patients should be treated with $T_4$. In this controversial area, some have argued that patients with serological evidence of anti-thyroid antibodies are likely to develop clinical hypothyroidism and should be treated.

## Other forms of thyroiditis

The term thyroiditis is a term applied to a number of conditions that arise as a result of inflammation of the thyroid gland and, as has been seen, Hashimoto's chronic lymphocytic thyroiditis is the most common. Others are thought to result from infections and give rise to very different clinical features.

Bacterial or fungal infections may precipitate acute thyroiditis whilst subacute thyroiditis, such as De Quervain's, has been attributed to a viral illness. De Quervain's is usually self-limiting, but with a tendency to recur and the diagnosis is made on clinical features (general malaise and a painful thyroid gland). If fine-needle aspiration cytological examination (FNA, see *Box 3.33*) is performed it may reveal the presence of inflammatory cells. The disease process is associated with evidence of an acute phase reaction (a non-specific reaction leading to the high erythrocyte sedimentation rate) and the release of thyroid hormones from damaged cells. It is not due to hyperfunctioning thyroid tissue and [99mTc] scans show reduced or absent iodine uptake (*Box 3.6*) and thiocarbamides play no part in treatment.

Some affected patients (approximately 50%) may have some symptoms of hyperthyroidism and, in a later phase of the illness, a temporary period of hypothyroidism may be experienced. During the acute phase, anti-inflammatory oral glucocorticoids (e.g. prednisolone) bring about rapid symptomatic relief.

Riedel's thyroiditis is not associated with features of inflammation but has additional features of fibrotic reaction elsewhere (e.g. retroperitoneal fibrosis in the abdomen). Like Hashimoto's disease, it results in progressive destruction of the thyroid gland that may necessitate $T_4$ replacement therapy.

## Secondary hypothyroidism

Less often, hypothyroidism may result from a loss of trophic stimulation due to damage or disease of the hypothalamic-pituitary axis. Thus, in the absence of the TRH and/or TSH drive, thyroid function is reduced. *Clinical Case 3.4* illustrates some of the clinical features of hypothyroidism and indicates how secondary hypothyroidism can be distinguished from primary hypothyroidism.

### Clinical Case 3.4:

A 28-year-old man was seen in the outpatient clinic with his wife. He had noted gradually worsening tiredness and fatigability, making his job difficult to maintain. He had gained weight (approximately 3 kg) and his wife had noted that he had worn an extra sweater during the winter months. His feet had been cold in bed and his hair and skin dry. His wife has had to take time off from work to bring her husband to the clinic (because her husband's car was being repaired following damage to both the near- and offside wings) and was naturally keen to see things sorted out quickly. The blood tests showed that the serum $T_4$ was low and the TSH was normal. Thyroid autoantibodies were negative.

This patient had clinical features typical of hypothyroidism. Whilst autoimmunity is the commonest cause of both primary hyper- and hypothyroidism, two noteworthy features indicate that this was not the cause of the hypothyroidism seen in this case. First, the patient was a young male and second, the serum TSH concentration was normal in the face of a low $T_4$ concentration. Thus, in the absence of raised concentrations of TSH with low concentrations of thyroid hormones (as seen in primary hypothyroidism) the cause lay at the level of the hypothalamus or pituitary gland. The fact that the patient had damaged both front wings of his car was another clinical indicator. He has a visual field defect (see *Box 7.1*) caused by a large benign pituitary tumor that extended above the pituitary fossa and pressed on the optic chiasm. The patient had secondary hypothyroidism due to hypopituitarism.

**Treatment of secondary hypothyroidism**

*Clinical Case 3.4* raised the clinical problem of how much $T_4$ should be given to replace a deficit. Over the last 20–30 years (and as assays for TSH have improved), the daily dose of $T_4$ has been reduced from 300–400 µg to about 125–175 µg (approximately 1.5 µg/kg ideal weight in adults). In a patient with primary hypothyroidism, there is general agreement that the amount of thyroxine given should be titrated against measurements of the serum TSH, aiming to keep this parameter within the normal range. This, of course, assumes normal function of the enzyme that converts $T_4$ to $T_3$ and is important in mediating the feedback effects of thyroid hormones on the pituitary gland. However, in a patient without an intact feedback loop and in the absence of a cheap, reliable measure of $T_3$ action in peripheral tissues, the replacement dose is generally guessed in the range 100–200 µg. The question of combined $T_3$ and $T_4$ replacement (mimicking the natural secretion of the thyroid gland) is under active discussion.

## Hypothyroidism in infancy and childhood

*Clinical Case 3.3* illustrated the dramatic effects of hypothyroidism during pubertal development. However the effects are worse (and permanent) when hypothyroidism occurs in fetal, neonatal and early childhood. An athyroidal or hypothyroidal neonate occurs in approximately 1:4000 live births and, since thyroid hormones are essential for normal development of the nervous and skeletal systems, neonatal screening programmes are used (*Box 3.24*). These involve measuring serum concentrations of TSH by a sensitive immunoradiometric assay (*Box 3.25*) and such tests ensure that all

## Box 3.24:
### Neonatal thyroid screening

- Screening is performed on capillary blood that is also used for phenylketonuria screening (the Guthrie test).
- Thyroid 'function' is assessed by measuring circulating TSH concentrations using an IRMA assay (see *Box 3.25*).
- Note that marked changes in thyroid physiology occur immediately after birth:
  - Circulating TSH increases to approximately 70 mU/l within minutes
  - $T_4$ and $T_3$ secretions consequently rise over the next 24h
  - There is a gradual decrease in the concentration of these hormones during infancy and childhood.
- The test results are, therefore, dependent on the time after birth when it is performed together with factors such as prematurity and illness.
- It does not diagnose cases of secondary hypothyroidism (low TSH due to hypothalamic or pituitary dysfunction).

affected neonates receive $T_4$ replacement as early as possible after birth.

The most severely affected infants will, however, be left with a permanent decrease in psycho-neurological function, probably reflecting intrauterine events. If there is any doubt about thyroid status (for example, with borderline results), it is better to replace thyroxine up to the age of, say, 2 years when treatment can be stopped under supervision and reassessment performed. The usual dose given is up to ten times the adult mean dose calculated on surface area. In childhood, acquired hypothyroidism (usually autoimmune) characteristically presents, as has been seen, with poor growth, epiphyseal dysplasia or poor school attainment. All features respond very well to $T_4$ replacement.

Goitrous hypothyroidism in childhood may be due to defects in the synthesis of thyroid hormones. The best recognised of these is Pendred's syndrome that is associated with congenital deafness and a defect in the synthesis of a protein (pendrin) thought to be involved in anion transport.

# Thyroid hormone resistance

The inability of target cells to respond to a hormone is known as hormone resistance and this is a common cause of endocrine disorders. Resistance can result from a reduction or loss of hormone receptors, or an aberrant receptor or signaling molecule.

Thyroid hormone resistance does exist but, compared to the millions of people exhibiting insulin resistance, the number of people showing resistance to thyroid hormones is minute. Complete resistance to thyroid hormone has never been recorded (it may be incompatible with life) and mutations causing resistance have only been found in the TR-β receptor (*Box 3.9*).

The key clinical features of thyroid hormone resistance are attention deficit hyperactivity disorder, developmental delay, learning disability, deafness and impaired growth in children with goiters. Patients with a generalized resistance and with signs and symptoms of hypothyroidism are treated with doses of thyroxine that facilitate normal growth and development. Paradoxically, some patients with thyroid hormone resistance exhibit symptoms and signs of hyperthyroidism. This may result from relatively greater resistance at the pituitary gland than in peripheral target tissues resulting in TSH secretion inappropriately high for these tissues. In such patients, beneficial effects have been seen with TRIAC (see *Box 3.29*) or with the D isomer of $T_4$ that have a higher affinity for the thyroid hormone receptor than $T_3$.

# Non-thyroid illness ('sick euthyroid' syndrome)

Measurements of serum thyroid hormone and/or TSH concentrations are often abnormal in patients hospitalized for acute illness (*Box 3.26*). These are usually reversible disturbances detected by biochemical assays but without associated symptoms of hypo- or hyperthyroidism. Such a condition has

## Measurement of serum TSH concentrations — immunoradiometric (IRMA) and enzyme-linked immunoabsorbent assays (ELISA)

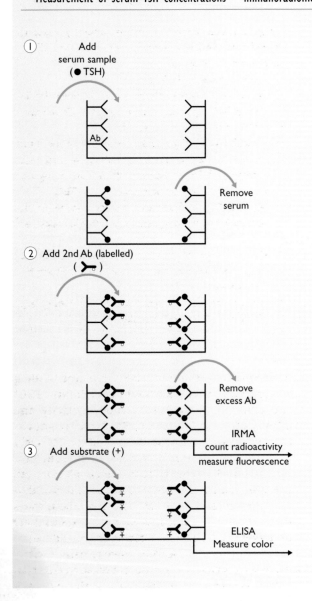

① Add
serum sample
(● TSH)

Ab

Remove
serum

② Add 2nd Ab (labelled)
( >● )

Remove
excess Ab

IRMA
count radioactivity
measure fluorescence

③ Add substrate (+)

ELISA
Measure color

These assays use two mouse monoclonal antibodies. They are very sensitive and specific.

① The first antibody (Ab), attached to the sides of the incubation well, captures TSH in the serum sample.

② A second Ab labelled with a radioactive, fluorescent or enzyme marker binds to a second site on the TSH molecule.

③ When the second antibody carries an enzyme marker, a substrate is added and the enzyme will induce a color reaction.

④ The concentration of the hormone will be directly proportional to the amount of radioactivity (IRMA), fluorescence or color intensity (ELISA).

There is an international standard for human TSH so the reliability and reproducibility of the assays can be monitored world-wide.

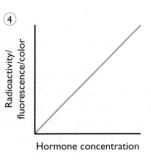

④

Radioactivity/
fluorescence/color

Hormone concentration

been termed 'sick euthyroid' syndrome, although a better term is 'non-thyroid illness'. It is considered to result from the effects of acute illness and/or the drugs treating the illness (*Box 3.27*) on the synthesis, transport and metabolism of hormones. To understand these it is necessary to discuss the transport and metabolism of thyroid hormones and the concept of 'total' and 'free' circulating hormone concentrations.

## Box 3.26:
### Non-thyroid illness

**Definition:** Disturbances in the circulating concentrations of thyroid hormones and TSH assays arising in systemic non-thyroid illnesses and normalizing after recovery.

**Classification:**

- Low serum $T_3$, normal $T_4$. The most common biochemical abnormality, it is seen in approximately 70% hospitalized patients. $T_3$ reduced by about 50%, $rT_3$ increased (except in renal failure) due to its decreased clearance as a result of reduced activity/production of 5' mono-deiodinase Type I.
- Low serum total $T_3$ and $T_4$. Usually seen in severely ill patients. Free $T_4$ is normal owing to inhibition of $T_4$ binding or production of altered TBG.
- High serum total $T_4$, normal total $T_3$. Seen in patients with liver disease producing increased quantities of TBG. Free $T_3$ low or low-normal, $rT_3$ high.
- Increased serum total $T_4$ and TBG, normal $T_3$ and paradoxical decreases in $rT_3$. Seen in patients with HIV infection.

**Clinical considerations:**

- Drugs, used to treat the severely ill, affect thyroid physiology (see *Box 3.27*).
- Radiology investigations of sick patients may utilize radiographic agents containing high concentrations of iodine.
- Diagnosis of 'true' thyroid disease in severely ill patients is difficult; no single investigation is reliable. A serum TSH >20mU/l is indicative of primary hypothyroidism (particularly when autoantibodies are present) and a TSH <0.05mU/l is suggestive of hyperthyroidism.

## Box 3.27:
### Drugs and the thyroid gland

Drugs can alter thyroid hormone status by affecting thyroid hormone synthesis, transport or metabolism. They act at a number of sites to:

- Block $I^-$ uptake, e.g. lithium.
- Decrease iodination of the tyrosine molecules in thyroglobulin, e.g. some sulfonamides and sulfonylureas.
- Inhibit hormone secretion, e.g. lithium
- Alter thyroid binding globulin concentration and, thus, concentrations of 'free' thyroid hormones, e.g. estrogens, clofibrate increase TBG whilst androgens, glucocorticoids and L-asparginase decrease TBG.
- Alter binding to TBG or transthyretin, e.g. salicylates, phenytoin and some non-steroidal anti-inflammatories such as fenclofenac.
- Decrease conversion of $T_4$ to $T_3$, e.g. glucocorticoids, propranolol, amiodarone, some iodinated radiographic contrast agents.
- Increase hormone degradation or excretion, e.g. phenytoin, carbamazepine, cholestyramine.

transthyretin (previously called thyroxine-binding prealbumin), thyroxine-binding globulin (TBG) and albumin. These vary in their capacity and affinity for $T_3$ and $T_4$ (*Box 3.28*); about 70% of circulating thyroid hormones are bound to TBG. Only a tiny fraction (<0.5%) of released thyroid hormones exist in a free form in the circulation and this is in equilibrium with the bound forms of thyroid hormones. The free-hormone hypothesis states that it is only the free thyroid hormones that act on target cells. The bound forms are considered to act as a circulating reservoir. There remains controversy as to whether the ratio of bound to free hormone changes as blood passes through the capillary bed of an organ.

Assays for thyroid hormones (see below) may measure the 'total' $T_4$ or $T_3$ or the respective 'free' fractions. Any reduction of serum TBG concentration (e.g. reduced synthesis in liver disease or increased loss in kidney disease) reduces the concentrations of total $T_4$ and total $T_3$. The feedback loop 'senses' changes in free hormone concentra-

# Transport and metabolism of thyroid hormones

The iodothyronines are virtually insoluble in water and, once released from thyroglobulin, they are very rapidly bound to the plasma proteins,

- Over 99% circulating thyroid hormones are bound to plasma proteins of which about 70% is bound to TBG, 10–15% to transthyretin and 15–20% to albumin. Only a tiny fraction is in the 'free' form.
- The interaction of $T_4$ with TBG can be expressed by the following equation:

$$T_4 + TBG \rightleftharpoons T_4.TBG$$

where $K_a$ is the equilibrium constant (a measure of affinity) and TBG the unoccupied binding sites. Thus:

$$K_a = \frac{[T_4.TBG]}{[T_4 + TBG]}$$

- Binding of hormones to plasma proteins provides a reservoir of active free hormone and delays metabolism of hormones.
- Changes in the concentration of binding proteins alters total hormone concentration and free hormone concentration.

Comparison of the serum concentrations of $T_4$ and $T_3$

|  |  | $T_4$ | $T_3$ |
|---|---|---|---|
| Serum concentration | Total | 100 nmol/l | 2 nmol/l |
|  | Free (%) | 20 pmol/l (0.02%) | 5 pmol/l (0.4%) |

tion and TSH secretion is modulated to maintain this. Similar compensations occur when TBG concentrations increase, most commonly as a result of pregnancy or estrogen administration.

Eighty per cent of the total thyroid hormones secreted each day is $T_4$ but this is relatively inactive at nuclear receptors and, thus, considered to be a prohormone. Approximately 70–80% of released $T_4$ is converted by deiodinases to the biologically active $T_3$, the remainder to reverse $T_3$ ($rT_3$) which has no significant biological activity. Deiodinases are unusual selenium-containing enzymes that are present in a number of tissues and are responsible for the metabolism of thyroid hormones (*Box 3.29*).

Removal of an iodine atom from the 5th carbon atom (5') of the outer tyrosine ring of $T_4$ by Type 1 and Type 2 deiodinases produces $T_3$ whilst deiodination of the inner (5) tyrosine ring by Type 1 and Type 3 deiodinases produces $rT_3$. Further deiodinations at the 3rd and 5th carbon atoms of both outer and inner tyrosine rings produce increasingly inactive diiodo- and monoiodo-thyronines and at the same time conserving iodine. Iodothyronines are excreted in the urine although some $T_3$ and $T_4$ is conjugated with glucuronide and excreted via the bile in the feces.

The decreased circulating concentrations of $T_3$ in the severely ill may be due to a reduction in 5' deiodinase activity as a result of the low calorie intake and the raised glucocorticoid secretions in response to stress. This reduces the conversion of $T_4$ to $T_3$ and, concomitantly, the conversion of $T_3$ to $T_2$.

The term 'sick euthyroid syndrome' presupposes that the results of all the biochemical changes are neutral with regard to thyroid hormone function. There is, in fact, little evidence to support this. However, it can be said that generally thyroid hor-

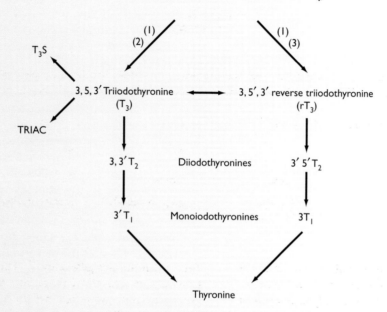

**3,5,3'5'-Tetraiodothyronine (thyroxine, or T$_4$)**

- Thyroid hormones are metabolized by a series of deiodinations which involve three types of deiodinases (indicated by numbers in brackets)

  Type 1: deiodinates at both the 5' and 5 carbon atoms and is found in the liver, kidney, thyroid, pituitary gland and central nervous system. With a high K$_m$ for T$_4$, it is the only isoenzyme inhibited by PTU. Its activity is increased in hyperthyroidism and reduced in hypothyroidism.

  Type 2: deiodinates only at the 5' position and is found in brain, brown fat, placenta and pituitary gland. With a lower K$_m$ than Type 1, it is considered to maintain intracellular concentrations of T$_3$. This is important in the negative feedback actions of T$_4$ on the pituitary gland. Its activity is decreased in hyperthyroidism and increased in hypothyroidism.

  Type 3: deiodinates only at the 5 position and is found only in brain and placenta. As it is incapable of converting T$_4$ to the active T$_3$, it may protect the brain and fetus from excess active T$_3$.

- Some T$_4$ is metabolised by being sulfated, decarboxylated, deaminated or conjugated with glucuronide (other pathways).

- Some T$_3$ may be sulfated (T$_3$S) or converted to the acetic acid derivative triiodoacetic acid (TRIAC) that is more potent than its parent T$_3$.

- Serum half lives: T$_4$ – 7 days, T$_3$ – 1 day, rT$_3$ – 4 hours.

mone treatment for the severely ill does not bring any clinical benefits.

## Biochemical measurements of thyroid hormone status

Assays of circulating thyroid hormone concentrations are usually referred to as 'thyroid function tests', often abbreviated to 'TFTs'. It is clear that they do not measure thyroid 'function' since this implies a measure of the effectiveness of thyroid hormone on peripheral tissues, but they are used as surrogate measures. Total (bound plus free) thyroid hormones can be measured by a competitive binding assay after chemically removing the binding proteins. As discussed above, this measurement may not reflect the physiological state since changes in the concentration of binding proteins alter the total hormone concentration. It is possible to measure the concentration of free thyroid hormones in serum samples by an indirect assay method (*Box 3.30*).

It is to be emphasized that, in the presence of an intact feedback loop, serum TSH concentration reflects the effects of thyroid hormones on the pituitary gland. For this reason serum TSH concentration has been recommended as first-line assay of 'thyroid function'.

The results of the biochemical tests obtained in the clinical cases may now be interpreted. In *Clinical Case 3.1* (iodide-induced hyperthyroidism), the concentrations of circulating thyroid hormones were high (total $T_4$ 310 nmol/l, NR 55-150 nmol/l) and, as a result of negative feedback, the peripheral concentration of TSH was low (<0.05 mU/l, NR 0.5-4.0 mU/l). There were no detectable anti-thyroid autoantibodies. In *Clinical Case 3.2* (Graves' disease), the concentrations of thyroid hormones were again high (total $T_4$ 320 nmol/l, NR 70-150 nmol/l) and the serum TSH concentration suppressed (<0.05 mU/l, NR 0.5-4.0 mU/l). The autoantibody titers (measured by the binding assay – see *Box 3.15*) were high, not only those against the TSH receptor but also to thyroid peroxidase and thyroglobulin. In *Clinical Case 3.3* (primary hypothyroidism), the operative hypothalamo-pituitary feedback loop led to high circulating TSH concentrations (>110 mU/l, NR 0.5-4.0

mU/l) in response to the unmeasurable total $T_4$ (<5 nmol/l, NR 70-150 nmol/l). In contrast, *Clinical Case 3.4* (secondary hypothyroidism) the loss of the feedback loop resulted in a normal circulating concentration of TSH, 2.5 mU/l (NR 0.5-4.0 mU/l), despite low circulating concentrations of thyroid hormones (free $T_4$ 4 pmol/l, NR 11-23 pmol/l).

## Thyroid growth

It has been seen that activation of the TSH receptor (whether by the hormone itself or by autoantibodies) is a potent stimulator to thyroid growth; since the receptors are present on every follicular cell, such growth tends to be diffuse.

Experimental studies, however, have shown that numerous cytokines and growth factors can affect thyroid function and these may have clinical implications. For example, they may exert overall inhibitory effects on the hypothalamo-pituitary-thyroid axis and could account for some of the effects seen in non-thyroidal illness. Cytokines may also be involved in the etiology of autoimmune responses and it is noteworthy that the thyroid gland produces more cytokines than any other endocrine gland. Like cytokines, growth factors are present at all levels of the axis and there is evidence that insulin-like growth factor potentiates TSH action on thyrotrophs. This could account for the growth of some nodules.

## Nodular thyroid disease

In contrast to diffuse goiters, sometimes focal abnormalities arise that affect only certain cells in the thyroid gland and give rise to nodules. These may be 'hot' (i.e. take up radioactive iodine and show increased thyroid hormone synthesis) or 'cold' (i.e. non-functional) (see *Box 3.6*).

### Clinical Case 3.5:

A 53-year-old woman came to the outpatient clinic. She had no symptoms but gave a history of a lump in her neck being noticed by her primary care physician during a routine 'well-woman' check. There was no family history of thyroid disease and she had a blameless past medical history. She was a nonsmoker and was on no medication apart from estrogen replacement therapy for menopausal hot flushes. She had not noticed any change in her voice, or difficulty swallowing or breathing. Examination was entirely normal except for a $3 \times 2$ cm single nodule in the left lower thyroid pole. Blood tests showed that her total $T_4$ was 196 nmol/l (NR 70–150nmo/l), free $T_3$ 7.8 pmol/l (NR 4.0–8.1pmol/l), TSH 2 mU/l (NR 0.5–4.0 mU/l) and thyroid autoantibodies were not present in serum.

In this patient, the serum total $T_4$ was raised whilst free $T_3$ and TSH were normal, indicating that she was euthyroid. The high concentration of total $T_4$ was due to an estrogen-induced increase in TBG. Estrogen increases glycosylation of this protein and, thus, reduces its metabolism. This resulted in an increase in bound $T_4$ and a consequent increase in $T_4$ secretion to maintain normal concentrations of 'free' $T_4$. The $^{99m}$Tc scan showed normal uptake of the radioactivity but with an area of decreased uptake in the region of the nodule (*Box 3.6*). This indicated that the nodule lacked the iodide symporter and, thus, it was a non-functional or 'cold' nodule.

### Prevalence and etiology of benign nodular disease

Studies of populations (such as Whickham in Northern England or Framingham in the US) have indicated that multinodular thyroids occur in around 5% of the population with a marked female preponderance (10:1). Autopsy studies have indicated a much higher incidence of nodular thyroid disease, indeed up to 50%, with multinodular disease outnumbering single nodules by about 4 to 1. The incidence increases markedly in people over 50 years of age. It is much higher in areas of iodine deficiency indicating the importance of iodine in the etiology of nodularity.

The etiology of benign nodular disease is not well understood although in some cases it is due to activating mutations of the TSH receptor or G-protein signalling system (*Box 3.12*). When such acti-

vating mutations of the TSH receptor are in the germ line (which is very rare) these will be passed on to succeeding generations appearing as familial hyperthyroidism.

The clinical index of a nodule, which makes no assumption of the underlying pathology, is the ability to detect one by palpation. Generally, (fat necks notwithstanding) this needs a lump 1 cm in diameter before it can be felt. However, if ultrasound scanning is used, it is more often than not that nodules some 2–3 mm in diameter are detected. The clinical relevance of such micronodularity detected on an ultrasound scan is very doubtful. However, the detection of a thyroid nodule(s) by palpation raises the important clinical question; is the lump malignant?

## Thyroid cancer

Tumors of the thyroid gland may be primary (arising from cells within the thyroid gland) or secondary due to malignant cells which have spread from other tissues (*Box 3.31*). Those arising from parafollicular cells which secrete calcitonin (giving rise to medullary cell carcinomas) are discussed on page 212. Lymphomas may arise from infiltrating lymphocytes and, though they are much more common in Hashimoto's disease, they are still very rare. Other tumors such as sarcomas from smooth muscle cells within the gland are also exceedingly rare.

The majority of primary tumors arise from epithelial cells of the thyroid gland and are, therefore, termed adenomas if benign and carcinomas if malignant. The epithelial cell tumors are sub-classified as either papillary or follicular according to their histological appearance. These tumors are found more often in women (2 to 4 fold more often than men), aged 45–50 years. In areas with adequate iodine intake, the commonest tumor is papillary, accounting for some 80% of all tumors. Where iodine intake is low there is a relative increase in follicular and anaplastic carcinomata, though no overall increase in frequency. A number of factors, both genetic and environmental has been implicated in the etiology of epithelial tumors (*Box 3.32*).

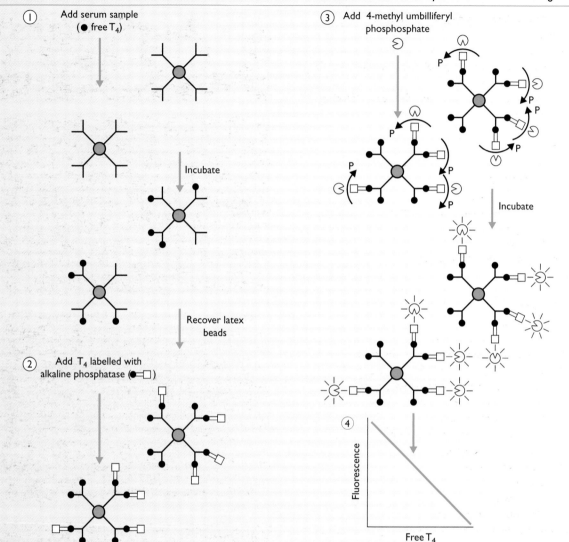

① Add serum sample
(● free T₄)

Incubate

Recover latex beads

② Add T₄ labelled with alkaline phosphatase (●—□)

③ Add 4-methyl umbilliferyl phosphosphate

Incubate

④

Fluorescence

Free T₄

① Free $T_4$ in patient's serum is captured on antibodies attached to latex beads, and hormones bound to plasma globulins are removed. Latex particles are recovered by binding to an inert glass fiber matrix.

② Latex particles are incubated with $T_4$ labelled with alkaline phosphatase. The $T_4$ binds to any unoccupied antibody binding sites on the latex particles. Excess $T_4$ is removed.

③ Latex particles are incubated with 4-methylumberlliferyl phosphate which fluoresces when its phosphate group is removed by the alkaline phosphatase on the $T_4$.

④ The intensity of fluorescence is indirectly proportional to the concentration of free hormone in the serum sample and comparison of the results with those from tubes containing known amount of $T_4$ allows calculation of the original concentration of free hormone.

**Note**

- There is no international standard for $T_4$ or $T_3$ assays.
- The direct measurement of <u>free</u> $T_4$ and $T_3$ requires physical removal of bound hormones by dialysis or unfiltration. Such assays are expensive and labor intensive and, though used for research studies, are not suitable for routine laboratory use.
- Total serum concentrations of $T_3$ and $T_4$ are measured by direct competitive binding assays.

These are classified according to histological features

**Primary**

Adenomata

- Follicular – including colloid, Hurthle cell and other variants
- Papillary – this may include some follicular elements
- Teratoma

Carcinomata

- Differentiated

    Papillary

        Pure papillary

        Mixed papillary and follicular

        Follicular

    - Undifferentiated

Other – e.g. lymphoma, fibrosarcoma

**Secondary**

**TNM Grading**

T – primary tumor

- T0 – no palpable tumor
- T1 – single tumor confined to the gland
- T2 – multiple tumors confined to the gland
- T3 – tumor extending beyond the gland
- N – regional lymph nodes
    - N0 – no palpable nodes
    - N1 – moveable nodes on one side
    - N2 – moveable bilateral nodes
    - N3 – fixed nodes
- M – distant metastases
    - M0 – none
    - M1 – distant metastases

Clinically, the dominant factor in governing prognosis in thyroid epithelial cell cancer is age. Others factors include size of primary tumor, degree of invasiveness, histological grade and the presence of metastases. Of these, all except histological grade are incorporated into the TNM classification.

These images are available in color on the website.

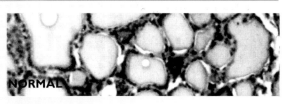

NORMAL

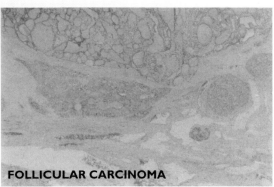

**FOLLICULAR CARCINOMA**

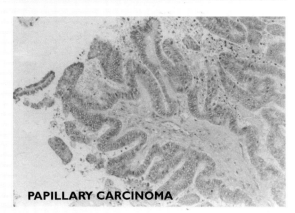

**PAPILLARY CARCINOMA**

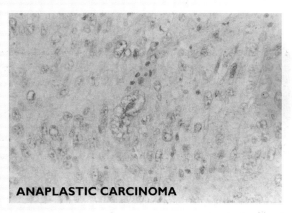

**ANAPLASTIC CARCINOMA**

## Etiological factors in thyroid cancer

**Growth factors** – the role of such known thyroid growth factors as TGF-$\alpha$, EGF, VEGF and IGF-I in neoplasia remains uncertain.

**Oncogenes** –

- *ret* is a gene coding for a tyrosine kinase receptor for neurotrophic growth factor. It is not normally expressed in thyroid follicular cell tumors. The *ret* genes express C-terminal fragments of the receptor which leads to unregulating signalling. *Ret* oncogenes have been designated *ret/ptc1*, *ret/ptc2*, *ret/ptc3* (where ptc stands for papillary thyroid carcinoma). The rearrangements of *ret* are particularly seen in patients who have had tumors after irradiation e.g. papillary tumors post-Chernobyl. *ret* is also a factor in medullary cell carcinoma of the thyroid gland.

- *ras* is a membrane associated monomeric G protein involved in signal transduction processes. Activating mutations of *ras* genes are found with a similar frequency in follicular adenomas and carcinomas.

- *p53* is a tumor-suppressor gene. Mutations of *p53* are seen in anaplastic cancers.

**Thyroid irradiation** – External irradiation dose-dependently increases the incidence of thyroid cancer and is marked in younger patients. Therapeutic doses of radioiodine do not appear to result in an increased risk of thyroid malignancy.

**Other** – Familial cases of thyroid cancer have been reported in familial adenomatosis coli, Gardner's disease and Cowden's syndrome. There is controversy over the association with certain histocompatibility antigens.

## Thyroid cancer conundra

There are three conundra. The first is that, whilst nodular thyroid disease is common in the general population, only about 30 people in a million are diagnosed clinically with thyroid cancer annually and 6 people in a million die each year of the disease. This is a minute fraction of all cancer deaths and the risk of thyroid cancer causing death is extremely low.

The second conundrum arises because it is difficult to differentiate benign from malignant primary epithelial tumors by their histological appearances. The commonly used criteria of histological malignancy are invasion of blood vessels or lymphatics and breach of the capsule containing the nodule cells. When thyroid glands are examined at autopsy the histological features of papillary cancer are seen in 5 to 25% of thyroid glands examined. Thus, thyroid nodules and histological appearances of thyroid cancer are extremely common yet clinical disease is rare.

Clinical suspicion of malignancy may be raised by the speed of growth of a nodule or the involvement of the esophagus, trachea or recurrent laryngeal nerve (giving a hoarse voice and difficulty in breathing or swallowing). However, the only certain clinical benchmark is the behavior of the tumor; if it spreads (or metastasizes) it is malignant.

Differentiating the few malignant tumors from a large number of benign nodules has exercised clinicians for many years and, though various imaging techniques have been used, most centers now use fine needle aspiration cytological examination (*Box 3.33*). Typically, FNA cytology is used to separate diagnoses into five categories.

The third conundrum arises because death rates from differentiated thyroid cancer are extremely low and distinguishing malignant from benign nodules is problematic; how should individual patients be treated? Prognosis is the most important consideration and whilst various staging systems have been used to predict this, none seems better than the long established Tumor (T), Node (N), Metastasis (M) or TNM classification (*Box 3.31*). In general, the bigger the tumor, and the less well differentiated it is the worse the prognosis. Age is the other very important factor and patients under about 45 years have a better prognosis.

There is no general agreement on the degree of surgery and post-operative radioiodine or radiotherapy but, given the risks of thyroid surgery (*Box 3.19*), it has been argued that low risk patients should have less aggressive surgery (e.g. lobectomy rather than total thyroidectomy). Although the experimental data were obtained from studies on rodents, there is general agreement that patients with differentiated thyroid cancer are treated with $T_4$ to suppress TSH secretion (via the negative feedback effect). Measurements of serum thyroglobulin

This technique has transformed the investigation of thyroid nodules and has largely replaced ultrasound and $^{99m}$Tc scans . It is easy to perform in the out-patient clinic and well accepted by patients.

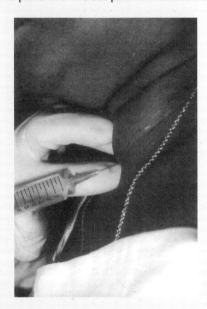

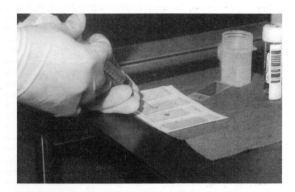

- A hypodermic needle is inserted into the nodule and cells in the nodule are aspirated by negative pressure in the hypodermic syrings as the needle is passed repeatedly through the nodule.

- Aspirated material is discharged onto glass slides, spread thinly, dried then fixed and stained. The stained cells are examined under the microscope for diagnosis and subsequent clinical management.

| Diagnosis | Suggested management |
|---|---|
| Benign | Follow up. Possible thyroxine therapy* |
| Probably malignant | Surgery |
| Follicular neoplasm | Surgery. Recommended since distinguishing between benign and malignant follicular cells is difficult on histological grounds alone |
| Technically unsatisfactory | Reaspirate |
| Cyst | Aspiration may cure |

*Evidence for efficacy is poor.

- False positive and negative rates are usually given as about 5%.
- FNA itself can cause abnormalities in the morphology of thyroid cells that may make histological examination of subsequently removed surgical material difficult to interpret.

(an index of TSH stimulation on the thyroid gland) may be used to monitor the effects of exogenous $T_4$.

The patient in *Clinical Case 3.5* underwent FNA. Cyst fluid was removed with resolution of symptoms. Cytological examination showed no evidence of malignancy.

# CLINICAL CASE QUESTIONS

The following are examples of applied pathophysiology and these clinically based questions can be answered with the information provided in this chapter. Answers and additional material are available on the website.

## Clinical Case Study Q3.1

A 43-year-old old female nurse was referred to the endocrine clinic. She weighed 110 kg and was 1.67 m tall. Her primary care physician had taken her blood for routine tests and had found the total $T_4$ to be 257 nmol/l (NR 70–150 nmol/l) with a free $T_3$ of 12.7 pmol/l (NR 4.0–8.1 pmol/l) and a TSH of <0.05 mU/l (NR 0.5–4.0 mU/l). There was no family history of any endocrine disease and her serum thyroid autoantibodies were normal. The primary care physician had treated the patient for several months with carbimazole 30 mg daily with no change in her biochemical tests of thyroid function. He therefore stopped the carbimazole and referred the patient for further investigation. A $^{99m}Tc$ scan of the thyroid gland was performed 4 weeks after cessation of the carbimazole (see Box Q3.1a).

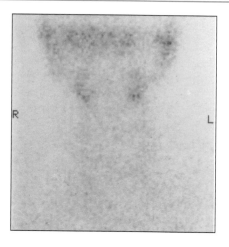

Box Q3.1a. This $^{99}Tc$ scan of Clinical Case Study Q3.1 taken at a time when the patient denied taking any medications for several months. (Compare the image with a normal scan (shown in Box 3.6).

**Question 1:** Using your knowledge of the hypo-thalamo-pituitary-thyroid axis feedback loop, how may the serum assays be interpreted and what are the possible diagnoses?

**Question 2:** How would you distinguish between these possibilities?

## Clinical Case Study Q3.2

A 59-year-old old Pakistani woman was admitted via the Emergency Room with a 4-week history of fever (with profuse night sweats), malaise, nausea, but no vomiting. Her symptoms had not responded to two courses of antibiotics prescribed by the primary care physician. Over the same time, she had noted a sore throat with pain radiating to the ears. There was a strong family history of type 2 diabetes mellitus and no family or contact history of TB. On examination, she had a temperature of 38.5°C, a pulse rate of 120 beats/min and a tender diffuse goiter (*Box Q3.2a*). She was noted to be mildly anemic (Hb 10.9g/dl) with an elevated peripheral blood white cell count (14.3 x 10⁹/l). A number of investigations were performed to find a source of infection to no avail. Her free T4 was 55 pmol/l and the serum TSH was unmeasurable (<0.05 mU/l). (*Box Q3.2a*) ⁹⁹ᵐTc scan of the thyroid was performed (*Box Q3.2b*).

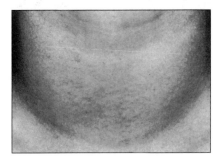

Box Q2.3a. The small diffusely enlarged thyroid gland.

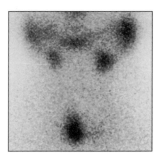

Box Q3.2b. The ⁹⁹ᵐTc scan of the patient performed during her admission.

**Question 1:** Given the clinical features and the serum assay results, what is the most likely diagnosis?

**Question 2:** In light of your answer to question 1, how should the ⁹⁹ᵐTc scan of the thyroid be interpreted?

**Question 3:** How should she be treated?

## Clinical Case Study Q3.3

A 34-year-old patient on the post-natal ward requested that her midwives send urgently for the duty pediatrician because of concerns for her 5-h-old baby. He was feeding poorly and his respiratory rate was rapid. Five years previously she had been treated for Graves' disease with courses of carbimazole and later radioactive iodine. The pediatrician found her son (*Box Q3.3*) to have a characteristic facial appearance with staring eyes, a marked tachycardia and fever.

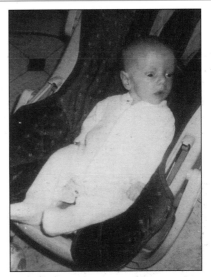

Box Q3.3. Photograph of the child in *Clinical case study Q3.3* taken by his mother a few weeks after birth

Question 1: What is the diagnosis and how is it related to the mothers previous medical history?

Question 2: How can it be confirmed and treated?

Question 3: Could it have been predicted and what is the likely prognosis?

# The adrenal gland

## Chapter objectives

*Knowledge of*

1. Synthesis of adrenocorticosteroids and its regulation
2. Metabolism of adrenal steroids
3. Physiological roles of adrenocorticosteroids
4. Clinical sequelae of disorders of steroid synthesis and secretion
5. Synthesis of catecholamines and its regulation
6. Metabolism of catecholamines
7. Physiological roles of catecholamines
8. Clinical sequelae of disorders of catecholamine synthesis and secretion
9. Investigation and treatment of adrenal disease

*"The naming of Cats is a difficult matter,*
*It isn't just one of your holiday games;*
*You may think at first I'm as mad as a hatter*
*When I tell you that a cat must have three different*
*names."*
*The Naming of Cats in Old Possum's Book of Practical*
*Cats, TS Eliot.*

All steroid hormones are synthesized from choles-terol and are categorized in the human into six dif-ferent classes or families according to activity determined in early bioassays. Like T.S. Eliot's cats, each has three different names (*Boxes 4.1 & 4.2*). The 'classical' steroid-producing endocrine glands (notwithstanding the kidneys that produce the active steroid metabolite of vitamin D) are the adre-nal cortex and the gonads.

The major secretions of the adrenal cortex (*Box 4.2*) are cortisol (the main member of the glucocor-ticoid family in humans), aldosterone (a mineralo-corticoid), and the 'weak' androgens androstenedione and dehydroepiandrostenedione (DHEA). Cortisol is an important metabolic hor-mone; aldosterone a hormone involved in salt and water homeostasis whilst the androgens are regard-ed as having little physiological significance when gonadal function is normal.

The first two clinical cases illustrate the potency of the effects of adrenocortical hormones and their different biological activities.

---

### Clinical Case 4.1:

A 52-year-old lady had been attending another hospital for some years with diabetes mellitus and systemic hypertension. She was a non-smoker but enjoyed a sherry in the evenings. There was no family history of diabetes mellitus or hypertension and she had never been pregnant, though the causes of this primary infertility had not been investigated. She had asthma and eczema and had been referred because of concern that she was becoming cushingoid (*Box 4.3*) as a result of her steroid treatment for these conditions.

---

115

**Box 4.1:**
**Steroid terminology**

Ⓐ

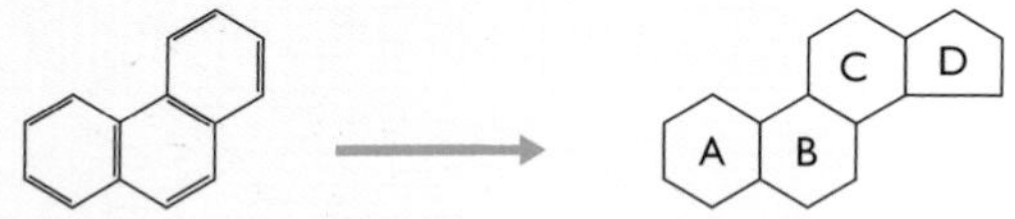


Phenanthrene — Cyclopentanoperhydrophenanthrene

Ⓑ

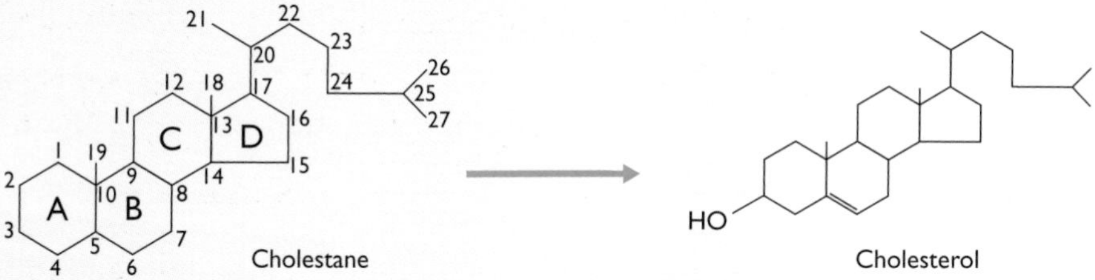


Cholestane — Cholesterol

Ⓒ

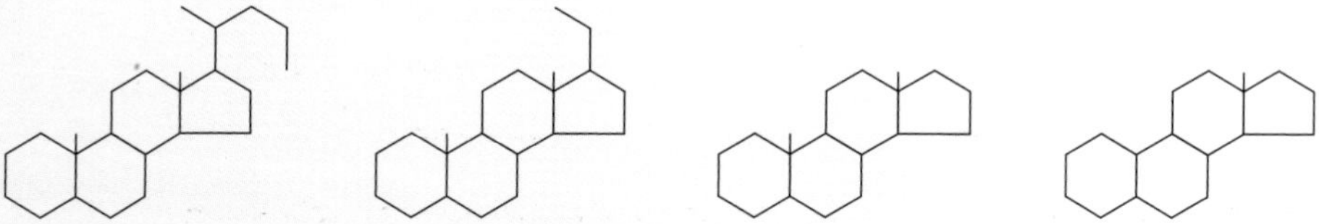

| Cholane | Pregnane | Androstane | Estrane |
|---|---|---|---|
| **C-24** | **C-21** | **C-19** | **C-18** |

Ⓐ The basic structure to the steroids is a phenanthrene ring to which a pentano ring has been added. Thus, the basic skeleton is a cyclopentanoperhydrophenanthrene made up of four rings (labeled A to D) and in which there is rigid code of numbering for the carbon atoms.

Ⓑ The parent hydrocarbon, and from which cholesterol is derived, is termed cholestane. By truncation, this C-27 compound is converted into the *pater familias* steroids:
cholane (C-24) – the parent of bile acids
pregnane (C-21) – the parent of progestins, glucocorticoids and mineralocorticoids
androstane (C-19) – the parent of androgens
estrane (C-18) – the parent of estrogens.

Ⓒ The five major endocrine families of C-21, C-19 and C-18 steroids in man are shown in *Box 4.2*.

## Box 4.2:

Five major endocrine families* derived from the *pater familias* steroids, pregnane, androstane or estrane

4-ene-3-one

**Progesterone**

**Cortisol**

**Aldosterone**

**Testosterone**

**Estradiol**

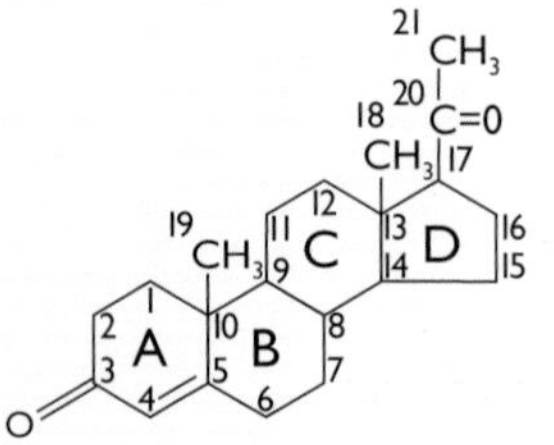

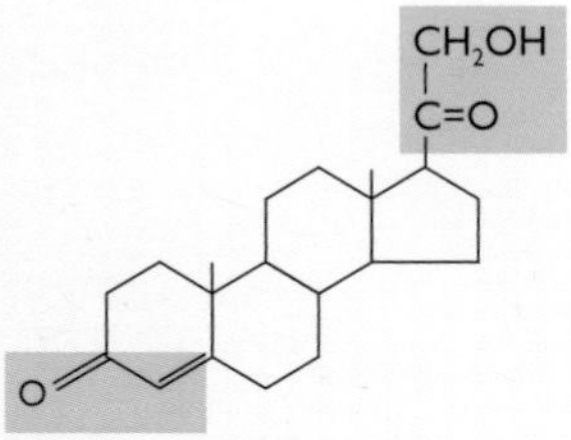

Shaded boxes show structural requirements for glucocorticoid and mineralocorticoid activity.
Hatched boxes show additional structural requirements for specific glucocorticoid or mineralocorticoid activity (see text).

| **Family** | **Principal active steroid in the family** | | |
|---|---|---|---|
| | **Trivial name** | **Systematic name** | **Common name** |
| Progestins (C-21) | Progesterone | Preg-4-ene-3,20-dione | P4 |
| Gluco-corticoids (C-21) | Cortisol | 11β,17,α,21-trihydroxy-pregn-4-ene-3,20-dione | F |
| Mineralo-corticoids (C-21) | Aldosterone | 11β,21-dihydroxy-3,20-pregn-4-ene,18-al | Aldo |
| Androgens (C-19) | Testosterone | 17β-hydroxy-androst-4-ene-3-one | T |
| Estrogens (C-18) | Estradiol | 3,17β-dihydroxy-1,3,5[10]-estratriene-diol | E2 |

- Common names were usually very empirical in origin. Thus compounds E, F (cortisol) and S were the 5th, 6th and 19th steroids to be isolated from the adrenal cortex.
- The systematic names look exceedingly complex. For those wishing to interpret the 'shorthand' nomenclature this is given on the Website.

*The sixth, vitamin D, features in *Box 5.6*.

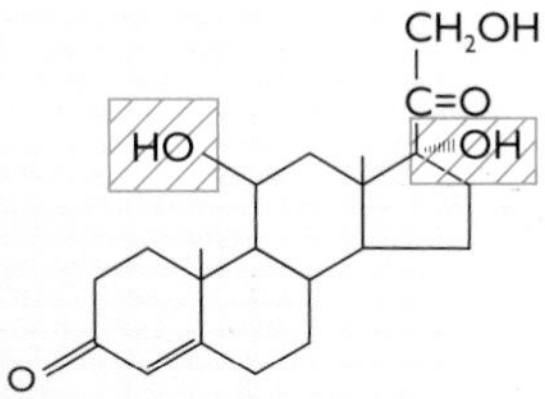

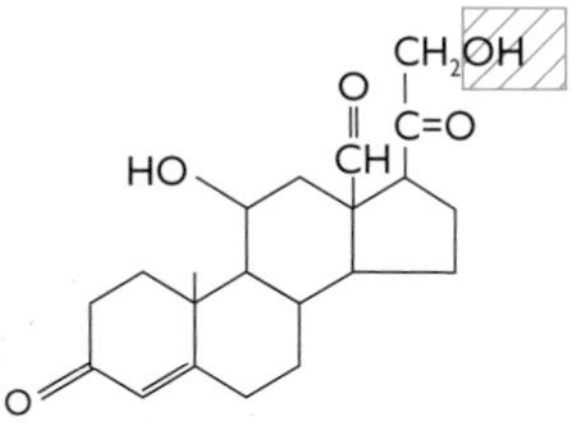

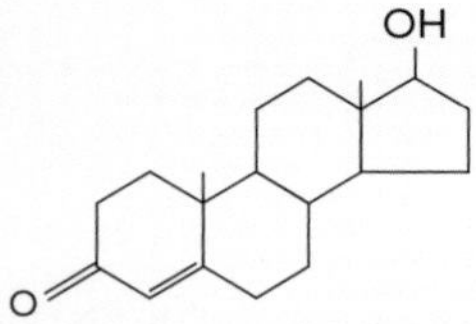

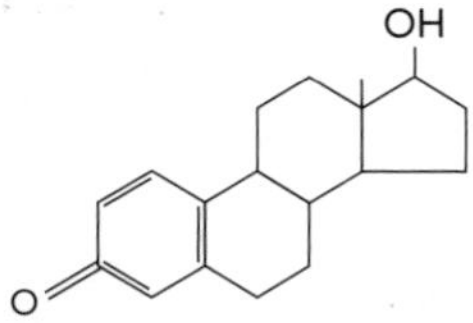

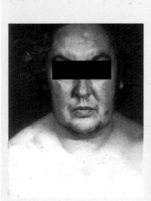
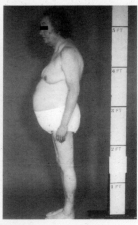
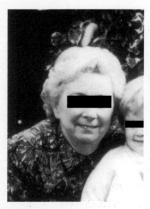
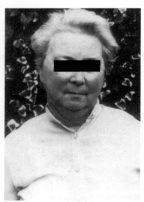

Clinical photographs of *Clinical Case 4.1*

These images are available in color on the website.

Family album pictures of *Clinical Case 4.2* taken approximately 2 years apart in front of the same ivy-covered wall.

## Clinical Case 4.2:

A 63-year-old woman had been previously treated at another hospital at the age of 44 years for carcinoma of the right breast. This involved removal of the breast (mastectomy), removal of both ovaries (termed bilateral oophorectomy) and chemotherapy. Two years later, local recurrence had been treated by further surgery. After a further local recurrence, some 8 years after the original diagnosis, she had received surgical treatment, with subsequent radical radiotherapy and the estrogen receptor antagonist tamoxifen. Six years later, the tamoxifen had been stopped and treatment with 600 mg medroxyprogesterone daily started. Over the subsequent 2 years, she had noted increased appetite with weight gain, abdominal swelling, easy bruising and poor healing of minor trauma. She had been treated with diuretics for newly diagnosed hypertension and had developed a plethoric face over 2 years (*Box 4.3*).

It is self-evident that patients with endocrine diseases are bioassays of circulating hormones. Clearly, there are some similarities in these cases: both are female, middle-aged and being treated with synthetic steroids. Both patients manifest the typical effects of excessive glucocorticoid action; centripetal obesity and relatively thin arms and legs. Whilst *Clinical Case 4.2* shows some minor changes in hairline, *Clinical Case 4.1* shows marked features associated with excessive androgen action; excess facial hair growth (hirsutism) with acne, greasy skin and male pattern temporal baldness (*Box 4.3*). She had been taking inhaled and topical synthetic glucocorticoids, whilst *Clinical Case 4.2* was prescribed an oral synthetic progestagen as secondary treatment for her breast cancer. To compare and contrast the clinical problems suffered by these patients, it is necessary to examine the biological effects of the different hormones secreted by the adrenal cortex and also those used therapeutically in these Clinical Cases.

# Specificity of the biological effects of adrenal steroid hormones

The different classes of steroid hormones are all generated by the enzymatic modification of the cholesterol nucleus and the structures of steroid hormones in two-dimensional drawings appear very similar (*Box 4.2*). This raises the question of how different steroids exert specific actions in target cells. Specificity first requires structural differences between steroid hormones.

A number of empirical studies over many years has established that the basic structural requirement for a steroid to possess glucocorticoid or mineralocorticoid activity is that it should be a carbon 21 (C-21) compound with a –CO-CH$_2$OH side-chain attached at C-17. In addition, there must be an unsaturated bond between C-4 and C-5 (sometimes referred to as Δ4) and a keto group (-C=O) at C-3 of ring A, together termed 4-ene-3-one (or Δ4, 3-keto). Specific glucocorticoid activity requires a hydroxyl group at C-11 and this activity is enhanced by a similar group at C-17. Mineralocorticoids, on the other hand, require a hydroxyl group on C-21 whilst the presence of hydroxyl groups at C-11 and C-17 *decrease* mineralocorticoid activity.

Androgenic effects are generated by C-19 compounds containing a 17β-hydroxyl group. The latter is very important since oxidation to 17-keto results in marked loss of activity and it is also stereospecific since steroids containing a 17α-hydroxyl group have little or no androgenic activity. The presence of either a 4-ene-3-one configuration or a 3-keto group in ring A is also necessary. The naturally occurring progestagens are, like cortisol and aldosterone, also 21-carbon molecules and possess keto groups on C-3 and C-20 for biological activity.

The second way in which specificity of steroid hormone action may be generated is, in large part, via the evolution of receptors that have much higher affinity for the active hormones than for metabolites or structurally similar steroids. This appears to be the case for estradiol and 1,25-dihydroxyvitamin D, the structures of which differ most from the other steroids. However, glucocorticoids, mineralocorticoids, progestagens and androgens have closer structural similarities and their specificities are markedly reduced. For example, the affinity of the mineralocorticoid receptor for cortisol is the same as that of the glucocorticoid receptor.

# Cholesterol and steroid synthesis in the adrenal cortex

Cholesterol is either obtained from the diet or synthesized from acetate by a CoA reductase enzyme. Approximately 300 mg cholesterol is absorbed from the diet each day and about 600 mg synthesized from acetate. Cholesterol is insoluble in aqueous solutions and its transport from the main site of synthesis, the liver, requires apoproteins to form a lipoprotein complex. Circulating lipoproteins were first characterized by centrifugation and as a result are grouped by density.

In the adrenal cortex, about 80% of cholesterol required for steroid synthesis is captured by receptors which bind low-density lipoproteins (LDL) although recent evidence has shown that high-density lipoprotein (HDL) cholesterol may also be taken up by adrenal cells. The remaining 20% is synthesized from acetate within the adrenal cells by the normal biochemical route. The cholesterol can be stored as esters in lipid droplets or utilized directly (*Box 4.4*).

The first stage in the synthesis of adrenal steroids is the hydrolysis of cholesterol esters and the active transfer of free cholesterol to the outer membrane of the mitochondria by a sterol transfer protein (*Box 4.4*). The transfer of hydrophobic cholesterol to the inner mitochondrial membrane is chaperoned by a *s*teroidogenic *a*cute *r*egulatory (StAR) protein where the first enzymatic process in steroid hormone synthesis occurs. The enzyme, known as side chain cleavage enzyme, P450$_{scc}$, (which also has 20,22 desmolase activity), converts cholesterol to pregnenolone. Indeed, most of the subsequent steps in steroid hormone synthesis also involve cytochrome P450 heme-containing enzymes, so-called because light is maximally absorbed at 450 nm when the proteins are complexed with CO. The genes coding for the *cy*tochrome *P*450 enzymes are abbreviated to CYP

Diagrammatic outline of the synthesis of cortisol from cholesterol in the adrenal cortex (see text and *Box 4.5* for details)

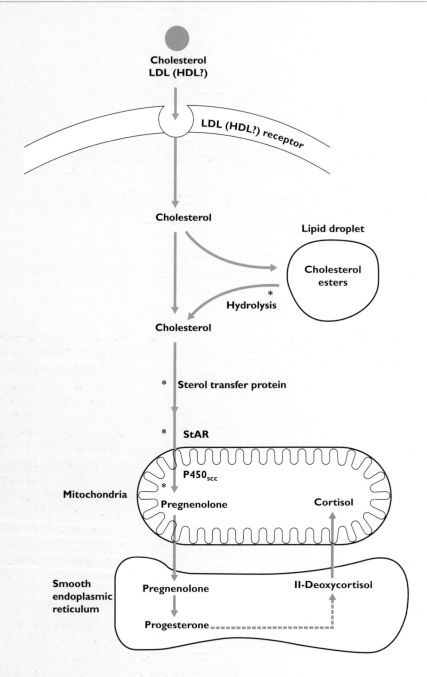

*Activities known to be regulated by ACTH.

**Box 4.5:**

Synthesis of the major steroid hormones secreted by the adrenal cortex

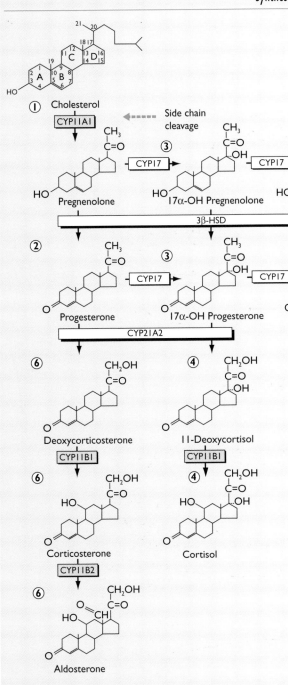

① The genes coding for the P450 enzymes are abbreviated to CYP and the first step in the synthesis of hormones is the 6 carbon unit side chain cleavage of cholesterol. Many of the subsequent steps also require P450 enzymes which activate oxygen and induce hydroxylations.

② Conversion of pregnenolone to progesterone requires oxidation of the 3-OH group and isomerization of the $\Delta^5$ double bond to $\Delta^4$ by 3β-hydroxysteroid-dehydrogenase (HSD).

③ Synthesis of cortisol and androgens requires C-17 hydroxylations of pregnenolone or progesterone.

④ Cortisol is formed by the subsequent hydroxylations at C-21 and C-11.

⑤ DHEA (+ sulfated form) and androstenedione are formed by removal of the two-carbon side chain at C-17.

⑥ Aldosterone is formed from progesterone by subsequent hydroxylations at C-21 and C-11 followed by oxidation of the C-18 methyl group ($CH_3$) to an aldehyde (CH=O).

Synthesis of steroid requires trafficking between mitochondria and smooth endoplasmic reticulum. Shaded boxes indicate mitochondrial enzymes. All others are in the smooth endoplasmic reticulum.

121

(*Box 4.5*) and they catalyze hydroxylations of the steroid molecule.

Pregnenolone is then shuttled from the mitochondria to the smooth endoplasmic reticulum where it is converted to progesterone or to 17α-hydroxypregnenolone. Through subsequent hydroxylations, progesterone can be converted to corticosterone (another glucocorticoid that is only released in small amounts in the human) and then aldosterone, whilst 17α-hydroxypregnenolone can be converted to androgens and cortisol (*Box 4.5*). There is, however, considerable interconversion between these two pathways and it should be noted that the final stage in cortisol synthesis takes place back in the mitochondria.

In functional terms, the adrenal cortex is, therefore, not a single endocrine gland since it secretes different steroids with widely different activities and functions. This is achieved by differential expression of enzymes resulting in functional zonation that has anatomical correlates.

## Anatomical and functional zonation in the adrenal cortex

Each adrenal gland weighs approximately 4 g and sits in close proximity to a kidney (in the UK, adrenal whilst, in the US and France, reference is made to a position above the kidney, viz suprarenal and sûrrénale (*Box 4.23*)). The cortex forms about 90% of its mass, the remaining core being the adrenal medulla. In the adult, it can be divided morphologically and functionally into three layers (the glomerulosa, fasciculata and reticularis (*Box 4.6*)). Each layer has a distinct histological appearance and secretes different steroid hormones (aldosterone, cortisol and androgens, respectively). A fourth or fetal zone is present during development. The inner 10–20% of the gland is the adrenal medulla secreting catecholamines. In the UK, these hormones are called adrenaline and noradrenaline; but the terms epinephrine and norepinephrine are also used for the same hormones.

Embryologically, the adrenal gland develops from two cell types (*Box 4.7*). The innermost layers of the gland contain most of the apoptotic and senescent cells indicating that this is where the cells die, supporting the concept that cortical cells originate from the outer layers of the cortex and move inwards. In addition, the arrangement of blood flow within the gland appears to be crucial in developing and maintaining the morphological and functional zonation of the gland (*Box 4.6*). The arrangement is such that blood vessels supplied from branches of the aorta, phrenic and renal arteries flow from the outer cortex to drain inwardly into venules of the adrenal medulla. Thus, glomerulosa cells differentiate on the arterial side and reticularis cells on the venous side.

The enzyme 17α-hydroxylase (CYP 17) is not present in the outer layer of the cortex and, thus, cortisol and androgens cannot be formed in this layer. Steroids and their metabolic by-products (notably lipid hydroperoxides) are released into the adrenal circulation and inhibit critical enzymes in subsequent layers through which the blood flows. As a result, no aldosterone can be synthesized by cells below the outer glomerulosa layer. In the inner layer, 17α-hydroxyprogesterone cannot be converted to cortisol but is shunted into the formation of androgens. Interestingly high cortisol concentrations reaching the adrenal medulla stimulate the synthesis of phenylethanolamine-*N*-methyltransferase which catalyzes the conversion of norepinephrine to epinephrine (see *Box 4.39*). Thus, the structural relationship between the cortex and medulla and its blood supply has additional functional implications within the medulla.

## Glucocorticoid receptors

Glucocorticoids are essential to life and after removal of both adrenals humans will not survive for long without glucocorticoid replacement. Cortisol has a wide range of actions, many of which are considered 'permissive'. This is because it does not always initiate processes but allows them to occur by increasing the activity of enzymes, inducing enzymes or augmenting/inhibiting the action of other hormones.

Receptors for glucocorticoids (GRs) are usually intracellular and unlike thyroid hormones they usually exist in the cytoplasm, not the nucleus, and are associated with heat shock proteins (*Box 4.8*).

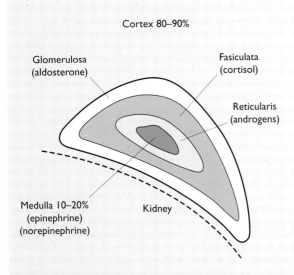

Diagrammatic representation of the different zones of
the adrenal gland and their hormone secretions

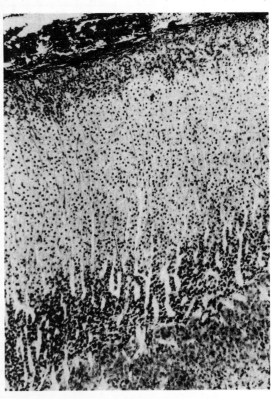

Low power photomicrograph of a cross-sectional view
of the adrenal gland

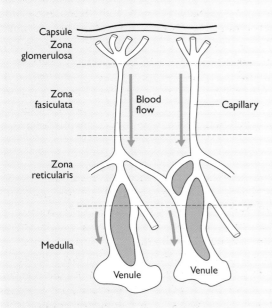

Highly schematic diagram showing the blood flow within
the adrenal gland. Arterial blood is supplied by the
phrenic, renal and aortic arteries. Venules of the medulla
drain into the vena cava from the right adrenal gland and
into the renal vein from the left gland

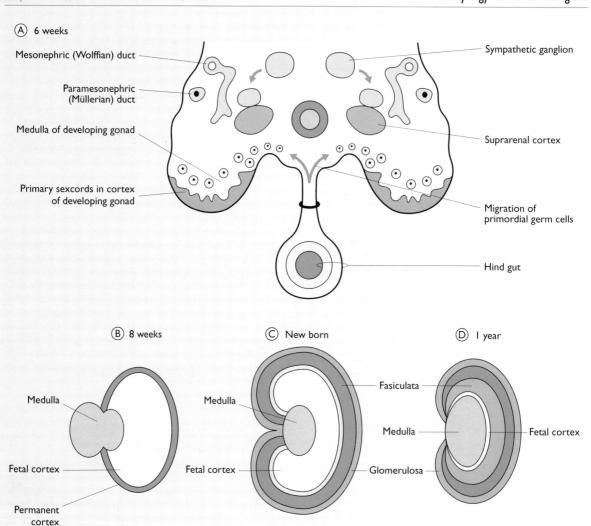

Ⓐ 6 weeks

Mesonephric (Wolffian) duct

Paramesonephric (Müllerian) duct

Medulla of developing gonad

Primary sexcords in cortex of developing gonad

Sympathetic ganglion

Suprarenal cortex

Migration of primordial germ cells

Hind gut

Ⓑ 8 weeks

Medulla

Fetal cortex

Permanent cortex

Ⓒ New born

Medulla

Fetal cortex

Fasiculata

Medulla

Glomerulosa

Ⓓ I year

Fetal cortex

Ⓐ Two-dimensional diagram of a transverse section of the caudal region of a 6-week embryo. The fetal suprarenal cortex is derived from mesodermal cells. The medulla is formed from an adjacent sympathetic ganglion that is derived from neural crest cells. The diagram also shows the development of the gonads at this time (see *Box 6.3*)

Ⓑ After the neural crest cells have migrated they are engulfed by the fetal cortex and they differentiate into the secretory cells of the adrenal medulla. More mesodermal cells surround the fetal cortex and these will eventually form the permanent adult cortex.

Ⓒ At birth the adrenal gland is relatively much larger than the adult gland due to the extensive size of the fetal cortex. The zona glomerulosa and fasiculata are differentiated.

Ⓓ After I year the fetal cortex has all but disappeared but the zona reticularis is not recognizable until the end of the 3rd year after birth.

The glucocorticoid receptor and activation by cortisol

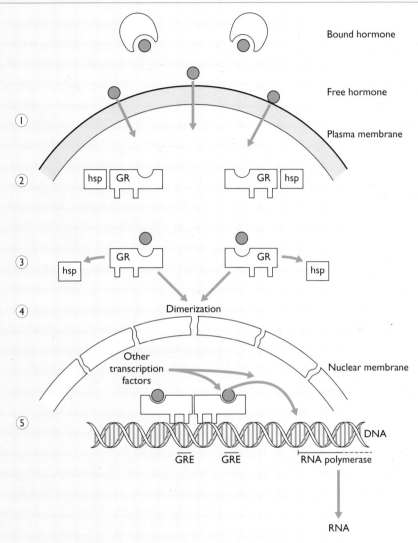

① Unbound, lipophilic cortisol readily crosses cell membranes and in target tissues will combine with the glucorticoid receptor (GR).

② Like the androgen and progesterone receptors, but unlike thyroid hormone receptors, unliganded GRs are located in the cytoplasm attached to heat shock proteins (hsp-90, hsp-70 and hsp-56).

③ When hormones bind to these receptors hsps are released and, through an energy-dependent process, the hormone receptor complexes translocate to the nucleus.

④ These complexes form homo- or heterodimers and the zinc fingers of their DNA-binding domains slot into the glucocorticoid response elements (GREs) in the DNA helix.

⑤ Together with other transcription factors, such as NF-κB or c-jun and c-fos, they initiate RNA synthesis (activation of RNA polymerase) downstream of their binding.

These are displaced when cortisol diffuses across the cell membrane, and binds to these receptors in target cells. Subsequent phosphorylation of the receptors facilitates translocation of the hormone-receptor complex into the nucleus where it forms a homo- or heterodimer with another hormone-receptor complex. The effects of heterodimeric forms may differ from those of the homodimers.

The zinc fingers in the DNA-binding domain of the dimerized receptors interact with specific grooves of the DNA helix containing a consensus sequence. The site of receptor binding on the DNA is known as the hormone response element (HRE) – in this case the glucocorticoid response element (GRE). In association with other transcription factors, the GRs stimulate or suppress gene transcription that is usually initiated down-stream of the GRE. The structural similarities of the DNA-binding domain of glucocortiocoid, estrogen, androgen and progesterone receptors are such that they can all bind to the same hormone response element, a consensus 15 nucleotide sequence. Additionally, cortisol has equal affinity for the aldosterone receptor in the kidney tubules but its rapid inactivation to cortisone in these cells normally prevents binding.

The expression of GR is ubiquitous and it occurs in two forms, GR-α and GR-β. The latter does not bind glucocorticoid and probably acts as a ligand-independent regulator of glucorticoid activity. Cortisol may also exert effects via membrane receptors as do other steroid hormones. The serum protein that transports cortisol, cortisol-binding globulin (CBG), can also bind to cell surface receptors. Cortisol may then bind to the CBG-receptor complex and activate adenylate cyclase, thereby providing a mechanism by which cortisol exerts non-genomic actions.

## Actions of glucocorticoids and clinical features of Cushing's syndrome

Cortisol, like the thyroid hormone $T_3$, has potent metabolic effects on many tissues (*Box 4.9*). These are essentially anabolic in the liver and catabolic in muscle and fat; the overall effect is to increase blood glucose concentrations. Thus, like growth hormone, epinephrine and glucagon, cortisol is also considered diabetogenic. It does this by opposing the action of insulin in peripheral tissues (decreasing glucose uptake via GLUT4 receptors) and increasing glucose production and release from the liver. The latter is accomplished through gluconeogenesis using amino acids (from the catabolic actions on muscle) as the primary carbon source (*Box 4.9*). Thus, *Clinical Cases 4.1* and *4.2* had thin arms and legs caused by the catabolic actions of excess glucocorticoids on peripheral muscle. Patients with Cushing's syndrome tend to have a particular weakness of the muscles around the hips and shoulders, termed a proximal myopathy.

Although cortisol has some minor lipolytic activity, this effect is overshadowed in a patient with Cushing's syndrome by the increased insulin secretion in response to the diabetogenic actions of cortisol. Insulin has a strong lipogenic action (see *Box 2.8*) and, thus, the excess glucocorticoids seen in *Clinical Cases 4.1* and *4.2* increased fat deposition. The reason for the centripetal distribution of fat is not fully explained but probably results from metabolic differences between adipocytes in the omentum and those situated in subcutaneous tissues.

Bruising, scarring and purple striae around the abdomen are other classical signs of Cushing's syndrome (*Box 4.10*). Cortisol inhibits fibroblast proliferation and also the formation of interstitial materials such as collagen. Excess glucocorticoids result in a thinning of the skin and the loss of connective tissue support of capillaries. This makes them more susceptible to injury and leads to bruising. Bones are also affected by excess glucocorticoids. Cortisol decreases osteoblast function and decreases new bone formation; osteoclast numbers increase and measures of their activity increase. Furthermore, glucocorticoids decrease gut calcium absorption and decrease renal calcium reabsorption, thus adversely affecting calcium balance. Overall, excess glucocorticoids cause osteoporosis.

Glucocorticoids have other diverse actions including those on the cardiovascular system, central nervous system, kidney and the fetus. In the cardiovascular system, it is required for sustaining

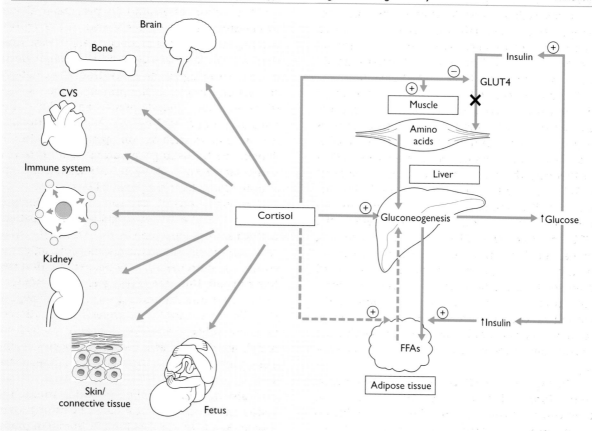

- Cortisol stimulates the release of amino acids from muscle. These are taken up by the liver and converted to glucose.
- The increased circulating concentration of glucose stimulates insulin release. Cortisol inhibits the insulin-stimulated uptake of glucose in muscle via the GLUT4 transporter.
- Cortisol has mild lipolytic effects. These are overpowered by the lipogenic action of insulin secreted in response to the diabetogenic action of cortisol.
- Cortisol also has varied actions on a wide range of other tissues (see text for details).

normal blood pressure by maintaining normal myocardial function and the responsiveness of arterioles to catecholamines and angiotensin II. In the CNS, cortisol can alter the excitability of neurons, induce neuronal death (particularly in the hippocampus) and can affect the mood and behavior of individuals. Depression may be a feature of glucocorticoid therapy. Furthermore, depressed patients may show increased cortisol secretion with alteration in the circadian rhythm of cortisol secretion.

In the kidney, cortisol increases glomerular filtration rate by increasing glomerular blood flow and increases phosphate excretion by decreasing its reabsorption in the proximal tubules. In excess, cortisol has aldosterone-like effects in the kidney

Common[*]

- Moon face (with plethora) (~100%)
- Weight gain, central obesity (~100%)
- Hypertension (~80%)
- Mental changes (~80%)
- Impaired glucose tolerance/diabetes mellitus (~70%)
- Hypogonadism – menstrual irregularity/infertility in women, loss of libido in men (~70%)
- Hirsutism in women (~70%)
- Purple striae (~60%)
- Acne (~60%)
- Osteopenia/osteoporosis (~50%)
- Easy bruising (~50%)
- Proximal myopathy (~50%)

Less common

- Poor wound healing (~30%)
- Polycythemia (~10%)
- Renal stones (~10%)
- Headache (~10%)
- Exophthalmos (~10%)

[*]Compare with the photographs in *Box 4.3* and in color on the website.

causing salt and water retention. This is because the capacity of 11β-hydroxysteroid dehydrogenase type 2 enzyme that converts active cortisol to inactive cortisone in the kidney tubule is overwhelmed. Cortisol is then available to interact with the aldosterone receptor for which it has equal affinity (*Box 4.11*). This may be a factor in the hypertension seen in patients with Cushing's syndrome.

Cortisol also facilitates fetal maturation of the central nervous system, retina, skin, gastrointestinal tract and lungs. It is particularly important in the synthesis of alveolar surfactant which occurs during the last weeks of gestation. Babies born prematurely may suffer respiratory distress syndrome and mothers with pre-term labor may be treated with glucocorticoids to stimulate fetal synthesis of surfactant.

One of the most important actions of glucocorticoids is on inflammatory and immune responses (*Box 4.12*) and it is these actions which led to the development of a multi-million dollar pharmaceutical industry in synthetic glucocorticoid preparations. Inflammation (increased capillary permeability, attraction of leukocytes etc.) results from injury and these effects are mediated by several factors the production of which is inhibited by cortisol.

Some of these factors are synthesized from arachidonic acid and cortisol inhibits the synthesis and release of arachidonic acid by inducing lipocortin which inhibits phospholipase $A_2$. This enzyme releases arachidonic acid from phosphatidyl choline and, thus, the availability of arachidonic acid for the synthesis of inflammatory mediators is reduced. In addition, glucocorticoids stabilize lysosomes, preventing the release of proteolytic enzymes. They inhibit the proliferation of mast cells, production of cytokines and also the recruitment of leukocytes to the site of infection or trauma. They also affect the numbers and functions of circulating neutrophils, eosinophils and fibroblasts. In addition, glucorticocoids reduce the number of circulating thymus derived lymphocytes (T- cells) and as a result the recruitment of B lymphocytes. The net result is to reduce both cellular and humoral immunity.

## Adrenal cortical androgens

The two steroids produced in greatest quantities by the adrenal cortex, DHEA and its sulfate, have an ill-defined role in normal physiology. Together with androstenedione, they are generally termed 'weak androgens' and have a much lower affinity for the androgen receptor than testosterone. These adrenal androgens are, however, converted peripherally to the more active testosterone (*Box 4.13*). In males, the amount released from the adrenal glands and converted to testosterone is physiologically insignificant compared to the amount secret-

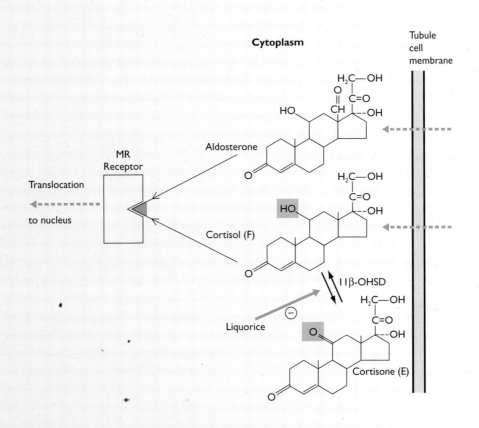

- Cortisol and aldosterone have equal affinity for the mineralocorticoid (MR) receptor.
- Circulating concentrations of cortisol are 100 times higher than aldosterone but it does not normally interact with the aldosterone receptor because cortisol is rapidly metabolized to inactive cortisone by 11β-hydroxysteroid dehydrogenase (11β-OHSD) type 2.
- From a scientific point of view this is a novel method of achieving hormonal specificity and from the medical point of view it involves the observation that eating large amounts of liquorice causes hypertension.
- The active component of liquorice is glycyrrhetinic acid which inhibits 11β-OHSD.
- Cortisol, in excess, can saturate the activity of 11β-OHSD and then interacts with the aldosterone receptor.

ed by the testes but, in females, adrenal-derived testosterone is important in maintaining normal pubic and axillary hair.

After the menopause, adrenal androgens may also be an important source of estradiol, again due to peripheral conversion. Adrenal androgen hyper-secretion does not cause any clinical signs in adult males but is detectable in females by signs of hirsutism and masculinization. These effects are examined in more detail in *Clinical Case 4.3* and the role of adrenal androgens in the adrenarche of puberty is discussed on page 238.

To understand the biochemical investigations of *Clinical Cases 4.1* and *4.2* it is not only important

Box 4.12:
### Major effects of glucocorticoids on inflammation and immune responses

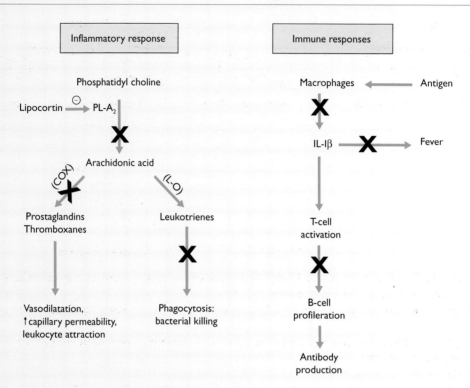

- Glucocorticoids inhibit the conversion of phosphatidyl choline to arachidonic acid by inducing the production of lipocortin (now termed annexin) which inhibits phospholipase-A$_2$ (PL-A$_2$).
- They inhibit the production of inflammatory prostaglandins and thromboxanes by inhibiting cycloxygenase (COX).
- They inhibit the production and action of leukotrienes which are also formed from arachidonic acid by lipo-oxygenase (L-O).
- They block cytokine (IL-1$\beta$) production, reduce the number of circulating T cells and so reduce antibody production.
- x = inhibitory effects of glucocorticoids.

to know the actions of adrenal cortical hormones, but also the control of their secretions.

## Hypothalamic control of adrenocortical steroid synthesis – CRH and vasopressin

Corticotrophin-releasing hormone (CRH) is a 41-amino-acid peptide secreted by neurosecretory cells predominantly located in the paraventricular nucleus of the hypothalamus (*Box 4.14*). Released from nerve terminals in the median eminence, this peptide is transported to the anterior pituitary corticotrophs in the hypophyseal portal capillaries where it acts on a G-protein linked receptor to stimulate an increase in cAMP. The subsequent signal transduction pathways stimulate both the synthesis and release of adrenocorticotrophin (ACTH).

The action of CRH on pituitary corticotrophs is potentiated by arginine vasopressin (AVP), also

**Box 4.13:**
Peripheral metabolism of adrenal androgens

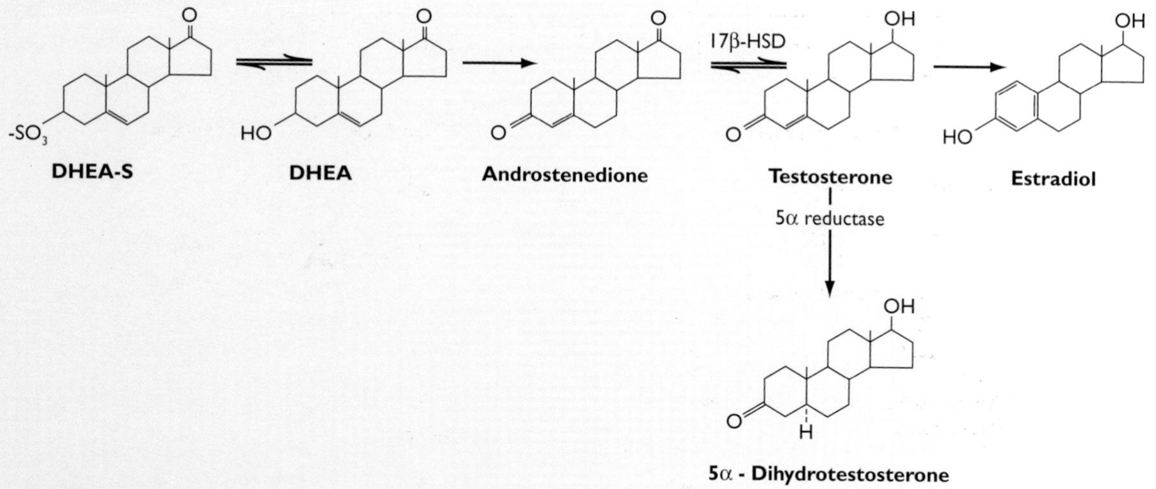

- Androstenedione, DHEA and its sulfate DHEAS are metabolized to the more potent testosterone by 17β-hydroxysteroid dehydrogenase via androstenedione.
- In some target tissues, testosterone is 5α-hydroxylated to the more potent 5α-dihydrotestosterone or converted to estradiol.
- Most androgens are conjugated prior to excretion in the urine. Testosterone and androstenedione are cleared three times more rapidly in men than women.
- DHEAS can be excreted unchanged.
- Androstenedione may be metabolized to androsterone or etiocholanolone and, thence, 17β reduced, conjugated and excreted.
- 5α-dihydrotestosterone is reversibly inactivated by 3α-reduction and a smaller amount is converted to 5α-androstanedione.

known as antidiuretic hormone (ADH). AVP, secreted by parvocellular (small) neurosecretory cells in the supraoptic and paraventricular nuclei of the hypothalamus, is also released into the hypophyseal portal capillaries. This contrasts with the magnocellular (large) neurosecretory cells in the same nuclei whose axons terminate in the posterior pituitary and release AVP into the general circulation (see *Box 7.43*).

Recent evidence has shown that there are at least two types of CRH receptors that differ in their anatomical location and in their pharmacology. It may well be that these two receptors mediate different functions of CRH. For example hyperactivity of CRH neurons both in the hypothalamus and other brain regions may not only activate the increased ACTH/adrenal activity associated with stress but also certain associated behavioral symptoms such as depression, sleep and appetite disturbances and psychomotor changes. CRH is also produced in the placenta, as is a specific binding protein, CRH-BP. This binding protein may modulate the paracrine effects of CRH within the placenta and its reduced production at term suggests that CRH/CRH-BP may play a role in parturition. CRH synthesis and CRH receptors have also been identified in immune cells and there is evidence that CRH may not only be anti-inflammatory through its central action on glucocorticoid secretion but also pro-inflammatory through direct effects of peripherally released CRH. Thus, CRH is not simply a neurohormone that controls the secretion of ACTH.

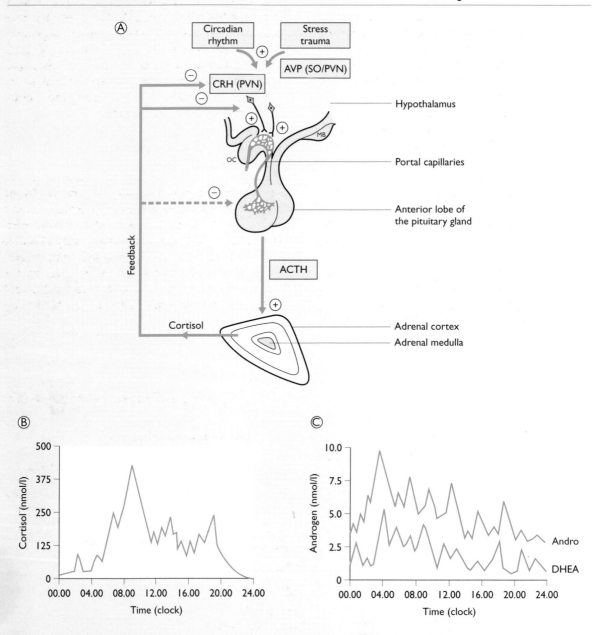

A  Diagram depicting the factors which control the secretion of cortisol. B  24 h secretory pattern of cortisol. C  24 h secretory patterns of androstenedione (Andro) and dehydroepiandrostenedione (DHEA).

Abbreviations: CRH, corticotrophin releasing hormone; AVP, vasopressin; PVN, paraventricular nucleus; SO, supraoptic nucleus; OC, optic chiasm; MB, mamillary bodies.

## Pituitary control of adrenocortical steroids – ACTH

ACTH is derived from a large precursor molecule pro-opiomelanocortin (POMC) that is cleaved by the action of specific peptidase enzymes (*Box 4.15*). Whilst this prohormone can give rise to numerous hormones, including opioid peptides and melanocyte stimulating hormone (MSH), the main product of POMC cleavage in the corticotroph cells is ACTH. In the brain, other products predominate.

The main action of ACTH on the adrenal cortex is to stimulate the synthesis and release of glucocorticoids and androgens via cAMP-dependent mechanisms via a G-protein coupled receptor. The immediate actions of ACTH on steroid synthesis are to increase cholesterol esterase, the transport of cholesterol to and across the mitochondrial membrane, cholesterol binding to $P450_{SCC}$ and, hence, an increase in pregnenolone production (*Box 4.4*). Subsequent actions include the induction of steroidogenic enzymes and conspicuous structural changes characterized by hypervascularization, cellular hypertrophy and hyperplasia. This is particularly notable when excess ACTH is secreted over prolonged periods of time (e.g. pituitary-dependent Cushing's). Whether androgen synthesis and secretion is under some other control remains uncertain. In contrast, the primary stimulus for aldosterone secretion is through the renin-angiotensin system (see *Box 4.33*).

## Feedback control of glucocorticoids

The production of glucocorticoids is controlled by a classical negative feedback loop in which neurons in the hypothalamus detect circulating concentrations of glucocorticoids and consequently stimulate or inhibit the release of CRH and AVP from the parvicellular neurons (*Box 4.14*). AVP secreted by the magnocellular neurons is controlled by different stimuli, namely serum osmolarity and blood volume.

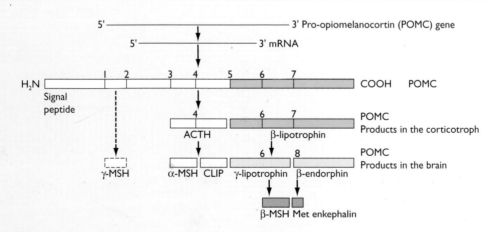

The pro-opiomelanocortin (POMC) gene codes for a large pro-hormone plus signal sequence that is subsequently cleaved at the numbers indicated into smaller active molecules under the action of peptidases. The processing of POMC is tissue-specific as indicated on the diagram.

This feedback loop can, however, be over-ridden by both internal and external factors. Human biological clocks (normally entrained to the light–dark cycle) produce a circadian rhythm in the release of ACTH and, consequently cortisol, with peak concentrations of these hormones in the early morning and a nadir in the evening (*Box 4.14*). Thus, for patients requiring cortisol replacement therapy a larger dose of the steroid is given in the morning with a lower dose in the evening to simulate the normal endogenous rhythm. Stress, whether generated by physical or emotional trauma, is also a potent stimulus to cortisol secretion and can over-ride negative-feedback effects.

In addition to ACTH drive of the adrenal cortex, there is also evidence for non-ACTH-mediated regulation that could partly explain why, in some clinical situations, there is a dissociation between ACTH and cortisol secretions. The nerve supply of the adrenal cortex may modulate adrenocortical function and activation of the adrenomedullary system, that releases both catecholamines and peptides, is also implicated as a local control mechanism. In addition, immunomodulatory peptides such as cytokines, which can be released within the gland or by circulating leukocytes, also stimulate cortisol secretion. This could, in part, account for the rise in cortisol seen during chronic infection and sepsis.

The control of glucocorticoid production is, indeed, complex, but patients with suspected Cushing's syndrome are investigated using the physiological principles inherent in the control system.

# Excess glucocorticoids: biochemical investigation of Cushing's syndrome

Once suspected, the diagnosis of Cushing's syndrome requires biochemical confirmation and elucidation of its cause. Endogenous causes may be primary (due to adrenal dysfunction) or secondary due to excess secretion of ACTH either from the pituitary gland or another (termed ectopic) source (*Box 4.16*). Alternatively therapeutic glucocorticoids may be the cause.

---

**Box 4.16:**
**Causes of Cushing's syndrome**

**Common (~ 99%)**

- Exogenous therapeutic glucocorticoids

**Uncommon (~ <1%)**

- Anterior pituitary adenoma
- Ectopic ACTH
- Adrenal adenoma

**Rare (~ <0.01%)**

- Adrenal carcinoma
- Ectopic CRH
- Alcoholic
- Bilateral multinodular hyperplasia

---

*Clinical Case 4.1* not only showed signs of excess glucocorticoid but also of excess androgen secretion. Thus, it is highly unlikely that her cushingoid symptoms were the outcome of her steroid treatment. These were inhaled beclomethasone and topical betamethasone, both of which are 'pure' glucocorticoids, without androgenic effects (*Boxes 4.17 and 18*). Thus, the cause of her cushingoid symptoms is likely to be endogenous rather than exogenous. There are a variety of tests to investigate and confirm the different causes of Cushing's secretion; these include measurements of cortisol and ACTH secretion and dynamic functional tests.

# Measurements of cortisol in blood, urine and saliva

Random measurements of peripheral blood cortisol concentrations are generally unhelpful in the diagnosis of Cushing's because the diurnal rhythm in cortisol secretion together with inter-individual differences makes interpretation of the results difficult. However, since the diurnal rhythm in cortisol secretion is lost in *any* endogenous cause of Cushing's syndrome, measurements of serum corti-

Structures of various immunosuppressive steroids compared with those of progesterone and cortisol

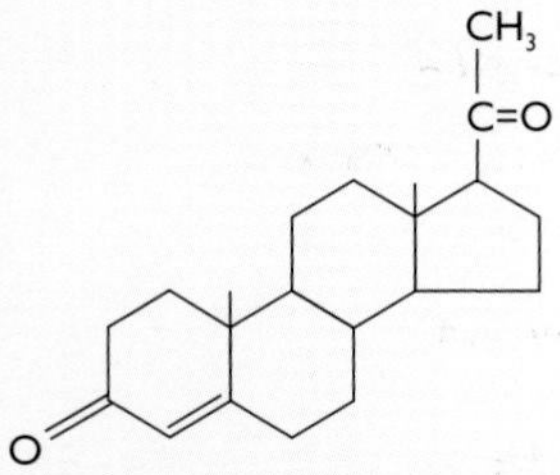

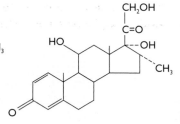

**Progesterone**

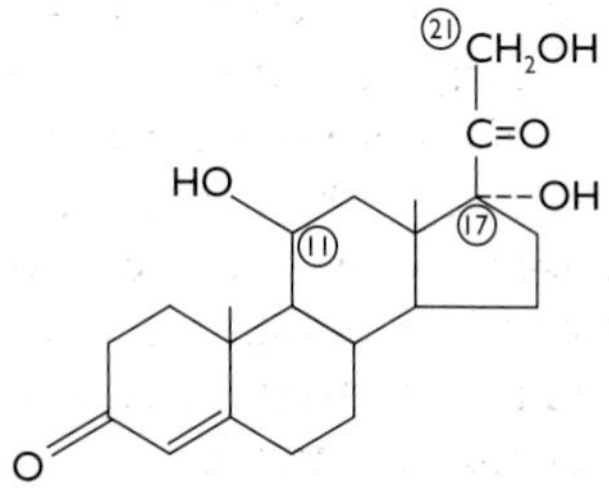

**Cortisol (hydrocortisone)**

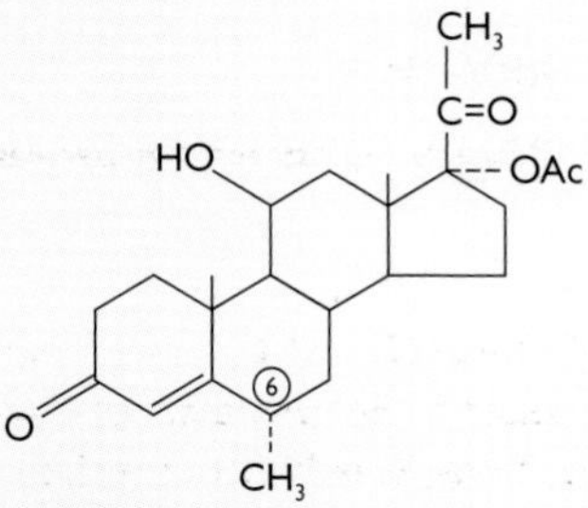

**Medroxyprogesterone acetate**

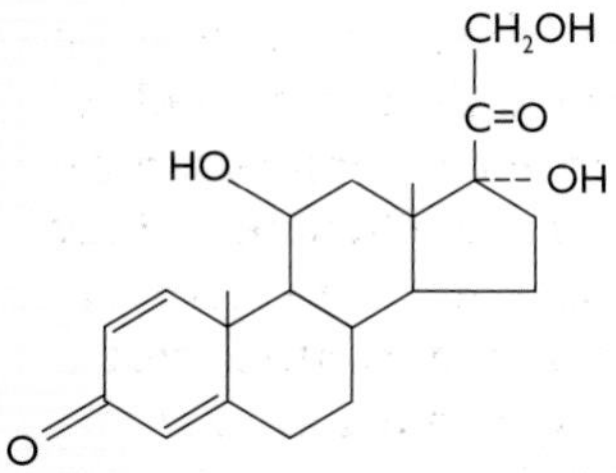

**Prednisolone**

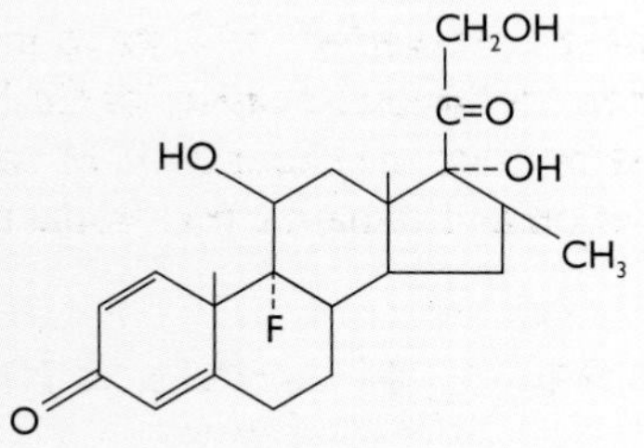

**Betamethasone (topical)**

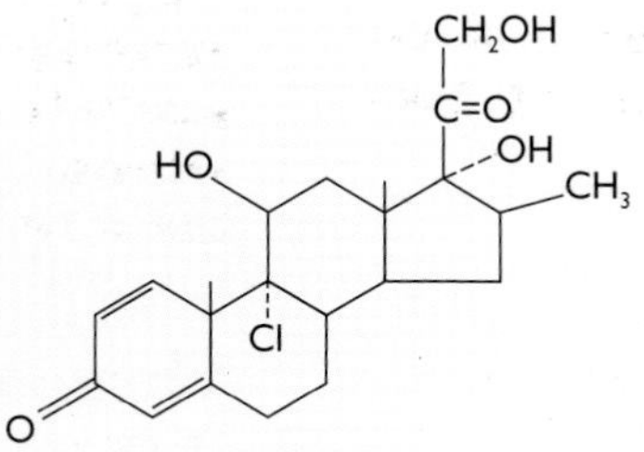

**Beclomethasone (inhaled)**

**Dexamethasone**

All these steroids are C-21 or C-22 compounds with the 4-ene-3 keto core typical of all adrenal corticosteroids. Different side chains determine the potency and effective routes of administration.

Approximate relative activities of adrenal steroids and synthetic steroids

| Steroid | Activity | | |
|---|---|---|---|
| | Mineralocorticoid* | Glucocorticoid† | Androgen§ |
| Cortisol | 1 | 1 | |
| Aldosterone | 600 | 0.3 | |
| Fludrocortisone | 200 | 10 | |
| Prednisolone | 0.8 | 4 | |
| Methylprednisolone | 0.5 | 5 | |
| Betamethasone | 0 | 25 | |
| Dexamethasone | 0 | 30 | |
| Medroxyprogesterone | 0 | 0.5 | |
| Testosterone | | | 1.0 |
| Dihydrotestosterone | | | 2.0 |
| Dehydroepiandrosterone | | | 0.1 |
| Androsterone | | | 0.1 |
| Androstenedione | | | 0.25 |
| Androstanediol | | | 0.65 |

*Mineralocorticoid assay based on salt-retention and cortisol given arbitrary potency of 1.

†Glucocorticoid assay based on anti-inflammatory activities and cortisol given arbitrary potency of 1.

§Androgenic potency with testosterone given arbitrary value of 1.

sol at 09.00 to give a 'peak' value and those at 24.00 to give 'trough' values can be useful in the diagnosis (*Box 4.19*). It is important that the midnight sample is taken with the patient unstressed. Since, however, this test requires hospital admission, a more frequently used alternative is to measure salivary cortisol in which concentration is independent of saliva flow rates due to its lipid solubility. This allows patients to collect their own samples in the comfort of their own homes.

*Clinical Case 4.1* showed no diurnal variation in her cortisol secretion, mean concentrations being 1031 nmol/l and 915 nmol/l at 09.00 and midnight respectively and the corresponding mean plasma ACTH concentrations measured with a two site IRMA (see *Box 3.25*) were 30 and 12 pmol/l. These measurements indicate that the cause of the Cushing's is ACTH-dependent and not due to primary adrenal over-activity that would have suppressed ACTH due to negative feedback effects.

Another way of estimating cortisol secretion is to measure the small fraction of unmetabolized, unconjugated cortisol that is excreted in the urine over a 24 h period. Termed urinary free cortisol, this measurement allows assessment of total cortisol secretion throughout the day. The 24 h urinary free cortisol excretions measured by radioimmunoassay (see *Box 6.14*) for two consecutive days were 1245 and 1456 nmol/d (NR 100–220 nmol/d) for *Clinical Case 4.1* whilst those for *Clinical Case 4.2* were low, at 42 and 34 nmol/d.

Box 4.19:
The investigation of the cause of Cushing's syndrome

- In iatrogenic Cushing's syndrome due to the ingestion of synthetic or natural glucocorticoids, the concentration of cortisol in blood and urine is low and often unmeasurable (unless the offending steroid interferes in the cortisol assay), as is the ACTH concentration.
- In all causes of endogenous Cushing's syndrome the daily secretion is increased and the circadian rhythm is lost. (Blood concentrations of cortisol may *not* be outside the normal range for the 09.00 cortisol concentration but are inappropriate for the time of day.)

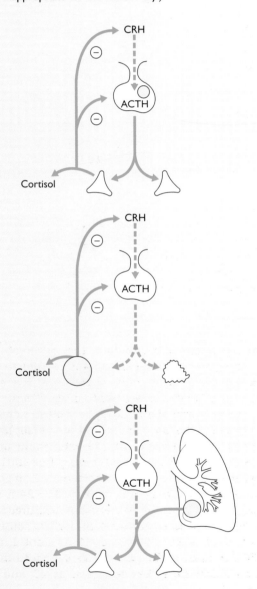

**In pituitary Cushing's disease:**
Circulating concentrations of cortisol and ACTH are elevated for the time of day.
Cortisol secretion is ACTH-dependent and therefore:
- cortisol concentration shows an exaggerated rise in response to CRH
- 11-deoxycortisol increases in a metyrapone test
- feed-back loop is intact but reset so that the 09.00 h cortisol concentration is suppressed during a high-dose (but not low-dose) dexamethasone test

**In the case of an adrenal tumor:**
Circulating concentration of cortisol is elevated and ACTH is suppressed and usually unmeasurable
Cortisol secretion is ACTH-independent and therefore:
- 09.00 h cortisol concentration is not suppressed during a dexamethasone test
- cortisol concentration does not rise in response to CRH
- 11-deoxycortisol does not increase in a metyrapone test

**In ectopic ACTH production:**
Circulating concentrations of cortisol and ACTH are elevated for the time of day.
Cortisol secretion is ACTH-dependent but the feed-back loop is destroyed and therefore:
- cortisol concentration shows no response to CRH
- 11-deoxycortisol fails to fall or shows a subnormal increase in a metyrapone test
- 09.00 h cortisol concentration is not suppressed during a dexamethasone test

In conjunction with cortisol and ACTH measurements, dexamethasone, metyrapone and CRH tests are used to confirm the cause of Cushing's syndrome (*Box 4.19*).

## Dynamic tests of endocrine function

Dexamethasone is a potent synthetic glucocorticoid with negligible mineralocorticoid action and it is administered to suppress the endogenous release of ACTH and cortisol. 'Low' doses (i.e. 2 mg/day) suppress ACTH and cortisol in normal subjects and the overnight low-dose dexamethasone test is used to screen patients initially before deciding on a more formal investigation. Given that hypertension is associated with obesity and that obesity is epidemic, there is a relatively large number of obese hypertensive patients in whom Cushing's syndrome is suspected. The vast majority of these obese, hypertensive people have 09.00 cortisol concentrations that suppress normally (e.g. to <50 nmol/l, *Box 4.19*).

'High'-dose dexamethasone (i.e. 8 mg/day) suppresses ACTH and cortisol secretion in patients with pituitary dependent Cushing's, an effect that will not be seen in patients who have Cushing's syndrome due to an ectopic source of ACTH. Patients with primary adrenal overactivity have unmeasurably low ACTH concentrations and cortisol concentrations that are unaffected by dexamethasone at high or low dose.

Metyrapone is a drug that inhibits the final C-11 hydroxylation in the synthesis of cortisol (*Box 4.5*) and is used in a test in which the peripheral blood concentration of 11-deoxycortisol, the immediate precursor of cortisol, is measured. In pituitary-dependent Cushing's disease, metyrapone reduces serum cortisol concentrations and consequently increases ACTH secretion due to reduced negative feedback. The increased ACTH drive leads to an increase in serum 11-deoxycortisol concentration. This is not seen in cases in which the Cushing's syndrome is due to ectopic ACTH (there is no increase in ACTH secretion) nor when it is due to an adrenal tumor (cortisol production is independent of ACTH).

The CRH test investigates the functional capacity of the pituitary gland using measurements of ACTH or cortisol response to an injection of CRH. Cortisol is often measured because the assays are less expensive than those for ACTH. Alternatively, ACTH measurements can be made from venous drainage of the anterior pituitary gland by simultaneous bilateral catheterization of the inferior petrosal sinuses; many regard this as the definitive investigation of Cushing's syndrome. As a less invasive test, an overnight low-dose dexamethasone test followed by a CRH test has received recent support.

Other biochemical information can also be used to help diagnosis. For example, when both ACTH and its precursors are measured, the ratio of precursors to ACTH is higher in ectopic ACTH secreting tumors (e.g. small cell tumors of the lung) than in pituitary tumors. Similarly, when urine is subjected to specialized (gas–liquid) chromatographic analysis, the ratio of adrenal steroid precursors to products may be higher in cases of adrenal tumors than in ACTH-driven disease. In addition, the clinical features may vary. For example, adrenal tumors are associated with a greater degree of androgenization than ACTH-driven disease.

These tests were not performed in *Clinical Case 4.1* because the results of the high-dose dexamethasone test (ACTH suppression) and CRH tests (an exaggerated response) were conclusive and confirmed that she had Cushing's disease as a result of an ACTH-secreting pituitary tumor. This is the commonest cause of endogenous Cushing's even though it has an incidence of only about 1 per million per year. It is three times more common in women and has a peak incidence between 20 and 60 years. The cause is not certain. Some have argued for a hypothalamic cause, others that it is due to the spontaneous development of pituitary tumors. These are often very small and, indeed, may not always be visible on MR scan.

*Clinical Case 4.2* had low urinary cortisol concentrations and, despite her cushingoid appearance, underactive adrenal glands had been suspected. She underwent a tetracosactrin test (*Box 4.20*) to investigate the functional capacity of her adrenal cortex. Thirty minutes after a 250 µg bolus

**These require the stimulation of the adrenal cortex and the assay of secreted cortisol**

- Tetracosactrin is the first 24-amino terminal amino acids of the native ACTH that has 39 amino acids. It has full biological activity.
- Cortisol is measured in peripheral venous blood before (i.e. at baseline) and at varying times after a tetracosactrin injection.
- In the 'short' test, serum cortisol is measured 30 minutes after a single injection of between 1 and 250 μg of peptide.
- In the 'long' test an intramuscular injection of a depot preparation of 1mg of tetracosactrin is given on more than one occasion (usually 3 days). The serum cortisol is measured on day 4.
- With loss of functional adrenal cortical tissue baseline concentrations of cortisol are usually low with little increment in response to tetracosactrin (maximum cortisol at 30 min <500 nmol/l) to either the 'short' or 'long' tests.
- In hypopituitarism, the cortisol response to the 'short' (30 min) tetracosactrin test is low because loss of endogenous ACTH drive has reduced the biosynthetic 'machinery' of the gland. (There is no storage of steroids.) The cortisol response to the 'long' test over several days is normal because the synthetic machinery is induced by many hours exposure to the synthetic ACTH drive so the serum cortisol rises >1000 nmol/l.

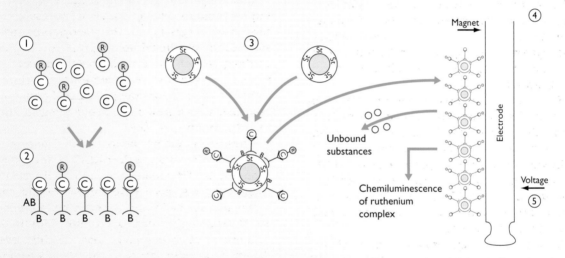

**An example of a commercial cortisol assay using an antibody based chemiluminescence technique**

1. Danazol is added to the serum sample to displace cortisol from the binding globulin. The cortisol © and a cortisol derivative labelled with a ruthenium complex ©–® are ...
2. incubated in the presence of a specific polyclonal antibody (AB) labeled with biotin (B). The two forms of cortisol bind competitively with the AB and then ...
3. particles coated with streptavidin (St) are added to the reaction mixture. The biotin on the AB forms a complex with streptavidin. The particles are aspirated into the measuring cell where ...
4. the microparticles are magnetically captured on the surface of the electrode. Unbound substances are then removed and finally ...
5. an electric voltage is applied to the electrode. This induces chemiluminescence (measured by a photomultiplier) of the ruthenium complex of the captured cortisol derivative.

The concentration of cortisol in the serum sample is inversely proportional to the intensity of chemiluminescence measured.

injection of tetracosactrin (the biologically active 24-amino terminal amino acids of ACTH) her serum cortisol concentration rose from 15 nmol/l to 120 nmol/l (NR >500 nmol/l). In view of this poor cortisol response and the low urinary cortisol excretion, she was started on hydrocortisone treatment (20 mg/day) and referred to the endocrine team.

The endocrine team reinterpreted the data in view of the clear discrepancy between the patient's appearance and the biochemical findings; no further tests were required. *Clinical Case 4.2* had been taking medroxyprogesterone acetate, a C-21 compound that has the 4-ene-3-one core structure. Whilst it lacks 11β,17α,21-trihydroxyl groups, the methylation at C-6 (*Box 4.17*) increases the glucocorticoid activity of prednisolone some six-fold. Thus, medroxyprogesterone whilst termed a progestagen, has approximately half the biological activity (per unit weight) of cortisol at the glucocorticoid receptor.

*Clinical Case 4.2* was taking 600 mg medroxyprogesterone daily. This is approximately equivalent to 300 mg of cortisol a day; some 30-fold the normal daily endogenous production of the hormone and 120 times the normal dose of medroxyprogesterone (5 mg) prescribed in many combined oral contraceptives. This suppressed ACTH secretion and reduced adrenal function, resulting in the poor response to tetracosactrin. In addition, medroxyprogesterone is thought to have some activity at the androgen receptor and this may account for the changes in hairline of this patient (note that they are much milder than those of *Clinical Case 4.1, Box 4.3*).

## Imaging the adrenal gland

In addition to biochemical investigations, a variety of scanning techniques is used to aid the diagnosis of Cushing's syndrome (*Box 4.21*). Though ultrasound is a cheap and non-invasive test, the best resolution of the adrenal glands is obtained by CT or MR scanning whilst MR imaging is preferred for the pituitary gland. It is to be emphasized that these techniques not only provide an anatomical diagnosis but also functional information. Thus, a single large adrenal in the presence of a contralateral small gland would point towards an adrenal tumor producing excess cortisol, suppressing ACTH leading to atrophy of the other gland. Bilaterally enlarged glands would tend to indicate ACTH-dependent disease, regardless of the source of the ACTH.

Information from imaging modalities must *always* be interpreted in the light of the results from endocrine investigations. For example, bilateral nodular hyperplasia of the adrenal glands can occur in the absence of excessive ACTH drive and both the pituitary and the adrenal glands are predisposed to the formation of 'incidentalomas'. This term is given to the radiological appearance of a tumor when no functional activity is clinically apparent. Published frequencies are approximately 5% for the adrenal gland and about 25% for the pituitary gland.

## Treatment of Cushing's syndrome

The most common cause (indeed, the *only* common cause) of Cushing's syndrome, is an exogenous, usually therapeutic, source of glucocorticoid steroid as seen in *Clinical Case 4.2*. The ideal form of therapy is simply to reduce the dose of the prescribed steroid and, if necessary, to use additional drugs to facilitate this reduction without flare-up of the underlying disease activity. It is essential to do this slowly and progressively to avoid precipitating acute glucocorticoid deficiency that may be fatal. This was done in *Clinical Case 4.2*, the dose of medroxyprogesterone being gradually tailed off over many months. Her clinical symptoms improved markedly.

Cushing's syndrome with an endogenous cause is one of the most difficult endocrine diseases to diagnose and treat accurately. On a statistical basis, the odds will be in favor of a pituitary adenoma accounting for some 80% of cases of endogenous Cushing's syndrome. Difficulties arise, however, with rare cases of alcoholic pseudo-Cushing's (as was suspected in *Clinical Case 4.1*), cyclical Cushing's, well-differentiated sources of ectopic ACTH, such as carcinoid, and vanishingly rare

The use of radiological techniques in the investigation of Cushing's syndrome

①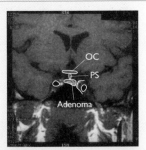

**MR pituitary**

**MR scan of the pituitary gland**
- The imaging technique of choice for the hypothalamus and pituitary gland, though relatively expensive and not as widely available as CT scanning
- Positive findings depend on the size of the tumor (~ 70%)
- OC, optic chiasm, PS, pituitary stalk

②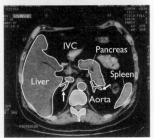

**CT adrenals, adrenals arrowed**

**CT scan of the adrenal gland**
- The imaging technique of choice with its wider availability and greater spatial definition. Ultrasound may be preferred in children
- Virtually 100% of tumors may be satisfactorily imaged
- IVC, inferior vena cava

③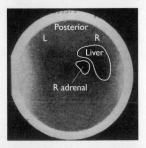

**CT adrenals, adrenal adenoma**

Chemical shift MR imaging of the adrenal gland is used to distinguish benign 'incidentalomas' from malignant tumors

④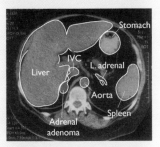

**Iodocholesterol scan**

**Radiocholesterol scan**
- Imaging with labeled cholesterol compounds (such as $^{75}$Se-cholesterol, $^{131}$I-19-cholesterol) lacks the spatial definition of CT and MR but is non-invasive and may best be used for examination for ectopic steroid-producing tissue

⑤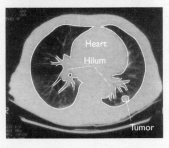

**CT chest**

**CT scan of the chest**
- May be useful in the search for non-pituitary ACTH-dependent disease

These clinical images are available on the website

causes of Cushing's syndrome associated with food intake or ectopic CRH production (*Box 4.22*).

The preferred treatment of endogenous Cushing's syndrome (whether it is caused by overactivity of the adrenal gland or increased secretion of ACTH from the pituitary gland or an ectopic source) is usually surgical removal of the cause (*Boxes 4.23* and *4.24*). It can be difficult, however, to locate pituitary or ectopic tumors even with the best MR imaging equipment. Thus, radiation may be used as an adjunct to surgery or drugs such as metyrapone can be used to reduce activity of the adrenal cortex.

In some cases, when it is impossible to remove the ectopic source of ACTH (either because it cannot be located or because it has metastasized) bilateral adrenalectomy is performed. The surgical anatomy of the adrenal glands is complex (*Box 4.23*) and approaches to the adrenal gland include posterior, flank and anterior. Laparoscopic techniques have been developed and tend to be used for smaller tumors of the adrenal and for those considered benign.

Replacement hormone therapy after treatment of Cushing's syndrome will, of course, depend on the underlying diagnosis and the therapy used. Thus, in pituitary Cushing's when a small tumor has been removed, no replacement may be required in the long term. However, the remaining normal corticotroph cells will be atrophied as a result of the feedback inhibition and it may be some time before they recover. Thus, replacement may be required in the short term. Larger pituitary tumors may be associated with hypopituitarism requiring additional hormone replacement. Unilateral adrenalectomy will require no replacement therapy (though, again, it may be some time before the contralateral adrenal cells recover) but bilateral adrenalectomy will always require life-long glucocorticoid and mineralocorticoid replacement therapy.

---

**Box 4.22:**
Replacement hormone therapy after treatment
Problematic Cushing's syndrome[*]

**Alcoholic**

- Only a small proportion of alcoholics develop Cushingoid features: a genetic factor has been implicated. There is a poor correlation between clinical features and biochemical estimates of adrenal activity. The presence of concomitant depression or malnutrition may further complicate interpretation

- Evidence for causes in its development include:
  Acute ethanol administration activates the hypothalamo-pituitary-adrenal axis
  Animal studies show that ethanol can decrease hypothalamic sensitivity to glucocorticoid feedback with a resulting hypersecretion of CRH
  Liver effects of ethanol may decrease CBG synthesis and increase free cortisol concentrations

**Cyclical Cushing's**

- Spontaneously remitting and relapsing Cushing's is said to be more commonly seen in ACTH-dependent disease particularly carcinoid tumors secreting ACTH

- Diagnosis may be difficult with unexpected or 'inappropriate' results to biochemical tests

**Tumors producing ectopic ACTH or CRH**

- These cause particular problems when:
  They are metastatic (e.g. small cell cancers), or
  When they are small slow-growing occult carcinoids that cannot be localized

[*]Depression is associated with raised concentrations of cortisol with evidence of CRH overactivity and alterations in circadian rhythmicity. The results of dynamic tests may be difficult to distinguish from Cushing's syndrome.

**Box 4.23:**
## Surface and surgical anatomy of the adrenal glands

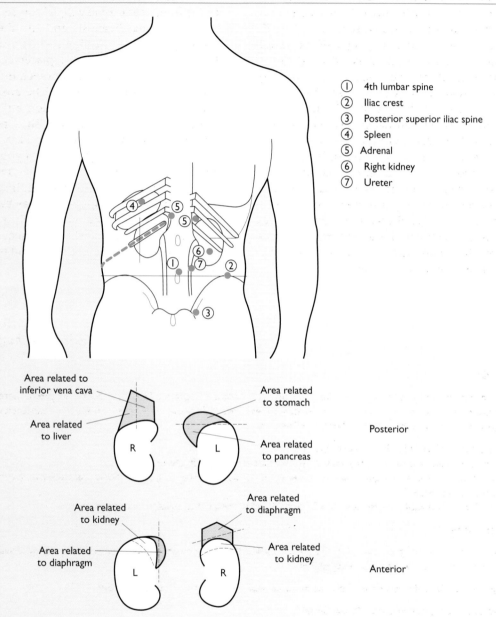

① 4th lumbar spine
② Iliac crest
③ Posterior superior iliac spine
④ Spleen
⑤ Adrenal
⑥ Right kidney
⑦ Ureter

Area related to inferior vena cava

Area related to liver

R

Area related to stomach

L

Area related to pancreas

Posterior

Area related to kidney

Area related to diaphragm

L

Area related to diaphragm

R

Area related to kidney

Anterior

- The adrenal glands are retroperitoneal structures
- Each gland has three arteries, a superior from the inferior phrenic, a middle from the aorta and an inferior from the renal artery
- Each has a single vein. The left drains into the left renal vein; the right is very short and drains into the inferior vena cava. Great technical expertise is required to avoid surgical trauma to the inferior vena cava.

**Medical**

| Drug | Use | Advantages | Disadvantages/side effects |
|---|---|---|---|
| **Adrenal inhibition**[*] | | | |
| Metyrapone | Any patient with endogenous hypercortisolism<br><br>May be used prior to surgery or where cardio-respiratory disease, or metastases preclude surgery | Cheap, effective Inhibits $P450_{11\beta}$ (mainly), $P450_{scc}$ and $P450_{aldo}$ | Increases the production of cortisol precursors, especially androgens and mineralocorticoids, exacerbating hypertension and hirsutism. Nausea and dizziness |
| Trilostane | as above | Inhibits $3\beta$-hydroxysteroid dehydrogenase | Relatively weak inhibitor. Gastrointestinal and neurological symptoms |
| Aminoglutethimide | as above | Inhibits $P450_{scc}$ | Proximal action leads to hypoadrenalism, necessitates glucocorticoid replacement. Sedation, depression, dizziness. Blocks thyroid hormone synthesis |
| Ketoconazole | as above | Inhibits $P450_{11\beta}$ and, at higher doses $P450_{scc}$ | Gastrointestinal symptoms, gynecomastia. Teratogenic. Liver damage. |
| Etomidate | as above | Inhibits $P450_{11\beta}$ and, at higher doses $P450_{scc}$ | Intravenous use. Sedative. |
| Mitotane (o'p'-DDD) | as above | Inhibits $P450_{scc}$, $P450_{11\beta}$, $P450_{18\beta}$ | Gastrointestinal and neurological symptoms |
| **Mineralocorticoid antagonist** e.g. Spironolactone | Block mineralocorticoid actions | Cheap, orally active | Gynecomastia, impotence, decreased libido. Hyperkalemia |
| **Inhibition of ACTH**[†] **secretion** e.g. valproic acid, cyproheptadine, bromocriptine | Pituitary Cushing's disease | Active in a few patients | No long-term or large studies with any of the drugs, some of which e.g. cyproheptadine have notable side effects |

Contd

## Nelson's syndrome

*Clinical Case 4.1* underwent bilateral adrenalectomy rather than removal of the pituitary tumor because she had previously undergone neurosurgery after a subarachnoid hemorrhage. Bilateral adrenalectomy in patients with pituitary-dependent Cushing's dis-ease may be followed by a marked enlargement of the ACTH-secreting tumor and the enlarged pituitary gland may cause pressure on the optic chiasm and result in visual loss. At the same time the increased ACTH secretion can cause marked skin pigmentation. This is termed Nelson's syndrome and there has been vigorous debate as to whether

**Surgical§**

| Procedure | Use | Advantages | Disadvantages/complications |
|---|---|---|---|
| Unilateral adrenalectomy | Patients with adrenal adenoma/carcinoma | Curative. May be done laparoscopically | Classical operations expensive and scarring. Mortality (~1–5%), hemorrhage (~0.5%), infection (~5%) |
| Bilateral adrenalectomy | Patients with adrenal multinodular hyperplasia or ACTH-dependent disease not amenable to other surgery (e.g. ectopic ACTH) | As above | Post-operative hypoadrenalism (~100%) Larger operation with higher rates of complications |
| Pituitary surgery (Box 7.28) | Pituitary Cushing's | Potentially curative | |

**Radiotherapy**

| Procedure | Use | Advantages | Disadvantages/complications |
|---|---|---|---|
| Cranial (Box 7.28) | Pituitary Cushing's | Avoids anesthetic and operative risks | Poorly effective in adults (~20%), better in children (~80%). |

*In ACTH-dependent pituitary disease the feedback loop produces an increase in circulating ACTH that tends to reduce the effect of these drugs.
†The use of these agents is in part predicated on the hypothesis that pituitary Cushing's disease results from hypothalamic overactivity perhaps mediated by residual tissue of the embryonic pars intermedia
§Outcomes and complications depend on a number of factors including technical expertise, tumor size and surgical approach.

these tumors are naturally aggressive or develop these tendencies on removal of feedback suppression from the adrenal glands. To prevent the development of Nelson's syndrome *Clinical Case 4.1* received prophylactic pituitary radiotherapy in addition to both glucocorticoid and mineralocorticoid replacement therapy.

# Excess adrenal androgens – congenital adrenal hyperplasia (CAH)

*Clinical Case 4.1* illustrates the effects of an excess of all adrenal steroid hormones under the control of ACTH and *Clinical Case 4.2* the more selective effects of an excess of exogenous steroid with glucocorticoid (and some androgenic) actions. *Clinical Case 4.3* illustrates the clinical circumstances in which there is a selective excess of adrenal androgens caused by a deficiency of an enzyme required for normal steroidogenesis.

## Clinical Case 4.3:

A 26-year-old woman was referred to the Endocrine clinic because of increasing facial hair. A nursery school teacher with Greek parents, she had her menarche at 11 years of age but had always noted irregular periods and a tendency to be overweight. When seen, she was 1.70 m tall with a weight of 87 kg. On examination, she was obese but had no clinical evidence of glucocorticoid or mineralocorticoid excess and her blood pressure was normal. She had, however, excess facial hair, areolar hairs on the breasts, male pattern pubic hair with an extension up the linea alba in the midline of the lower abdomen.

There was hair on the inner thighs but none on her back. There was no clitoral hypertrophy, breast atrophy or other signs of masculinization such as deep voice and muscular development. It had previously been suggested to her that the excess hair was a consequence of her Mediterranean origins and she was very resentful that her sister (a child of the same parents) was not similarly affected.

This young patient showed signs of mild androgen excess although 'mild' is not a word to use to a young female patient whose anxieties have driven her to seek medical attention. Excess hair growth may be distressing for young women, particularly in a culture where models in magazines appear with every body hair air-brushed away.

The majority of androgens in women originate from steroid precursors synthesized in the adrenal cortex (*Box 4.5*), rather than the ovaries, but in clinical practice attention should be paid to both glands. A gross excess of androgens after puberty leads to loss of female characteristics and masculinization, but assessing mild hyperandrogenism and hirsutism can be problematic. It is important to dis-tinguish the fine vellus hair that covers most of the body from the stiffer and thicker terminal hair whose growth and distribution is dependent on androgens (see *Box 6.22*). Low concentrations of androgens are required for terminal hair growth in the axillae, lower abdomen and upper thighs but higher concentrations cause growth at distances away from these areas. Pale skins and dark vellus hair may cause undue worry, although it is perfectly normal. There is also ethnic variation in the amount of body hair (particularly in ethnic groups around the equator) that should also be taken into consideration.

In this patient, baseline concentrations of androgens and the progesterone precursor were abnormally high; serum testosterone was 6.3 nmol/l (NR <2.5 nmol/l), androstenedione 39.2 nmol/l (NR 4–10.6 nmol/l), 17α-hydroxyprogesterone 150 nmol/l (NR <18 nmol/l). Thus, this patient has evidence of pathological production of androgenic steroids. *Clinical Case 4.3* has a loss of function mutation in the cytochrome P450 enzyme 21-hydroxylase (*Box 4.25*), an enzyme essential for the synthesis of glucocorticoids and mineralocorticoids. As a consequence, the loss of negative feed-

---

**Box 4.25:**
**Congenital adrenal hyperplasia (CAH) — CYP21A2 deficiency**

- 21-hydroxylase (CYP21A2) deficiency is the most common form of CAH accounting for 90% of all such cases. Common in Alaskan Eskimos (~1 in 700 live births) but less common in most Western countries (between 1 in 5000 and 1 in 15 000 live births).
- Clinical manifestations vary according to the sex of the patient but result from a loss of aldosterone and cortisol metabolism with precursors being shunted into androgen synthesis (see *Box 4.26* ①).
- Total ablation of enzyme activity (e.g. deletion or missense mutations) results in 'salt-wasting' disease (loss of aldosterone) and virilization and ambiguous genitalia of a female infant (increased testosterone production). Salt wasting results in severe dehydration in the first 14 days of life with hypotension and death if untreated
- Children with mutations resulting in 1–2% normal enzyme activity (e.g. missense mutations) have virilization but not salt-wasting
- Mutations resulting in 20–60% normal enzyme activity give the so-called 'non-classical' presentations similar to that of *Clinical Case 4.5*
- Boys without salt-wasting may present with precocious sexual development
- Treatment is with oral glucocorticoid therapy (monitored to result in suppression of the high concentrations of precursors such as 17α-hydroxyprogesterone) together with mineralocorticoids (monitored by blood pressure and by assays of serum renin)

back from glucocorticoids, an increased ACTH drive and an increased steroid synthesis shunted into the androgen pathway, leads to the increased production of adrenal androgens.

Several suppression and stimulation tests of the adrenal gland and the ovary are available to define the source of the excess androgens. In this case, the elevated 09.00 h 17α-hydroxyprogesterone concentration together with the observation that 3 days treatment with 2 mg dexamethasone daily suppressed serum testosterone to 1.1 nmol/l (NR <2.5 nmol/l) was evidence that the excess androgens were due to a disorder of adrenal steroid synthesis. The treatment is to remove the ACTH drive to androgen synthesis by giving exogenous glucocorticoid.

Whilst a loss of function mutation in the CYP 21A2 gene is the most common form of CAH, other enzyme deficiencies occur and the clinical features of CAH vary according to the enzyme affected, the severity of the defect and the sex of the patient (Box 4.26). The more proximal the deficiency in the steroidogenic pathway the more widespread the defect so both the adrenal glands and gonads will be affected (Box 4.26). Measuring the relative concentrations of precursor molecules will generally allow diagnosis of the specific enzyme defect. The 'milder' cases such as Clinical Case 4.3 are characterized by the retention of some enzyme activity and later presentation. These may require ACTH stimulation (a tetracosactrin test) or specialized chromatographic analysis of a 24 h collection of urine to make a biochemical diagnosis.

Whilst CAH is rare, a common cause of the associated features of obesity, menstrual irregularity and hirsutism is polycystic ovary syndrome (PCOS, see page 266). The etiology of this syndrome is poorly understood but is associated with hyperandrogenism. However, in almost all patients with CAH ultrasound scanning of the ovaries will reveal polycystic ovary (PCO) appearances. This was the case in Clinical Case 4.3 and this led to a marked delay in the true diagnosis. Her PCO had been considered the cause of her hirsutism rather than CAH inducing the symptoms of PCOS.

# Deficiency of adrenocortical secretions – Addison's disease

Worldwide, the most common cause of Addison's may still be tuberculosis but in Western countries autoimmune disease is a more common cause of adrenal failure (Box 4.27). A relatively recent development has been the effect of the human immunodeficiency virus (HIV). This has increased the incidence of hypoadrenalism due to infectious agents including viruses such as cytomegalovirus, fungi such as histoplasmosis, coccidiomycosis or blastomycosis, bacteria such as tuberculosis or the drugs that are used to treat these agents. AIDS itself may be associated (by an as yet unknown process) with generalized resistance to glucocorticoid effects of cortisol. Clinical Case 4.4 illustrates some of the clinical features of Addison's disease.

## Clinical Case 4.4:

A 43-year-old married woman was referred to the outpatient department with increasing skin pigmentation and weight loss (Box 4.28). There was no obtainable family history of any illness and, apart from lethargy, she denied any other problem. She had two healthy children. She was taking no medication. A forthright lady, she professed a hearty dislike for both medical and dental surgeries. She had a supine systolic blood pressure of 50 mmHg (that became unrecordable when standing) but adamantly refused hospital admission.

Taken together, the major features of this case indicate primary adrenal failure i.e. Addison's disease (Box 4.29). The low systolic blood pressure is indicative of a deficiency of both glucocorticoids and mineralocorticoids, weight loss, due to reduced appetite, is a consequence of cortisol deficiency and skin pigmentation is caused by excess ACTH (the result of loss of glucocorticoid negative feedback).

### Skin pigmentation

The pigmentation of Addison's disease is so noteworthy that few cases of primary hypoadrenalism

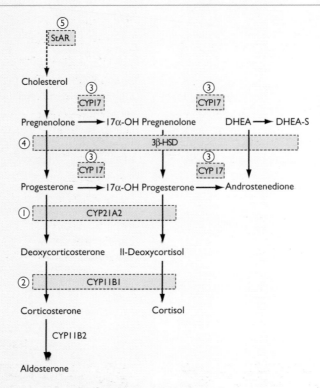

① See box 4.25

② CYP11B1 deficiency: very rare with an incidence of ~1 in 100 000 live births but as frequent as 1 in 5000 amongst Jews of Moroccan ancestry. Clinical presentation: virilization, similar to CYP21A2 deficiency but with additional hypertension, perhaps due to increased production of 11-deoxycortisol which has mineralocorticoid actions

③ CYP17 deficiency: extremely rare (approximately 200 cases in the world literature) and expressed in both adrenal gland and gonad. Clinical presentation: hypertension with hypokalemia due to excessive production of mineralocorticoids; failure of pubertal development in genetic females and genetic males presenting at puberty with female external genitalia and intra-abdominal testes

④ 3β-HSD2 deficiency: classical form leads to defective production of all steroids. Clinical presentation: adrenal failure in early infancy; moderate virilization in females; varying degress of genital ambiguity in males; mild, non-classical form may present with hirsutism and oligomenorrhea

⑤ StAR protein defect: loss of all steroidogenic capacity in adrenal gland and gonad. Clinical presentation: adrenal failure in early infancy; genetic males have female external genitalia (loss of androgens); frequently fatal if undiagnosed

reach the severity of that seen in *Clinical Case 4.4* although difficulties may arise in the case of Afro-Caribbeans or Asians where the increase in pigmentation may not be detected so easily. In conditions associated with high circulating concentrations of ACTH (e.g. primary adrenal failure or ectopic production), melanosome function within the melanocytes is stimulated. This is because ACTH is equipotent with melanocyte-stimulating hormone (MSH) at the G-protein linked melanocortin-1

## Box 4.27:
### Causes of hypoadrenalism

**Common** (~ >99%)

- Abrupt cessation of exogenous sources of glucocorticoids

**Rare** (~ <1%)

- Primary (Addison's disease)
  - Autoimmunity
  - Infection (e.g. tuberculosis or fungal infections)
  - Hemorrhage
  - Metastases
  - Drugs – e.g. etomidate, ketoconazole, metyrapone etc.
- Secondary (any pituitary disease causing hypopituitarism)
- Tertiary (any hypothalamic disease causing hypopituitarism)

## Box 4.29:
### Clinical features of Addison's disease

**Common**
- Weakness (~100%)
- Weight loss (~100%)
- Pigmentation (~95%)
- Postural hypotension (~25%)
- Anorexia (~95%)
- Nausea (~95%)
- Abdominal pain (~30%)

**Uncommon**
- Vitiligo (~20%)
- Salt craving (~15%)
- Hypoglycemia (in adults ~ <1%)
- Aches and pains (~10%)

## Box 4.28:
### Clinical features of Clinical Case 4.4

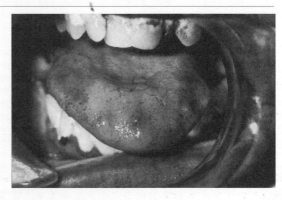

Above: Photograph of mouth showing marked pigentation of gums, buccal mucosa and tongue

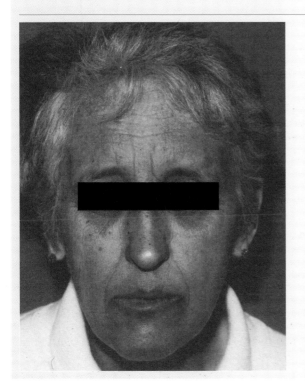

Left: Photograph of face at presentation

These clinical images are available in color on the website.

receptor. Thus, ACTH stimulates melanin production.

Skin color, along with religion, politics and wealth, is one of the most divisive factors in the human condition yet it is simply the interplay between the pigments melanin and hemoglobin. Constitutive skin color is determined by: the different ratios of eumelanin (brown/black) and pheomelanin (yellow/red) in the skin; the number of melanosomes; the rate of melanogenesis and the rate of transport of melanin from the melanocytes to the keratinocytes. Facultative skin color depends on the response of melanocytes to UV light and hormones (*Box 4.30*).

### Treatment of Addison's disease

Once suspected, it is imperative that Addison's disease is confirmed biochemically and that it is treated immediately. *Clinical Case 4.4* underwent biochemical confirmation using the short tetracosactrin test (*Box 4.20*). This showed a low basal serum cortisol concentration of 50 nmol/l and no response to this synthetic ACTH (the 30 min serum cortisol concentration was 55 nmol/l, NR >500 nmol/l). On completion of the test, she was given an intravenous injection of 100 mg hydrocortisone and an intravenous infusion of 1 liter of normal saline as she maintained her refusal to be admitted to hospital. She was given 9α-fludrocortisone 100 μg daily as mineralocorticoid replacement and 100 mg cortisol thrice daily tailing to a maintenance of 20 mg daily in divided doses. *Clinical Case 4.4* felt much improved within hours of receiving hydrocortisone.

# Aldosterone and the control of salt and water balance

The next clinical case is one in whom the biochemical changes in the concentration of plasma sodium were the most noteworthy feature, not skin pigmentation. It serves to introduce the functions and control of the mineralocorticoid, aldosterone.

## Clinical Case 4.5:

A 26-year-old man was admitted to hospital via the Emergency Room with extreme fatigue and malaise. Some 7 weeks earlier he had been seen in the same department following a road traffic accident in which he had been knocked off his bicycle by a car. He was normally employed in the computer industry and his fiancée reported a general decrease in his intellectual abilities. When examined, there were no focal neurological signs and an emergency CT scan of his head was normal. He was normotensive with no abnormal physical signs; his blood pressure was 120/80 mmHg both lying and standing. His serum sodium was reported to be 109 mmol/l (NR 135–145 mmol/l).

A low serum sodium concentration or hyponatremia is one of the commonest medical problems, affecting approximately 5% of all hospital inpatients. This man caused great diagnostic confusion and, as a result, his case is very educative. In brief, he had euvolemic hyponatremia (*Box 4.31*). That is, there was no evidence of depletion in circulating blood volume (such as postural hypotension, decreased skin turgor and sense of thirst) nor was there any sign of excess extracellular fluid (ECF) such as edema or ascites (accumulation of fluid in the peritoneal cavity). To interpret this case, a more detailed understanding of the control of salt and water is essential.

Aldosterone, secreted by the glomerulosa cells of the adrenal cortex, stimulates the active uptake of sodium (Na+), and consequently water, from the glomerular filtrate in the distal tubules of the kidney. Aldosterone synthesis and release is controlled by the renin-angiotensin system (*Box 4.33*). Smooth muscle cells in the afferent and efferent arterioles of the kidney synthesize, store and release renin. The release of this enzyme is stimulated by a reduced perfusion pressure in the kidney, increased activity of sympathetic nerves innervating the

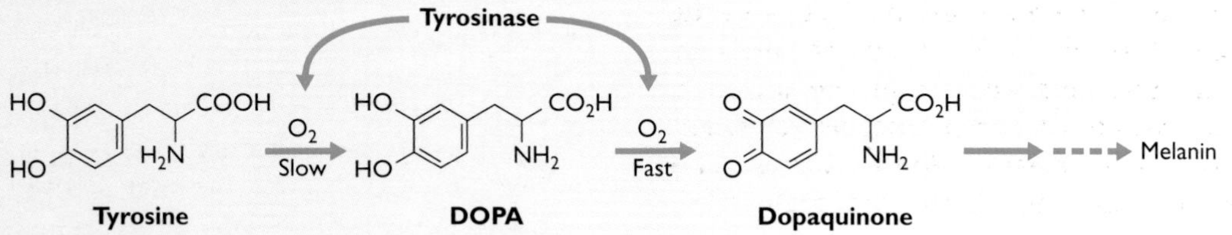

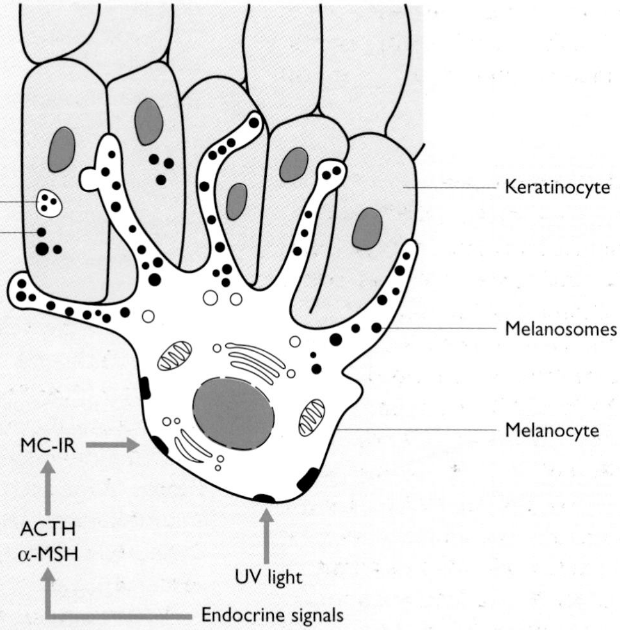

- Melanins are made from tyrosine. The initial reaction involves the enzyme tyrosinase; subsequent enzymic reactions form complex polymers. In the absence of cysteine, eumelanin (black) is formed, in the presence of this amino acid pheomelanin (yellow/red) is formed
- Each melanocyte is highly branched and functionally connected to approximately 35 keratinocytes through dendritic processes
- These reactions occur in specialized organelles of the melanocytes called melanosomes. These are transferred to the keratinocytes by a pinocytotic process where they fuse with acid lysosomes. With time the keratinocytes and melanocytes migrate to the surface of the skin and are shed
- Melanocyte numbers and melanin synthesis increase in response to UV as well as endocrine signals. The production of paracrine factors from the keratinocytes, including endothelin 1, α-MSH, ACTH, basic fibroblast growth factor, interleukin-1 and TNF-α affect human melanocyte proliferation and/or melanogenesis in experimental studies
- Sex steroids such as estradiol and testosterone increase pigmentation of genital skin and the areolae of nipples, for example during pregnancy. Locally synthesized vitamin D may also increase the melanogenic effects of UV radiation
- ACTH and α-MSH are equipotent at the melanocortin-1 receptor (MC-1R) that is expressed on the cell surface of melanocytes (see *Clinical Case 4.4*). The MC-1R is one of the family of 7-transmembrane G-protein coupled receptors. Activation of receptors increases intracellular cAMP and stimulates both proliferation of melanocytes and melanin synthesis. UV radiation increases MC1-R numbers on melanocytes

This classification is based on simple clinical signs.

**Hypovolemic**

- Patients are thirsty, have a low blood pressure (that falls still further on standing), a tachycardia, and decreased skin turgor

- There is a deficiency of total body water and an even greater deficit in extracellular sodium

- Urinary sodium concentration is low (<10 mmol/l), as a result of secondary hyperaldosteronism, except in cases due to renal loss

- The cause may be obvious such as diarrhea, vomiting, or fluid loss from extensive skin burns. It may be less obvious in salt-wasting renal conditions or when diuretics have been abused

**Hypervolemic**

- Patients have excess fluid in the legs (peripheral edema), in the abdominal cavity (ascites) or in the chest (pleural effusions)

- There is an increase in total extracellular sodium and a greater increase in total body water, as a result of secondary hyperaldosteronism

- The cause is usually due to failure of the heart, the liver or kidneys and, again except when the cause is renal, the urinary sodium concentration is usually low (<10 mmol/l).

**Euvolemic**

- Patients have, by definition, none of the signs of hypo- or hypervolemia

- The urinary sodium concentration is usually above 20 mmol/l

- The cause is usually obvious e.g. inappropriate prescription of intravenous fluids in a post-operative patient or endocrine (glucocorticoid deficiency or the syndrome of inappropriate antidiuresis, SIAD)

smooth muscle cells or a reduction in $Na^+$ delivery to the macula densa.

Once released, renin cleaves angiotensinogen to angiotensin I and this peptide is further converted by angiotensin-converting enzyme (ACE), found in the endothelial cells of the lung and kidney, to the octapeptide, angiotensin II. Angiotensin II then acts on the glomerulosa cells of the adrenal cortex to stimulate the production of aldosterone.

The action of aldosterone on the distal convoluted tubule cells of the kidney is mediated by cytoplasmic receptors that, like the glucocorticoid receptors, translocate to the nucleus of target cells after hormone binding (*Box 4.32*). The hormone-receptor complexes initiate the synthesis of proteins involved in active $Na^+$ uptake in the kidney through $Na^+$ selective ion channels. As a result of the sodium reabsorption, the transepithelial voltage is increased (tubular lumen negative) and there is a passive movement of $Cl^-$ from the lumen to the blood. Thus, both $Na^+$ and $Cl^-$ are retained, water follows down the osmotic gradient and ECF volume increases.

### Integrated endocrine control of salt and water balance

Aldosterone stimulates $Na^+$ and water retention, helping to maintain salt and water balance and, thus, blood pressure. The two other major hormones involved in this control are atrial natriuretic peptide (ANP) and arginine vasopressin (AVP), otherwise known as antidiuretic hormone (ADH) (*Box 4.34*).

ANP antagonizes the overall effects of aldosterone i.e. it promotes the excretion of sodium and, thus, reduces ECF volume. The 28 amino acid peptide is synthesized and stored in atrial myocytes. An increase in atrial tension caused by an increase in central venous pressure (CVP) stimulates ANP release. ANP inhibits $Na^+$ reabsorption in the distal convoluted tubules and collecting ducts via a cGMP-dependent mechanism. It also inhibits AVP, aldosterone and renin secretion and increases the GFR (hence, the sodium load delivered to the kidneys). The overall effect is to reduce the ECF volume.

Normally, $Na^+$ balance determines the ECF volume and thus blood pressure and the perfusion pressure within the vascular system. An increase in ECF stimulates $Na^+$ and water excretion through ANP release. A decrease causes $Na^+$ and water reten-

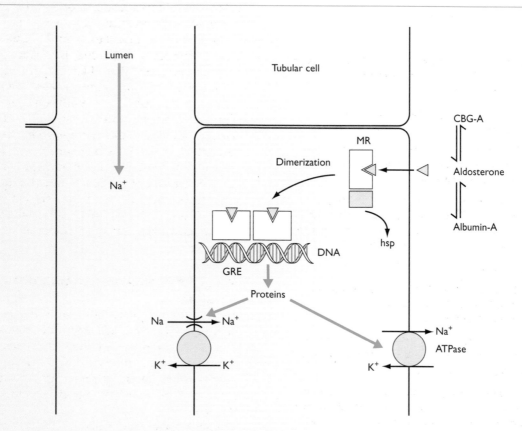

In the circulation aldosterone (A) is mainly bound to cortisol-binding globulin (CBG) or albumin. Free aldosterone enters the tubule cells of the kidney and binds to the mineralocorticoid receptor (MR). This induces release of a heat shock protein (hsp), dimerization of two MRs and translocation to the nucleus where it binds to a glucocorticoid response element (GRE) on the DNA and, along with other transcription factors, initiates protein synthesis. The aldosterone-induced proteins include factors that regulate the luminal $Na^+$ channel and components of the $Na^+/K^+$ ATPase pump. There is also evidence for rapid membrane effects of aldosterone on tubular cells.

tion through aldosterone secretion. Sodium salts are the major determinants of osmolality in the ECF since they are the most abundant solutes. Changes in sodium balance affect serum osmolality.

Regulation of serum osmolality is achieved by the action of AVP decreasing solute-free water clearance by the kidney (i.e. retention of water without electrolytes). Increases in osmolality are detected by osmoreceptors in the hypothalamus and these stimulate AVP secretion from the magnocellular neurosecretory cells in the supraoptic and paraventricular nuclei of the hypothalamus. AVP increases the reabsorption of water in the kidney by inserting water channels (aquaporins) into the membranes of tubular cells in the distal convoluted tubules and collecting ducts. Its secretion is inhibited by a reduction in serum osmolality resulting in reduced water reabsorption and increased excretion.

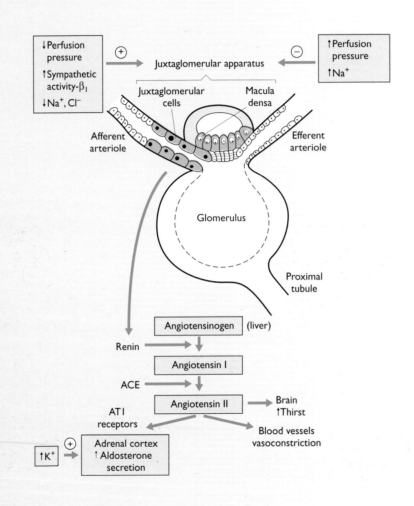

- Juxtaglomerular cells are modified smooth muscle cells that secrete renin
- The macula densa are tubular cells of the thick ascending limb of the loop of Henle that can detect circulating concentrations of sodium
- In response to the indicated stimuli, renin is secreted and converts angiotensinogen (synthesized in the liver) to angiotensin I
- Angiotensin-converting enzyme (ACE) converts antiotensin I →II which acts on AT I receptors in the adrenal cortex (glomerulosa), blood vessels and brain (via circumventricular organs)
- In addition to angiotensin II, high circulating concentrations of $K^+$ also stimulate aldosterone secretion

Simplifed diagram illustrating the integrated actions of aldosterone, arginine vasopressin (AVP) and atrial natriuretic peptide (ANP) in the control of salt and water balance

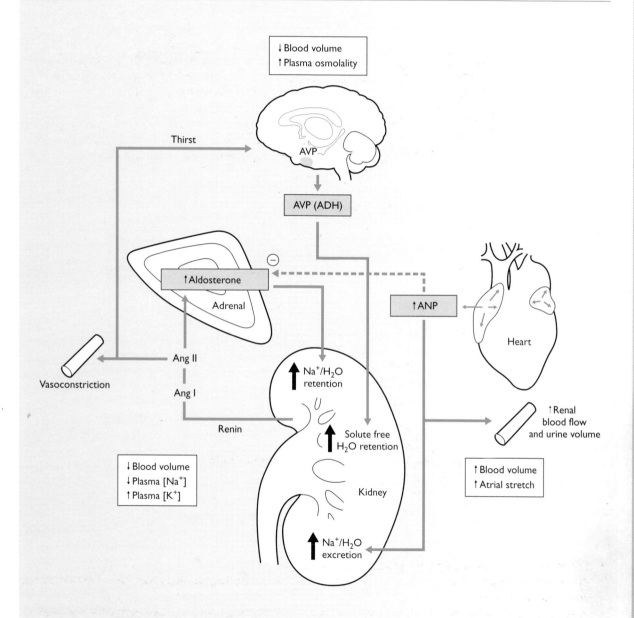

The renin/angiotensin system stimulates aldosterone secretion, and angiotensin II potentiates the release of AVP and stimulates thirst. Vasopressin secretion is also directly stimulated by hypothalamic osmoreceptors and volume receptors in the cardiovascular system. ANP is released in response to atrial stretch and also inhibits the synthesis and release of aldosterone, and inhibits renin production and AVP release.

AVP secretion is also stimulated by a reduced ECF volume. This is achieved through low-pressure volume receptors in the cardiac atria and pulmonary vessels. High-pressure sensors in the aortic arch, carotid sinus and the afferent arterioles of the kidney inhibit AVP secretion. Thus, whilst AVP controls solute-free water balance maintaining both osmolality and ECF volume, aldosterone and ANP regulate the ECF volume by controlling $Na^+$ balance. The relationship between $Na^+$ balance and ECF volume is complex, particularly under certain pathological conditions.

## Hyponatremia

Hyponatremia can be classified into hypo- hyper- and euvolemic and the classification is based on simple clinical signs (*Box 4.31*). It is evident that hyponatremia, as seen in *Clinical Case 4.5* can occur as a result of excess water intake, decreased water excretion, deficient $Na^+$ intake or excess loss of the cation. The abundance of $Na^+$ in the environment means that a deficient intake is virtually never seen. A deficiency can arise if doctors (unthinkingly or unwisely) replace the body's loss of salt-containing body fluids (e.g. diarrhea, sweat or plasma) with intravenous solutions containing only a sugar and water (e.g. 5% dextrose).

Since there was no evidence for a large oral intake of fluids or loss of any body fluid, the initial working diagnosis of *Clinical Case 4.5* was decreased water excretion due to the inappropriate secretion of AVP. This was thought to have resulted as a result of a head injury in the road traffic accident. The syndrome of inappropriate antidiuresis (SIAD) is incompletely understood but results from a defect in the excretion of free-water. It is generally seen in conditions affecting the nervous system or the chest and is diagnosed when patients have euvolemic hyponatremia, normal renal function and when other causes of decreased free water clearance (i.e. hypothyroidism and hypoadrenalism) have been excluded. In normal circumstances AVP, secreted by the parvicellular neurons, potentiates the action of CRH but in hypoadrenalism (with the loss of negative feedback) AVP secretion into the hypophyseal portal capillaries leads to an increase in AVP concentration in the general circu-

lation with secondary effects on renal free-water clearance.

After several days of fluid restriction (1000 ml/day) (*Box 4.35*) a short tetracosactrin test (*Box 4.20*) was performed on *Clinical Case 4.5*. The baseline serum cortisol concentration was low (45 nmol/l) and the response to tetracosactrin subnormal (30 min value 210 nmol/l, NR >500 nmol/l). A diagnosis of Addison's disease was made and he was treated with 10 mg hydrocortisone (cortisol) twice daily and referred to the Endocrine team.

The Endocrine team was concerned about the diagnosis because of the lack of family history of autoimmune disease and the absence of skin pigmentation. An alternative diagnosis of post-traumatic hypopituitarism was considered and pituitary function tests were performed. These

---

**Box 4.35:**
**Treatment of hyponatremia**

Two important principles should always be applied:
(1) An accurate diagnosis should be made and the underlying cause e.g. hypoadrenalism or hypothyroidism in the case of euvolemic or, say, cardiac failure in edematous states, treated
(2) The serum sodium should be corrected at a safe rate
  • Generally this means giving 0.9% saline infusions to the hypovolemic and restricting water intake to the euvolemic or edematous
  • The serum sodium should be corrected slowly if the hyponatremia developed slowly and the patient has few symptoms. The general recommendation is ≤0.5 mmol/l/h
  • A useful formula for calculating the required amount of sodium to correct serum sodium is:
    $Na^+$ deficit = 0.6 × lean body weight (kg) × (target serum $Na^+$ – current serum $Na^+$)
    But taken as a guide only: frequent estimations of serum $Na^+$ should be performed during treatment
Only rarely will additional therapy (such as loop diuretics, demeclocycline or lithium) be required to treat SIAD.

showed that he was also hypogonadal (serum testosterone 4.5 nmol/l, NR 9–25 nmol/l) with normal gonadotrophins (serum luteinizing hormone concentration 2.3 IU/l, follicle stimulating hormone 1.5 IU/l) and somatotrophin deficient (peak serum somatotrophin 5.6 mU/l after insulin induced hypoglycemia). A 'long' tetracosactrin test (*Box 4.20*) was, therefore, performed when the patient was taking 5 mg prednisolone daily rather than cortisol that would have been measured along with endogenous cortisol in the radioimmunoassay. This showed that the basal serum cortisol was unmeasurable and that over the succeeding 5 days it rose to 123 nmol/l (NR >1000 nmol/l, i.e. there was a poor cortisol response despite adequate stimulation with ACTH).

A diagnosis of primary hypoadrenalism was made and subsequently autoantibodies against the adrenal cortex were detected by immunofluorescence supporting a diagnosis of autoimmune Addison's disease. The hypogonadism and somatotrophin deficiency were considered to be the result of pituitary damage resulting from the head injury (i.e. secondary hypogonadism) even though the apparent injury had been quite minor. An MR scan of the pituitary gland was normal.

This patient was treated with androgens and given advice about his replacement glucocorticoids. However, his subsequent course revealed the difficulties associated with adequate patient education and the potent effects of glucocorticoid steroids on the brain.

He was admitted to hospital as an emergency some weeks later in a psychotic state. It transpired that he had developed a chest infection and had taken additional quantities of his cortisol as well as the prednisolone that had been prescribed by his primary care physician together with antibiotics for his infection. He had taken to doubling the steroid dose whenever he felt in the least unwell and on admission was taking in excess of 100 mg of prednisolone daily (roughly equivalent to 20 times the daily cortisol production) plus his replacement cortisol. The dose was reduced to normal over several weeks and his mental state improved.

It has been estimated that 5% of all hospital admissions are due to the unwanted effects of prescribed drugs and the next clinical case is a further example. It is used to illustrate the clinical importance of the transport and metabolism of adrenal steroids.

# Transport and metabolism of adrenocortical steroids

### Clinical Case 4.6:

A 36-year-old woman presented to hospital having suffered her first tonic-clonic epileptic seizure. She had fallen off a horse some 18 months previously while on holiday in Israel and had undergone neurosurgery to remove an intracranial hematoma. She had been told that her pituitary gland had been damaged by the head injury and had been treated with daily doses of hydrocortisone (15 mg), thyroxine (125 μg) and the synthetic AVP analog, desmopressin (20 μg). She was admitted and a CT scan of the brain confirmed structural brain damage presumed secondary to the previous injuries. She was discharged with the anti-epileptic medication, phenytoin, and the same doses of replacement therapy. Some 4 weeks later she was admitted with general malaise, vomiting and a low blood pressure of 70/40 mmHg. Her admission was precipitated by the initiation of her anti-epileptic medication.

Whilst thyroid hormones are stored, there is virtually no storage of steroids within the adrenal gland and, thus, their secretion requires an activation of the biosynthetic pathway. However, adrenocortical steroids share a number of features with thyroid hormones. They are relatively insoluble in aqueous solution and are bound to circulating proteins, with relatively small quantities of each steroid (<10%) circulating in a biologically active-free state.

The main glucocorticoid, cortisol, binds to corticosteroid-binding globulin (CBG or transcortin) whilst the main androgens (and estrogens) are transported attached to sex-hormone-binding globulin (SHBG). Both these specific transport proteins have high affinities for their respective hormones (*Box*

4.36) and normally carry 75–80% circulating hormones. A smaller percentage is bound to albumin that has a low affinity but a high capacity for the hormones. Like thyroxine-binding globulin (TBG), these proteins are synthesized by the liver and their concentrations in blood are altered by a number of factors, particularly by pregnancy and estrogen administration when their synthesis increases. The uptake of steroids by cells from capillary blood occurs by diffusion from the free hormone pool although, as with thyroid hormones, there is experimental evidence for specific transport mechanisms.

In the circulation, cortisol is in equilibrium with its biologically inactive 11-keto analog, cortisone. 11β-hydroxydehydrogenase type 2 inactivates cortisol whilst the type 1 enzyme converts inactive cortisone to cortisol. The enzymes are present in many tissues but of particular note is the inactivation of cortisol in kidney cells to prevent cortisol interacting inappropriately with aldosterone receptors (Box 4.11).

Both cortisol and cortisone are mainly metabolized in the liver (Box 4.37) and the reduced metabolites are conjugated and excreted in the urine as glucuronides. Measurement of cortisol metabolites in the urine provide a useful clinical index of cortisol secretion. Particularly useful are the 17-hydroxy-corticoids since these metabolites represent up to 50% of the total cortisol secretion. As discussed above, urinary free cortisol may be measured as a surrogate of daily secretion. The major androgens secreted from the adrenal cortex are androstenedione and dehydroepiandrostenedione (DHEA) and its sulfated form (DHEA-S). Androstenedione is reduced to androsterone in the liver prior to excretion whilst DHEA-S is excreted directly into the urine. Measurement of urinary or serum DHEA-S can indicate an adrenal abnormality.

In the case of *Clinical Case 4.6*, the patient was initiated on anti-epileptic medication with no change in the dosage of glucocorticoid replacement. The phenytoin led to the induction of liver enzymes involved in the metabolism of the steroids and subsequently to glucocorticoid deficiency. She responded well to an increase in hydrocortisone dose.

## Selective mineralocorticoid excess and deficiency

The most common causes of increased mineralocorticoid secretion, accounting for approximately 99% of all cases of hyperaldosteronism, are not due to a primary increase in aldosterone synthesis but to a secondary cause (Box 4.38). As has been seen,

**Box 4.36:**
Transport of steroids in plasma

| Steroid | Total conc. (nmol/l) | % unbound | CBG[*] | % bound to Albumin | SHBG[**] | $t_{1/2}$ in circulation (min) |
|---|---|---|---|---|---|---|
| Cortisol | 400 | 4 | 90 | 6 | 0.1 | 100 |
| Aldosterone | 0.4 | 40 | 20 | 40 | 0.1 | 10 |
| Progesterone | 0.6 | 2.4 | 17 | 80 | 0.6 | 5 |
| Testosterone[†] | 20 | 2.0 | 3 | 40 | 55 | 10 |
| Estradiol[§] | 0.1 | 2.0 | 0 | 68 | 30 | 20 |

[*]CBG = Cortisol-binding globulin – a glycosylated, 383 amino-acid α2-globulin (MW 59 000)
[**]SHBG = Sex-hormone-binding globulin – a glycoprotein MW 90 000 heterodimer of 373 amino-acid subunits
[†]In males
[§]In females

Unchanged cortisol

Tetrahydrocortisol (+5α)  Tetrahydrocortisone

0.5%  15%  15%

6β-Hydroxycortisol  1%

**CORTISOL**  Cortisone

5%  5%  10%

11β-Hydroxyetiocholanolone  Cortol (+β cortol)  Cortolone (+β cortolone)

18-Glucuronide  20%

**ALDOSTERONE**  35%

8%

3α-Hydroxy-5β-pregnone (11β-18),(18-20)-dioxide

Tetrahydroaldosterone (+ traces of isomers)

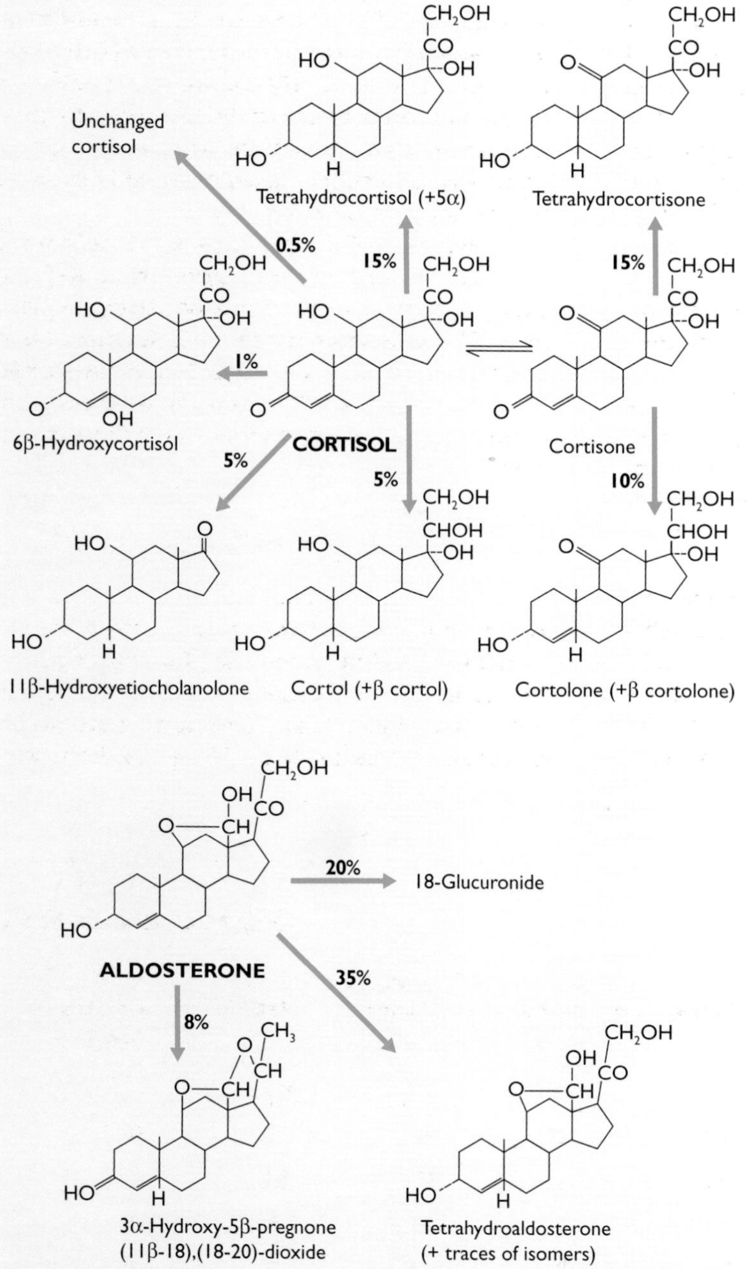

- Cortisol has a $t_{1/2}$ in the circulation of about 100 min. The small amount of cortisol excreted in the urine unchanged is representative of the daily secretion of cortisol. With high serum cortisol concentrations (about 700 nmol/l) the protein-binding capacity of serum is exceeded and more unchanged cortisol is excreted
- Reduction of the C-4–C-5 double bond is the rate-limiting step in cortisol metabolism. 5α-reductase produces a C-5 with the hydrogen below the plane of the A-ring whilst 5β-reductase produces a C-5 with the hydrogen above the plane
- Subsequent reduction of the 3-keto group by 3β-hydroxysteroid dehydrogenase leads to the production of tetrahydrocortisols, the majority of which is 3α,5β-tetrahydrocortisol
- Reduction of C-20 leads to cortols and cortolones
- 6β-hydroxylation is usually only a small proportion of daily excretion. However, in Cushing's syndrome other pathways may become saturated and this pathway may form a larger percentage of total excretion
- 11β-hydroxysteroid dehydrogenase type I has both dehydrogenase and oxoreductase activities. The formation of cortisol from cortisone predominates
- The vast majority (~95%) of C-19 and C-21 metabolites are excreted conjugated to glucuronide

- Aldosterone has a $t_{1/2}$ in blood of about 10 min and is virtually all removed in a single passage through the liver
- Direct conjugation of glucuronide at C-18 of unreduced aldosterone allows assessment of the excretion of the unreduced aldosterone
- The main pathway, like cortisol, involves reduction by a 5β-reductase and 3α-dehydrogenase.
- Note the different structure of aldosterone from that shown in Box 4.2. The hemi-acetal structure shown is more stable.

159

the secretion of large amounts of adrenocorticoids with mineralocorticoid actions (though not necessarily aldosterone itself) occurs *pari pasu* in Cushing's syndrome (probably accounting at least in part for the hypertension in *Clinical Case 4.1*) and in some of the syndromes of congenital adrenal hyperplasia.

Excessive production of aldosterone itself (termed primary hyperaldosteronism) is a rare disease that is clinically nondescript. Patients present with systemic hypertension and the only distinguishing feature of this disease is that serum analysis will usually indicate hypokalemia with an alkalosis. This is due to the excess aldosterone-induced sodium retention by the kidney in exchange for $K^+$ and $H^+$ that are lost in urine. Primary hyperaldosteronism is usually due to an adrenal adenoma (*Box 4.38*). Typically, patients are between the ages of 30 and 50 years and are more often female than male. They form much less than 1% of all cases of systemic hypertension in this age group but are important in having a surgically curable form of hypertension.

Once suspected, hyperaldosteronism can be confirmed by the measurement of 24 h urine aldosterone and by investigation of the feedback loop between renin and aldosterone. Thus, serum renin concentrations are suppressed and serum aldosterone concentrations cannot be suppressed by normal measures. A variety of tests has been used

**Box 4.38:**
Causes of mineralocorticoid excess

**Common (~99%)**
Secondary hyperaldosteronism[*]
Physiological
- Pregnancy
- Volume depletion of any cause e.g. hemorrhage, dehydration

Pathological: associated with normal or low blood pressure
- Congestive heart failure
- Nephrotic syndrome
- Cirrhosis
- Salt-losing syndromes of bowel or kidney or diuretic abuse

Pathological: associated with high blood pressure
- Renin-secreting tumour
- Renal artery stenosis
- Diuretic therapy in hypertension

**Uncommon (~<1%)**
Primary hyperaldosteronism
- Aldosterone-producing adenoma
- Bilateral or unilateral adrenal hyperplasia

Normal or suppressed endogenous aldosterone[†]
- Cushing's syndrome
- Congenital adrenocortical enzyme defect e.g. 11β- or 17α-hydroxylase deficiencies
- Exogenous mineralocorticoid
- Pseudo-hyperaldosteronism e.g. drugs inhibiting 11β-hydroxysteroid dehydrogenase

[*]Secondary hyperaldosteronism is not strictly a cause of mineralocorticoid excess since the increased secretion is compensating for underlying pathophysiological states.

[†]Cushing's syndrome or enzyme deficiencies may increase 11-deoxycortisol secretion; this has considerable mineralocorticoid activity.

to improve sensitivity in the detection of primary hyperaldosteronism in the at-risk hypertensive patient population. These include the use of aldosterone/renin ratios and the use of postural changes. It is important to emphasize that the sensitivity of many tests is reduced by a low-salt diet; investigation may require dietary supplementation with 6 g sodium chloride daily.

The same imaging techniques and analysis used for diagnosing Cushing's syndrome (*Clinical Cases 4.1* and *4.2*) also apply to hyperaldosteronism with CT or MR scans proving the most useful in detecting adrenal adenomas. It can either be treated surgically or medically with the aldosterone receptor antagonist spironolactone, the angiotensin II antagonists such as candesartan or losartan or the angiotensin-converting enzyme (ACE) inhibitors such as captopril or ramipril.

Mineralocorticoid deficiency occurs with glucocorticoid deficiency as a result of adrenal failure. Isolated hyporeninemic hypoaldosteronism occurs occasionally in diabetic patients with renal impairment. In severe cases, replacement therapy with fludrocortisone is required, though care is required to avoid inducing heart failure.

# The adrenal medulla and pheochromocytoma

The adrenal medulla forms part of the sympathoadrenal division of the autonomic nervous system. It has been known for over a hundred years that, when bilateral adrenalectomy is performed on experimental animals, replacement of adrenal cortical hormones is an absolute requirement for life. The same is not true of epinephrine and norepinephrine secreted by the adrenal medulla. One could conclude, therefore, that the adrenal medulla is not important clinically. Strictly speaking this may be true except for the rare tumors of the adrenal medulla that secrete excess catecholamines and often go undiagnosed.

The diagnosis of such pheochromocytomata is often made for the first time at post mortem and a study at the Mayo Clinic showed that nearly 80% of cases were unsuspected in life. The pathophysiology of the adrenal medulla is, thus, important in states associated with excess catecholamine secretion and this is illustrated in *Clinical Case 4.7.*

## Clinical Case 4.7:

A 45-year-old female university lecturer was admitted via the Emergency Room with a 2-year history of short-lasting episodes of right-sided upper abdominal pain and faintness. Her gastrointestinal and hepatobiliary systems had been repeatedly investigated to no avail. Numerous visits to the primary care physician had not provided a diagnosis and she vigorously refuted previous suggestions that the episodes were due to depression or associated with hyperventilation or panic attacks. On the day of admission, a particularly severe attack had been precipitated by the activities required to defrost her deep-freeze. When she was seen in the Emergency Room, examination of the abdomen was normal but her blood pressure was recorded as 120/80 mmHg supine, falling to 80 mmHg on standing.

The clinical presentation in this case may seem bizarre and, indeed, it is probably the reason the diagnosis was not made for several years. In order to understand the presenting symptoms, it is important to detail the synthesis and actions of catecholamines.

# Catecholamine synthesis and secretion

The adrenal medulla consititutes less than 20% of the adrenal gland. The cells are polygonal and arranged in cords. They receive blood either directly from medullary arterioles or from the venules of the cortex (rich in cortisol) that drain centripetally to medullary venules. Epinephrine and lesser amounts of norepinephrine are synthesized by and secreted from the chromaffin cells of the medulla in response to stimulation of pre-ganglionic (cholinergic) sympathetic nerves originating in the thoraco-lumbar lateral gray matter of the spinal cord. Chromaffin cells are so named because their *affinity* for *chrom*ium salts leads to characteristic staining. As modified post-ganglionic nerve cells, they are classical neurosecretory cells – neurons releasing hormones into the general circulation.

The catecholamines, like melatonin and thyroid hormones, are synthesized from tyrosine (*Box 4.39*) but unlike thyroid hormones, they are made from single tyrosine molecules. These are either synthesized from phenylalanine or imported from the circulation. The rate-limiting step in the synthesis of catecholamines is that catalyzed by tyrosine hydroxylase, converting tyrosine to dihydroxyphenylalanine (DOPA). Subsequent decarboxylations and hydroxylations oulined in *Box 4.39* con-

**Box 4.39:**
## Biosynthesis and control of catecholamines secreted by the adrenal medulla

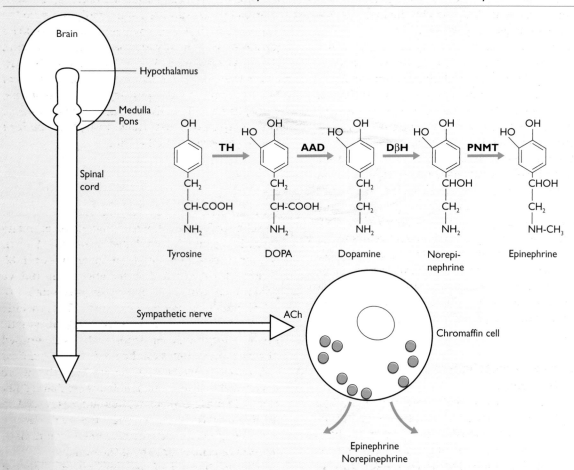

Stimuli from the hypothalamus, medulla and pons activate preganglionic cholinergic nerves that stimulate the release of epinephrine and smaller amounts of norepinephrine from the chromaffin cells of the adrenal medulla. All synthetic steps take place in the cytoplasm except the conversion of dopamine to norepinephrine which occurs in the secretory granules. Epinephrine is taken up into the secretory granules for storage and release.

Abbreviations: TH, tyrosine hydroxylase; AAD, amino acid decarboxylase; DβH, dopamine β-hydroxylase; PNMT, phenylethanolamine-N-methyltransferase.

vert DOPA to dopamine, norepinephrine and finally to epinephrine (catalyzed by the enzyme aromatic L-amino acid decarboxylase) results in the formation of dopamine. Further hydroxylation, catalyzed by dopamine β-hydroxylase takes place in secretory granules (unlike the other enzymatic processes) and results in norepinephrine. In some adrenal medullary cells, the synthetic process stops at norepinephrine but in most cells (and particularly those at the corticomedullary junction) it is converted to epinephrine by phenylethanolamine N-methyltransferase (PNMT). The activity of this enzyme is markedly increased by the high cortisol concentrations reaching the medulla.

Through an energy-requiring process, catecholamines are stored in secretory granules in association with ATP (four catecholamine molecules to one ATP) and a number of proteins, including adrenomedullin. Many functions of these proteins remain to be elucidated though some play a role in the storage mechanism since the intragranular concentration of catecholamine is such that they would cause osmotic damage if they existed free in solution. The output of the adrenal gland is controlled from nerve cells within the posterior hypothalamus which can ultimately stimulate acetylcholine release from preganglionic nerve terminals. This induces depolarization of the chromaffin cells and exocytosis of the catecholamine containing granules following a transient rise in intracellular calcium concentration. Once secreted their $t_{1/2}$ in the circulation is very short (approximately 1–2 min).

## Actions and metabolism of catecholamines

Catecholamines act on their target tissues through typical G-protein-linked membrane receptors. These receptors are classified as α or β on the basis of the physiological and pharmacological effects induced by hormone binding (Box 4.40). Further subclassification into $\alpha_{1A}$, $\alpha_{1B}$, $\alpha_{2A}$, $\alpha_{2B}$, $\beta_1$, $\beta_2$, $\beta_3$ is also made according to the activation or inhibition of different signal transduction pathways.

The physiological effects of the catecholamines are manifold and summarized in Box 4.40. They have been characterized as preparing us for 'flight or fight' with overall actions to increase heart rate and stroke volume, increase blood pressure, dilate bronchi, mobilize glucose and stimulate lipolysis. These actions are mediated by β-adrenergic receptors. Blood flow to the splanchnic bed is reduced by vasocontriction of arterioles. This effect is mediated by α-adrenergic receptors and it helps to divert blood flow to skeletal muscles.

Whilst most catecholamines released from sympathetic nerves are taken back up into the presynaptic terminal (termed uptake$_1$), catecholamines released into the circulation are taken up by non-neuronal tissues (uptake$_2$) and rapidly converted to deaminated products by monoamine oxidase (MAO) or to O-methylated products by catechol O-methyltransferase. The latter enzyme also catalyzes the meta-O-methylation of the products of MAO action – metanephrine, normetanephrine, epinephrine and vanilyl mandelic acid (Box 4.41). These may then be conjugated with glucuronide or sulfate and excreted in the urine.

# Diagnosis and treatment of pheochromocytomas

The clinical features of pheochromocytomas, many of which could be predicted from the known actions of catecholamines, are given in Box 4.42. Surges of catecholamine secretion can induce paroxysmal symptoms and many precipitants of catecholamine secretion are known. These include tumor palpation and drugs, particularly anesthetic agents. Operations on people with undiagnosed pheochromocytomas can be fatal. In Clinical Case 4.7, it seems likely that her particularly severe attack of abdominal pain and faintness that led her to seek immediate medical attention was caused by leaning over the edge of a chest freezer to remove ice. The pressure on the abdomen could have released catecholamines from the tumor.

The mechanism of her postural hypotension remains to be explained. Two mechanisms have been proposed, receptor down-regulation and the release of vasodilator peptides co-localized in the catecholamine secretory granules. Prolonged exposure of adrenergic receptors to high circulating concentrations of catecholamines reduces the number

Box 4.40:
Effects of catecholamines

**Cardiovascular**
- Increase in heart rate and force via $\beta_1$-receptors
- Increased venous return via $\alpha$-receptors
- Increased peripheral resistance via $\alpha$-receptors especially those in the subcutaneous, mucosal, splanchnic and renal vascular beds

**Visceral**
- Smooth muscle relaxation via $\beta_2$ actions and contraction via $\alpha$-mediated actions
- Modulation of fluid and electrolyte transport in the gut, kidney, gall bladder via $\alpha$ receptors

**Metabolic**
- $\beta$-receptor mediated glycogenolysis, lipolysis
- Increases in diet-induced and non-shivering thermogenesis via $\beta$ receptors

**Water and electrolyte metabolism**
- Decreased sodium excretion and glomerular filtration due to direct effects on the kidney
- $\beta$-receptor mediated effects on renin secretion leads to increased aldosterone production with effects on distal sodium handling
- Serum potassium may be increased as a result of $\alpha$-mediated effects on the liver but decreased as a result of $\beta_2$ receptor-mediated effects on muscle

**Hormone secretion**
- The sympatho-adrenal part of the autonomic nervous system modulates the responses of a number of endocrine systems, including:
  The renin-angiotensin-aldosterone system (*Box 4.33*)
  Increased secretion of glucagon and insulin via $\beta_2$-receptors: $\alpha_2$-mediated suppression is more important

of receptors (down-regulation) and also causes desensitization. Desensitization occurs by phosphorylation of the receptors and eventually a complete functional uncoupling of the receptor from its G-protein. Receptors can then be internalized into the cell. Thus, down-regulation and desensitization may lead to a reduction in the normal sympathetic vasoconstrictive tone ($\beta$-receptor mediated) and postural hypotension. In addition, peptides released with the catecholamines, notably adrenomedullin, are potent vasodilators and may also play a role in the hypotension observed in *Clinical Case 4.7*.

Overall, these tumors are rare (~1 per million per annum) and usually benign. They are found in the sexes equally and have a maximum incidence between the ages of 20 and 50 years, though they can occur at any age. In general, it is said that 10% are bilateral, 10% are extra-adrenal, 10% occur in childhood and that 10% are malignant. The majority of pheochromocytomas are sporadic and without known cause. Some occur in MEN type 1 (*Box 5.40*).

The first step in the diagnosis of these tumors is awareness of their possibility. The second is confirmation of the diagnosis biochemically. By and large, physicochemical analysis of catecholamine concentrations is performed using high-performance liquid chromatography (HPLC) with electrochemical detection. The assays with the lowest false negative rates are those for urinary and plasma catecholamine metabolites, metanephrines and normetanephrines. Chromatographic analysis of several 24 h urine collections from *Clinical Case 4.7* showed that her excretion of catecholamines was several times higher than normal.

Several stimulation and suppression tests are also available but the safest are the glucagon stimu-

## Catecholamine metabolism — diagnosis of pheochromocytoma

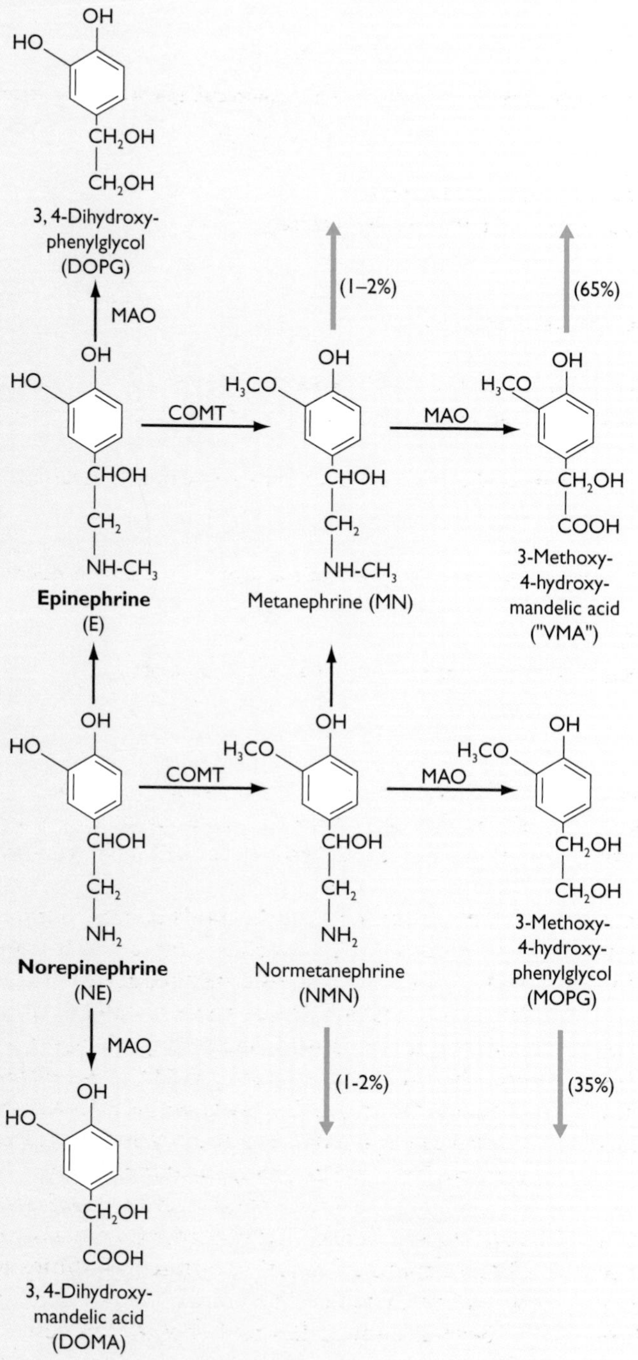

3, 4-Dihydroxy-phenylglycol (DOPG)

MAO

Epinephrine (E) — COMT → Metanephrine (MN) — MAO → 3-Methoxy-4-hydroxy-mandelic acid ("VMA")

(1–2%)  (65%)

Norepinephrine (NE) — COMT → Normetanephrine (NMN) — MAO → 3-Methoxy-4-hydroxy-phenylglycol (MOPG)

(1-2%)  (35%)

MAO

3, 4-Dihydroxy-mandelic acid (DOMA)

- Small quantities of free norepinephrine (~0.5%) or conjugated with sulfate (~2%) are excreted in the urine
- Catechol O-methyl transferase (COMT) converts the catecholamines to metanephrine and normetanephrine forming about 3% of total excretion
- Monoamine oxidase (MAO) produces aldehydes that are immediately metabolized to the corresponding carboxylic acid or alcohol by aldehyde or alcohol dehydrogenases
- MAO also catalyzes the metabolism of metanephrine and normetanephrine to vanilyl mandelic acid (VMA, ~65% of excretion) and the corresponding alcohol (MOPG, ~35% of excretion)

**Clinical importance:**

- The majority of DOPG comes from metabolism of neuronal norepinephrine that has not been released at synapses. Norepinephrine released into the circulation is not converted to DOPG. Thus, estimates of the excretion of non-metabolized catecholamines (i.e. epinephrine, metanephrine, norepine-phrine and normetanephrine) form a better diagnostic test for pheochromo-cytomas. Measurement of the ratio of DOPG to norepinephrine concentrations in blood may be a more sensitive way of detecting pheochromocytomas
- Assays for catecholamines use HPLC with electrochemical detection. This separates the different catecholamines and their metabolites according to their chemical structure
- Drugs that inhibit MAO have potentially disastrous effects on catecholamine metabolism, causing marked hypertension

## Box 4.42:
### Clinical features of pheochromocytoma

**Common**[*]

- Headache (~60%)
- Palpitations (~60%)
- Anxiety (~50%)
- Sweating (~50%)
- Abdominal pain (~25%)
- Glucose intolerance or diabetes mellitus (~40%).
- Hypertension – sustained or paroxysmal with or without postural hypotension (~50%)

**Uncommon**

- Weight loss (~10%)
- Chest pain (~20%)
- Tremor (~5%)
- Pallor (~5%)

[*]Note: Many of the features are paroxysmal, usually lasting less than 15 min. As a result, in an asymptomatic patient, normal urine or plasma catecholamines do NOT exclude the diagnosis.

## Box 4.43:
### MIBG scanning

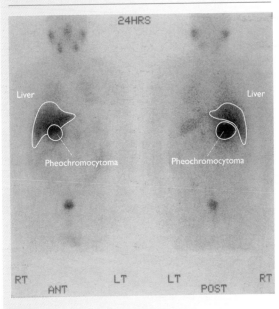

This image is available on the website.

---

lation and the clonidine or pentolinium suppression tests. These are based on the principles that catecholamine secretion from a pheochromocytoma (but not normal adrenal medulla) is stimulated approximately 2–5-fold by glucagon whilst catecholamine secretion from a pheochromocytoma is not suppressed by clonidine or pentolinium. These drugs suppress catecholamine secretion by at least 50% from a normal adrenal medulla.

The third step in the diagnosis of pheochromocytomata is their localization, usually with CT or MR scanning. These have sensitivities of about 98% and specificities of about 70%. 'Functional' scans can be performed using meta-iodobenzylguanidine (or MIBG). MIBG is taken up by the tumor by the uptake$_1$ process and the technique has a sensitivity of about 80% but nearly 100% specificity. The tumor of *Clinical Case 4.7* was localized to the right adrenal gland and lack of any other areas of uptake suggested that there were no functional metastases

(*Box 4.43*). Since pheochromocytomata may occur in a number of positions outside the adrenal glands MIBG scanning is extremely helpful when it is positive.

The only form of curative therapy (*Box 4.44*) is complete surgical removal of the tumor after initial medical treatment. The latter is required to reduce the risks of acute release of catecholamines in response to anesthetic drugs and surgical handling. The usual pre-operative treatment is initially with α-adrenegic blockade followed by combination α- and β-adrenergic blockade (*Box 4.44*). This avoids the increase in blood pressure that can be seen if β-blockade is initiated and there is unopposed α-adrenergic vasoconstrictive activity. Other treatments such as radiotherapy or chemotherapy are rarely successful but may be used as palliative therapy. More recently, large doses of radiolabeled MIBG have also been given for the palliation of metastatic disease.

## Medical

| Drug | Use | Actions/advantages | Disadvantages/side effects |
| --- | --- | --- | --- |
| Phenoxybenzamine | Any patient with endogenous source of catecholamines. Used prior to surgery or when cardiorespiratory disease, or metastases preclude surgery | Non-competitive $\alpha_1/\alpha_2$ antagonist. Cheap, effective. Dose titrated against blood pressure | Postural hypotension, nasal stuffiness |
| Doxazosin, prazosin | as above | Competitive $\alpha_1$ inhibitors | Effects on $\alpha_1$ receptors may be overcome during paroxysmal catecholamine secretion. No effects on $\alpha_2$ receptors |
| Labetalol | as above | Combined $\alpha$- and $\beta$-receptor antagonist | Ratio of 1:5 for efficacy at $\alpha$- and $\beta$-receptors respectively – effects on $\alpha$-receptors may be inadequate. Interferes in assay for catecholamines |
| Metyrosine | as above | Inhibits tyroxine hydroxylase | Sedation |
| Calcium antagonist (e.g. nifedipine) | as above | Peripheral vasodilator. Reduces catecholamine secretion | Less experience than with other drugs |

## Surgical*

| Procedure | Use | Advantages | Disadvantages/side effects |
| --- | --- | --- | --- |
| Unilateral adrenalectomy | Patients with adrenal pheochromocytoma | Curative. May be done laparoscopically | Expensive and scarring. Mortality (~3%), hemorrhage (~1%), infection (~2%) |
| Bilateral adrenalectomy | Patients with bilateral pheochromocytomata | Curative. Usually done in two procedures | As above but complication rates higher |

*Outcomes and complications depend on a number of factors including technical expertise, tumor size and surgical approach.

# CLINICAL CASE QUESTIONS

The following are examples of applied pathophysiology and these clinically based questions can be answered with the information provided in this chapter. Answers and additional material are available on the website.

---

**Clinical Case Study Q4.1:**

A 55-year-old woman presented with classical clinical features of Cushing's syndrome including hypertension, diabetes mellitus, central obesity and easy bruising. She denied previous depression or heavy alcohol intake and was not receiving any steroid containing medication.

---

**Question 1:** List the causes of Cushing's syndrome and discuss what initial investigations you would perform?

**Question 2:** In the light of these results, what additional tests would you perform?

**Question 3:** What is the likely cause of this patient's recurrent Cushing's and what further investigations should be performed?

---

**Clinical Case Study Q4.2:**

A 33-year-old Afro-Caribbean woman presented to the Emergency Room with a 3 day history of sore throat and anorexia and a 1 day history of strange behavior. In retrospect, she said she had needed to take six teaspoons of sugar in each tea and felt odd if she did not eat. She was admitted having been found in bed convulsing and incontinent of urine and feces. There was no history of previous illness nor was she taking any medication. On examination, there were no visible injection sites and she was pyrexial (temperature 39.8°C) with a blood pressure of 100/60 and pulse 88 min/l. Chest examination was normal and neurological examination made difficult by un-cooperativity. Investigations showed normal hemoglobin and white cell count, a serum sodium of 130 mmol/l (NR 135–145 mmol/l), potassium of 3.0 mmol/l (NR 3.5–4.7 mmol/l) and urea 5.6 mmol/l (NR 2.5–8.0 mmol/l) but the initial serum glucose was 0.6 mmol/l. The supine chest X-ray was reported normal as were CT head scan and lumbar puncture but blood cultures grew *Streptococcus viridans*.

**Question 1:** This patient has a *Streptococcus viridans* septicaemia and a tonic-clonic fit secondary to hypoglycemia. She was treated with high doses of intravenous penicillin and a glucose infusion. How would you investigate the cause of hypoglycemia in this patient?

**Question 2:** Given these findings, what further investigations would you perform?

**Question 3:** In the light of these results, what investigation would you perform?

**Question 4:** How do you account for the normal cortisol response to tetracosactrin?

## Clinical Case Study Q4.3:

A 64-year-old woman was seen in the Endocrine clinic because she had noticed increasing hirsutism for 6 years but worse over the last year. She had also noted increasing fatigability, and some left-sided abdominal pain. Her voice had become deeper but she had a normal appetite and no weight loss. She had a past history of mild hypertension and had had one child. She smoked 10 cigarettes a day. Examination revealed marked hirsutism with temporal recession of the hairline and a beard (Box Q4.3a). The blood pressure was 200/110 mmHg.

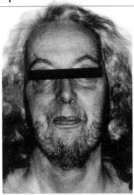

**Box Q4.3a**
Clinical photograph of the face of *Clinical Case Study Q4.3*

Note the marked male pattern balding and the beard.

Question 1: What initial investigations would you perform?

Question 2: Following the receipt of these results, what further investigations would you perform?

## CHAPTER 5

# The parathyroid glands and vitamin D

## Chapter objectives

*Knowledge of*

1. Physiology of the regulation of serum calcium and phosphate concentrations
2. Causes and clinical features of hypo- and hypercalcemia
3. Investigation and treatment of hypo- and hypercalcemia
4. Causes and clinical features of vitamin D deficiency
5. Investigation and treatment of vitamin D deficiency
6. Physiology of bone formation and its remodeling
7. Causes of osteoporosis, their investigation and treatment
8. Paget's disease and its treatment

*"Children, you are very little,*
*And your bones are very brittle;*
*If you would grow great and stately,*
*You must try to walk sedately."*
*A Child's Garden of Verses XXVII Good and Bad*
*Children, Robert Louis Stevenson.*

The calcium ion ($Ca^{2+}$) plays a fundamental role in a number of physiological functions including bone formation, muscle contraction, secretion, enzyme co-factor, stabilization of membrane potentials, blood coagulation and stimulus-response coupling (*Box 5.1*). Many of these effects are brought about by the binding of $Ca^{2+}$ to proteins altering their structures and, thus, functions.

Calcium is common, forming approximately 3.5% of the earth's crust and biosphere. In the adult human body there is about 1–2 kg calcium, 99% of which resides in teeth and bone as hydroxyapatite crystals. Of the remainder, approximately 1% is intracellular and a tiny fraction, less than 0.1%, is extracellular (*Box 5.2*). It is this small extracellular fraction of $Ca^{2+}$ that is homeostatically regulated by hormones and that determines calcium balance within the body.

> **Box 5.1:**
> **Functions of calcium and phosphate**
>
> **Functions of calcium**
> - Bone growth and remodeling
> - Secretion (exocytosis)
> - Excitation-contraction coupling
> - Stabilization of membrane potentials
> - Enzyme co-factor (e.g. in blood coagulation)
> - Second messenger
>
> **Functions of phosphate**
> Formation of:
> - High energy compounds e.g. ATP, creatinine phosphate
> - Second messengers e.g. cAMP, inositol phosphates
>
> Component of:
> - DNA/RNA
> - Phospholipid membranes
> - Bone
>
> Phosphorylation (activation/inactivation) of enzymes
> Intracellular anion

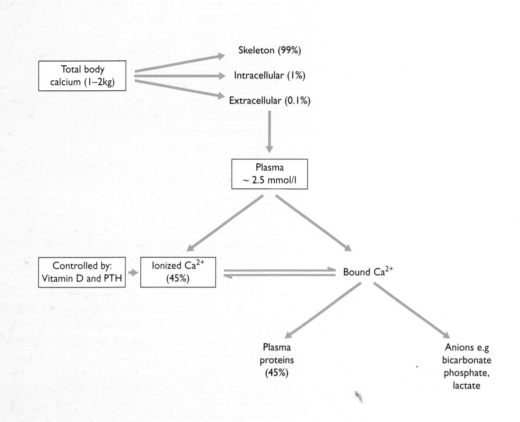

Phosphate forms about 0.09% of the earth's crust and biosphere. In the body at physiological pH, inorganic phosphate exists as $HPO_4^{2-}$ and $H_2PO_4^-$ (collectively referred to as $P_i$). Like calcium, it is critically important in physiological processes. Phosphate is an essential component of high-energy compounds (such as ATP and creatinine phosphate), second messengers (such as cAMP and inositol phosphates) and fundamental molecules including DNA, RNA and phospholipids. It is also an important intracellular anion to balance the charge of the cations $K^+$ and $Mg^+$ and enzymatic

phosphorylation of proteins alters their structure and function (*Box 5.1*). Bone contains 85% of the $P_i$ in the body with just under 5% in the intracellular compartment and less than 0.03% in the serum. Since the extracellular concentration of $P_i$ is inversely related to that of $Ca^{2+}$, and is also regulated by the same hormones, calcium and phosphate homeostasis are considered together.

Multiple symptoms arise when disease leads to hyper- or hypocalcemia and *Clinical Case 5.1* illustrates features of hypercalcemia.

## Clinical Case 5.1:

A 45-year-old woman presented to her primary care physician with general malaise, aches and pains, anorexia and weight loss of more than 3 months duration. Her only other symptoms had been polyuria and polydipsia, which, together with the weight loss, had suggested the diagnosis of diabetes mellitus. Her physician had, therefore, arranged for some biochemical tests to be performed. The fasting serum glucose concentration was normal (4.1 mmol/l, NR <3–6.0 mmol/l) but he was concerned when the laboratory staff phoned the surgery to report that her total serum $Ca^{2+}$ was high at 4.1 mmol/l (NR 2.2–2.6 mmol/l) with an albumin of 38 g/l (NR 38–40 g/l). Her serum urea and electrolyte concentrations were normal as were her routine hematological investigations.

Clinical Case 5.1 is a middle-aged woman suffering from the consequences of marked hypercalcemia, presenting with symptoms of polydipsia and polyuria. These, together with the weight loss, made her primary care physician suspect DM. However, this patient had anorexia whilst DM is much more commonly associated with a good appetite, despite weight loss. The polyuria resulted from the effects of hypercalcemia antagonizing the action of arginine vasopressin on the distal tubule and collecting ducts of the kidney (see Box 7.42). The resulting diuresis stimulated thirst and led to polydipsia. Her anorexia was due to the effects of hypercalcemia acting on the brain to reduce appetite.

To understand the pathophysiological mechanisms by which Clinical Case 5.1 developed hypercalcemia it is necessary to discuss the regulation of whole body calcium balance and factors controlling serum $Ca^{2+}$ concentration.

## Calcium and phosphate in serum and its measurement

Serum calcium ranges between 2.2–2.6 mmol/l although only about 1 mmol/l exists as free ionized $Ca^{2+}$ (Box 5.2). Serum proteins bind about 45% (mainly albumin and a smaller proportion to globulin) and approximately 10% is associated with inorganic anions such as lactate, phosphate and bicarbonate. The bound forms of calcium are in equilibrium with ionized $Ca^{2+}$ and so factors that affect calcium binding in the serum such as serum protein concentration, pH or phosphate affect serum $Ca^{2+}$ concentration. For example, a reduction in serum proteins reduces $Ca^{2+}$, as does alkalosis, whilst acidosis increases serum $Ca^{2+}$ concentrations. The total phosphate concentration in serum is normally between 0.8 and 1.45 mmol/l. Approximately 50% exists in free form (mainly $HPO_4^{2-}$), the remainder being bound to serum proteins (<10%), combined with $Na^+$ (30%), $Ca^{2+}$ or $Mg^{2+}$ (approximately 6%).

Serum calcium concentration is usually measured, as it was in Clinical Case 5.1, by a method developed some 30 years ago. This involves the addition of a chemical that displaces calcium from protein-binding sites. The total calcium concentration is then measured colorimetrically by its effect on an added dye (such as cresolphthalein). The ionized calcium (i.e. $Ca^{2+}$) concentration is not measured by all laboratories and no cheap automated assay exists. Various 'factors' have been used to 'correct' the serum concentrations of $Ca^{2+}$ when there are changes in serum albumin or, indeed, blood pH. Like calcium, the serum concentration of $P_i$ is also measured photometrically by the complex of phosphate ions with ammonium molybdate (and usually expressed in terms of phosphorus content).

## Intracellular calcium concentration

The intracellular cytosolic concentration of $Ca^{2+}$ is generally quoted as approximately 0.1 µmol/l, some four orders of magnitude lower than the extracellular concentration. This does not represent the total concentration because much of the intracellular calcium is sequestered in intracellular organelles such as the endoplasmic reticulum, sarcoplasmic reticulum (in skeletal muscle) and mitochondria. In response to a stimulus, the release of $Ca^{2+}$ from these intracellular stores, or its entry into the cells through $Ca^{2+}$ channels in the membrane, rapidly increases the intracellular concentration of $Ca^{2+}$ some 10–100 fold. Such a transient increase in intracellular $Ca^{2+}$ concentration is a ubiquitous signal transduction mechanism producing, for example, muscle contraction, secretion or enzyme activation. The latter includes the activation of a calcium-binding protein, calmodulin, that subsequently activates (by phosphorylation) protein kinase C, analogous to cAMP and diacylglycerol activating other specific protein kinases (*Box 5.3*). Protein kinase C may then activate cytoplasmic enzymes or affect gene transcription by phosphorylating further kinases such as those in the MEK–MAPK signalling pathway (see *Box 1.10*). Thus, intracellular $P_i$ is also important in signal transduction processes. As with $Ca^{2+}$, its actions are effected by its binding to intracellular proteins.

**Box 5.3:**
The role of calcium as a second messenger

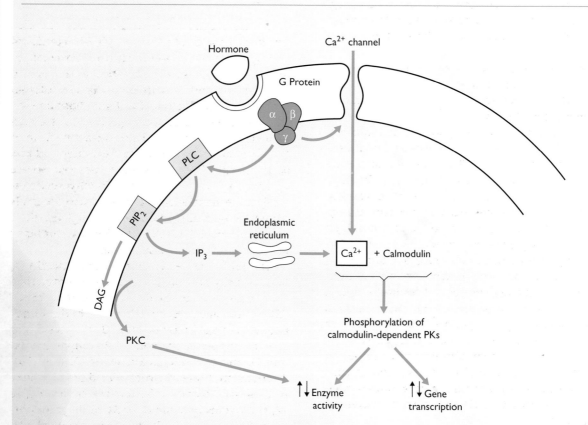

Intracellular concentrations of $Ca^{2+}$ increase as a result of either the opening calcium channels in the cell membrane or the release from intracellular stores such as that sequestered in the endoplasmic reticulum. The latter frequently involves the phospholipase C (PLC) activated hydrolysis of phosphotidylinositol 4,5-bisphosphate ($PIP_2$) to inositol trisphosphate ($IP_3$) and diacylglycerol (DAG). $IP_3$ releases stored $Ca^{2+}$ that combines with calmodulin. Both this complex and DAG can phosphorylate protein kinases (PKs) and thus initiate both cytoplasmic and nuclear actions.

# Calcium and phosphate balance

The daily turnover of calcium and phosphate for an adult is shown in *Box 5.4*. The net balance depends not only on the absorption of these minerals from the gut, their retention or excretion by the kidneys and loss in the feces, but also on bone turnover. The recommended intake of calcium is approximately 1000 mg/day although physiological states such as lactation and pregnancy increase requirements; these are also higher during childhood growth. The tendency to reduce the consumption of dairy products as a result of concern about serum cholesterol concentration or strict vegetarianism has led to a reduction in the daily intake of the vital element in some sections of the population.

The daily intake of $P_i$ is normally between 800–1500 mg, comfortably exceeding homeostatic minimum requirements. Homeostasis is primarily maintained by the kidneys which deal with the filtered $P_i$ by regulated reabsorption of approximately 80% of the total load. Any increase in the filtered load leads to $P_i$ excretion. Transport of $P_i$ across the luminal tubule membrane is mediated by $Na^+\text{-}PO_4^{3-}$ co-transporters, of which there are three families; two are expressed almost exclusively in the kidney. Transfer of $P_i$ across the basolateral tubule cell membrane is passive but regulated by an anion exchange mechanism. The maximal rate for $P_i$ reabsorption is variable; it decreases with a high-phosphate diet and increases with a low-phosphate diet. This variation in the rate of reabsorption is independent of parathyroid hormone (PTH, see below). Patients with chronic renal failure cannot excrete $P_i$ and, since gut absorption continues, $P_i$ accumulates in the body. The excess $P_i$ consequently complexes with $Ca^{2+}$ thus lowering ionized calcium concentrations. PTH secretion is, therefore, stimulated.

# Hormonal control of serum $Ca^{2+}$ and $P_i$ concentrations

Vitamin D, synthesized in the skin or obtained from the diet, and PTH, secreted by the parathyroid glands, increase serum $Ca^{2+}$ concentrations via actions on the gut, kidney and bone (*Box 5.5*). Calcitonin (secreted by the parafollicular cells of the thyroid gland) reduces serum $Ca^{2+}$ concentrations in experimental animal models. In the human, however, a marked reduction in the circulating concentration of this hormone (after, for example, total thyroidectomy) has no demonstrable effect on serum $Ca^{2+}$. Indeed, when its marked excess occurs in a clinical situation (see *Clinical Case 5.8*) it is notable for its lack of effect on calcium homeostasis.

# Sources, metabolism and transport of vitamin D

The dietary source of vitamin D ($D_3$ cholecalciferol and $D_2$ ergocalciferol) was the first to be recognized and, as a result, it was classified as a vitamin. However, vitamin $D_3$ is undoubtedly a secosteroid prohormone (see Website) for steroid hormone terminology) because even though it is not secreted by a classical endocrine gland, the active form of the hormone is released from the kidney and acts at distant sites, bone and kidney. The major source of vitamin D is synthesis from 7-dehydrocholesterol in the keratinocytes of the skin. Synthesis is stimulated by sunlight (*Box 5.6*) although the effect of near ultraviolet wavelengths (230–313 nm) may be reduced by melanin skin pigment.

The prohormones vitamin $D_2$ and vitamin $D_3$ have virtually no biological activity. However, they are hydroxylated in the liver at the carbon-25 (C-25) position and subsequently at C-1 in the kidney (and also in the placenta when this is present) to generate the active hormones 1,25-dihydroxyvitamin $D_2$ and 1,25-dihydroxyvitamin $D_3$ (*Box 5.6*). Alternatively, these 25-hydroxylated products may be C-24 or C-26 hydroxylated in the kidney to give 24,25-dihydroxyvitamin $D_2$ or 24,25-dihydroxyvitamin $D_3$ or the 25,26-dihydroxy equivalents. Whether these forms of vitamin D have any biological activity remains controversial, particularly in light of recent data from mice in which the 24-hydroxylase gene has undergone targeted disruption ('knock out'). Some argue that they are simply inactive alternatives to the 1,25-dihydroxyvitamin

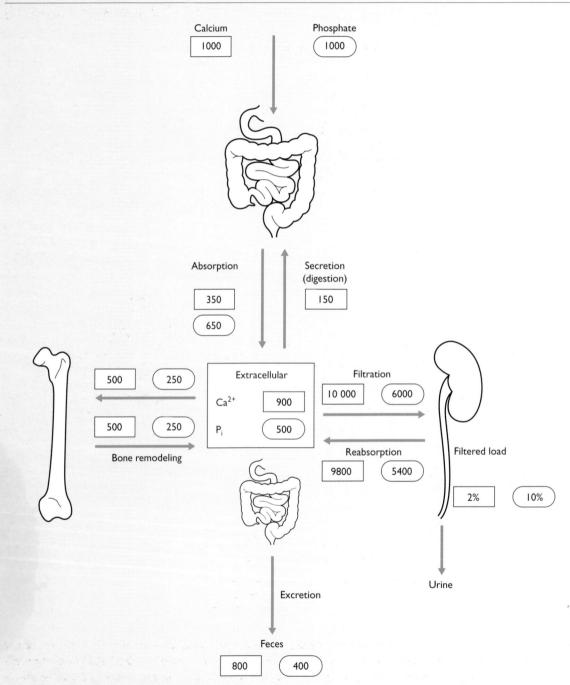

Daily turnover of calcium and phosphate in the human with a dietary intake of 1000 mg/day

Calcium
1000

Phosphate
1000

Absorption
350
650

Secretion
(digestion)
150

500    250

500    250

Bone remodeling

Extracellular

$Ca^{2+}$    900

$P_i$    500

Filtration
10 000    6000

Reabsorption
9800    5400

Filtered load

2%    10%

Urine

Excretion

Feces
800    400

Numbers are milligrams/day with those for calcium in squares and for phosphate in ovals.

Overview of the hormonal control of calcium and phosphate homeostasis by parathyroid hormone (PTH) and 1,25-dihydroxyvitamin D (1,25-(OH)$_2$D)

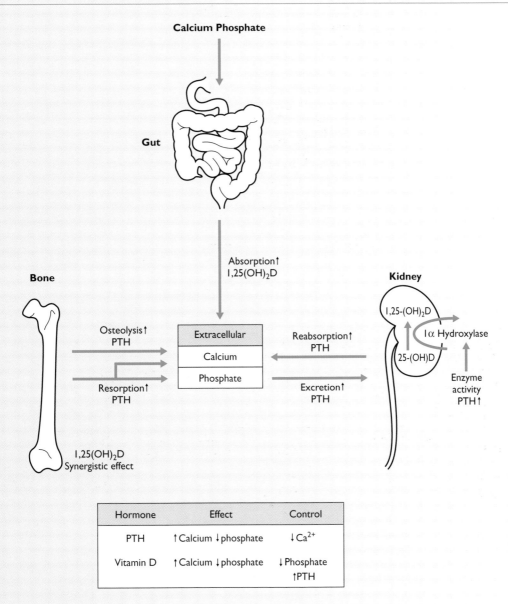

| Hormone | Effect | Control |
|---------|--------|---------|
| PTH | ↑Calcium ↓phosphate | ↓Ca$^{2+}$ |
| Vitamin D | ↑Calcium ↓phosphate | ↓Phosphate ↑PTH |

PTH stimulates the release of Ca$^{2+}$ from bone by increasing osteolysis and resorption, increases Ca$^{2+}$ reabsorption and phosphate excretion in the kidney and increases the conversion of inactive 25 hydroyxvitamin D (25-(OH)D) to the active 1,25-(OH)$_2$D. Its secretion is stimulated by a reduction in plasma Ca$^{2+}$ concentration. The main action of the active vitamin D, 1,25-(OH)$_2$D, is to increase Ca$^{2+}$ absorption in the gut and synergize with PTH on bone. Its production is increased by a reduction in circulating phosphate and increased PTH concentrations.

**Box 5.6:**
**Vitamin D synthesis**

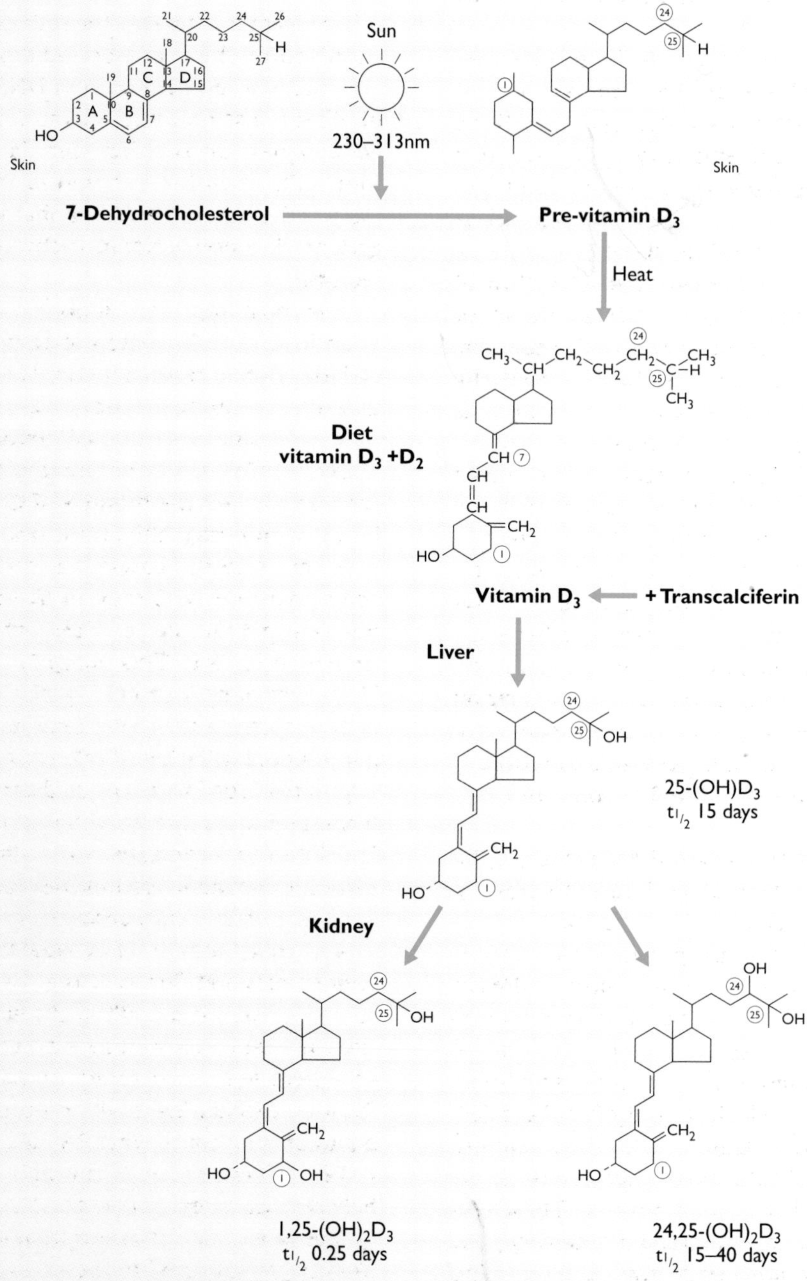
Sun
230–313nm
Skin
Skin
7-Dehydrocholesterol
Pre-vitamin D3
Heat
Diet
vitamin D3 +D2
Vitamin D3
+Transcalciferin
Liver
25-(OH)D3
t1/2 15 days
Kidney
1,25-(OH)2D3
t1/2 0.25 days
24,25-(OH)2D3
t1/2 15–40 days

Vitamin $D_3$ synthesis in the skin is stimulated by sunlight and subsequent hydroxylations in the liver (at C-25) and kidney (at C-1) produce the active form of the hormones. In the circulation vitamin $D_3$ is bound to transcalciferin with only a small fraction in free form. Approximate half-lives ($t_{1/2}$) in the circulation of the active and inactive metabolites are also shown.

D hormone. Thus, this pathway may be compared with the hepatic alternatives of 5'-outer ring or 5-inner ring deiodination of thyroxine to give active tri-iodothyronine ($T_3$) or inactive reverse $T_3$ (see *Box 3.29*).

Four important points should be emphasized regarding the synthesis of active metabolites of vitamin D. The first is that the hydroxylations progressively increase the polarity of the hormone so that it becomes more water soluble and less lipid soluble. The second is that C-25 hydroxylation in the liver is determined almost entirely by the concentrations of the precursors. A clinical consequence of this is that measurements of serum 25-hydroxyvitamin D are good indicators of body vitamin D status. The third is that the activity of the C-1 hydroxylase in the kidney is regulated by changes in the serum concentrations of PTH, $P_i$ and $Ca^{2+}$. Thus, a reduction in serum $Ca^{2+}$ concentration and the consequent increase in PTH secretion independently stimulate C-1 hydroxylase activity, as does a decrease in serum $P_i$ concentration. Note also that 1,25-dihydroxycholecalciferol regulates its own synthesis by decreasing the transcription of the C-1 hydroxylase enzyme. The fourth is that C-1 hydroxylation of 25-hydroxycholecalciferol occurs in other cell types (monocytes/macrophages and lymphocytes) but in these it is not regulated by the same factors.

Like all steroid and thyroid hormones, 1,25-dihydroxyvitamin D circulates bound to a globulin that is synthesized in the liver (in this case transcalciferin). A small proportion of vitamin D remains in a free form in the circulation and has a serum $t_{1/2}$ of about 5 h. Transcalciferin preferentially binds 25-hydroxylated molecules and so non-hydroxylated molecules are stored in adipose tissue. This has some clinical utility (see *Box 5.29*). Vitamin D is rapidly cleared by the liver and biliary metabolites of 1,25-dihydroxyvitamin D are more polar than the native hormone. These glucuronides and sulfates undergo an entero-hepatic circulation being absorbed from the gut and resupplied to the liver.

## Classical actions of vitamin D on intestine and bone

Vitamin D acts via receptors that dimerize with other receptors, notably the retinoic acid receptor. In this form, the ligand-bound dimerized receptor attaches to a specific region of DNA. With the help of other transcription co-activators or co-repressors, gene expression is either stimulated or inhibited (*Box 5.7*). As with other steroid and thyroid hormones, there is also evidence that vitamin D exerts actions via a non-genomic pathway via membrane receptors.

The most important action of 1,25-dihydroxyvitamin D is to increase the active absorption of $Ca^{2+}$ from the intestinal lumen of the gut (*Box 5.8*). Calcium is absorbed from the gut by several processes. The best studied involves: the active uptake of $Ca^{2+}$ from the luminal brush border of the enterocytes; the binding of $Ca^{2+}$ to a calcium-binding protein (CaBP); translocation of the complex across to the basolateral surface of the cell; active extrusion of $Ca^{2+}$ by an ATP-dependent calcium pump that pushes $Ca^{2+}$ out of the cell in exchange for $Na^+$. This pump is maintained by a $Na^+/K^+$ exchanger (pumping $Na^+$ back out of the cell) retaining a favorable sodium gradient. In the gut lumen, ionization of calcium occurs at low pH. Exposure of food to gastric acid and substances that form soluble complexes with $Ca^{2+}$ (e.g. amino acids and bile salts) increases absorption whilst those forming insoluble complexes (e.g. oxalate and long-chain fatty acids) decrease absorption.

$Ca^{2+}$ may also be absorbed from the gut by endocytosis and fusion of the particles with lysosomes containing a CaBP. At the basolateral surface, the calcium is released by a process of exocytosis that involves the opening of calcium channels. Another mechanism that has been proposed is via a paracellular route whereby calcium, bound to a CaBP, is transported through gap junctions between the enterocytes (*Box 5.8*).

The rate of calcium absorption across the duodenum is proportional to the number of CaBPs and 1,25-dihydroxyvitamin D increases the expression

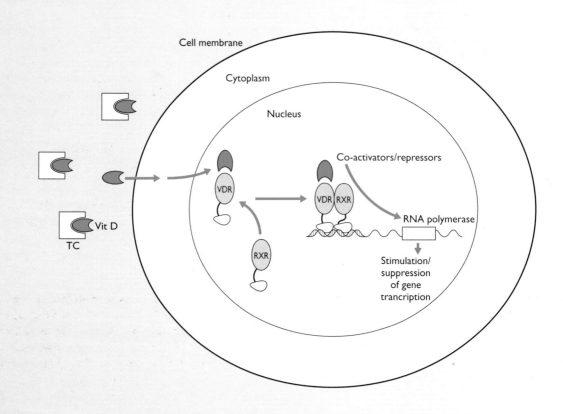

Cell membrane

Cytoplasm

Nucleus

Co-activators/repressors

VDR

VDR RXR

RNA polymerase

Vit D

TC

RXR

Stimulation/
suppression
of gene
trancription

In the circulation, vitamin D is bound to the globulin, transcalciferin (TC), with only a small fraction existing in free form. The free form crosses the cell membrane and the nuclear membrane where, in target cells, it interacts with a vitamin D receptor (VDR). This induces dimerization with the retinoic acid receptor (RXR), DNA binding and interaction of receptors with transcription factors resulting in stimulation or inhibition of gene transcription

of CaBPs. In addition to stimulating CaBP production in the gut, vitamin D increases the permeability of the brush border to $Ca^{2+}$, increases the number of $Ca^{2+}/Na^+$ exchange pumps in the basolateral membrane and may open $Ca^{2+}$ channels via activation of a membrane-bound receptor. Some of these effects may account for the rapid effects of vitamin D on calcium absorption before an increase in CaBP is observed. Finally, it should also

be noted that vitamin D also increases uptake of $P_i$ and $Mg^{2+}$ from the gut.

Within bone, 1,25-dihydroxyvitamin D has an effect synergistic with that of PTH stimulating bone resorption and, thereby, raising circulating $Ca^{2+}$ concentrations. The precise actions of 1,25-dihydroxyvitamin D on bone have not been clearly defined. It is thought that it induces differentiation of monocytic cells (originating in bone marrow)

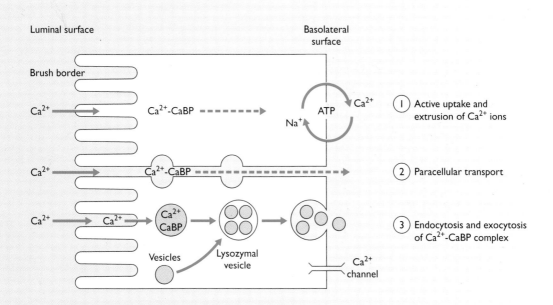

① Ca²⁺ enters the microvilli of the brush border through calcium channels, the opening and closing of which are regulated by the concentration of unbound Ca²⁺ in the microvilli. The ion is transferred across the enterocyte to its basolateral surface via a series of binding proteins (calmodulin, calbindin and a Ca⁺/Na⁺ pump) that have increasing affinities for calcium. In the absence of vitamin D, and hence calbindin, calcium absorption is impaired. Alternative mechanisms may involve a paracellular route ② or capture of Ca²⁺ in endocytotic vesicles ③. All transport mechanisms require calcium-binding proteins (Ca BPs), the synthesis of which is increased by vitamin D.

into osteoclasts and activates these bone-resorbing cells by stimulating the release of a paracrine signal from neighboring osteoblasts (see *Box 5.32*). Vitamin D also plays an important role in bone mineralization with clinically very important effects, discussed in relation to *Clinical Case 5.4*. Whether this is due to an increase in the extracellular supply of calcium and phosphate or the stimulation of bone formation by a direct effect is not defined.

# Parathyroid glands and PTH synthesis

The parathyroid glands develop embryologically from the 3rd and 4th branchial arches (see *Box 3.21*).

Typically, there are four parathyroid glands, one lying behind each of the upper and lower poles of the thyroid gland. Supernumerary glands in the neck or mediastinum (particularly within the thymus) are not uncommon and may cause considerable clinical problems in the search for sources of excessive PTH secretion. Six glands have been reported in approximately 2.5% of the normal population with even seven or eight glands in a few people. Each gland weighs approximately 30–50 mg and is supplied by blood from the thyroid arteries; these can easily be disrupted during thyroid surgery.

PTH is initially synthesized as a larger preprohormone and subsequently cleaved to a biologically active 84 amino acid peptide (molecular weight 9600, *Box 5.9*). This synthesis occurs in the

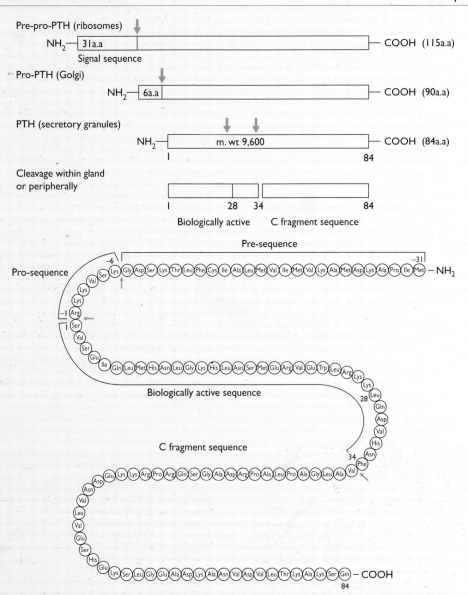

PTH is synthesized from the precursor molecule pre-pro-PTH containing 115 amino acids. As the peptide length increases inside the rough endoplasmic reticulum, the signal sequence is removed in two steps leaving pro-PTH with 90 amino acids. After transport to the Golgi apparatus, a further 6 amino acids are removed from the amino-terminal leaving PTH the full biological activity of which resides in the first 34 amino acids. Further cleavage of PTH to inactive fragments can occur either within the parathyroid glands or the circulation.

Parathyroid hormone related peptide (PTHrp), synthesized in many more tissues, has structural homologies with PTH (see *Box 5.19*).

more numerous chief cells of the parathyroid glands (*Box 5.10*). The less numerous oxyphil cells that appear at puberty secrete PTH only in certain pathological conditions. Full biological activity resides in the first 34 amino-terminal amino acids of the PTH molecule and cleavage of both the amino- and carboxy-terminals of the peptide leads to the production of truncated peptides with little or no biological activity. Cleavage of the first two amino acids from the amino terminal of the peptide markedly reduces bioactivity of PTH but leaves the ability of the hormone to bind to receptors unaltered. PTH does not have a serum-binding protein and the $t_{1/2}$ of circulating PTH is about 4 min; it is rapidly cleared by the liver and kidney.

Since the carboxyl terminal fragment of PTH is biologically inactive, assays that only measure the carboxyl terminal portion of the molecule may give aberrant results, especially in renal failure when there is accumulation of the truncated peptides. Modern assays use two different antibodies, one to recognize the amino-terminus and another the carboxyl-terminus and the principle of these two-site immunoradiometric assays has been described in detail (*Box 3.25*).

## Control of PTH secretion

Changes in circulating $Ca^{2+}$ concentrations are detected and alter PTH secretion via a negative feedback system. The chief cells detect circulating concentrations of $Ca^{2+}$ by a unique G-protein-linked calcium receptor. An increase in $Ca^{2+}$ binding stimulates phospholipase C and inhibits adenylate cyclase and the resultant rise in phosphatidylinositol trisphosphate ($IP_3$) and reduction in cAMP concentrations reduces PTH release. A decrease in the activation of this receptor reduces the generation of $IP_3$ and increases the generation of cAMP leading to an increase in PTH secretion (*Box 5.11*). As a result, PTH secretion is inversely proportional to serum calcium concentration (*Box 5.12*). The 'set point' for PTH secretion is around 1.3 mmol/l. Maximal rates of secretion are achieved at a serum $Ca^{2+}$ concentration of about 1.15 mmol/l. However, the secretion of PTH is never fully suppressed and hypercalcemia arises in the presence of hyperplastic parathyroid glands (*Box 5.16*).

In addition to this negative feedback control of PTH secretion, an increase in vitamin D concentration not only reduces transcription of the C-1 hydroxylase gene but also that of the PTH gene. Thus, vitamin D not only regulates its own conversion to its active metabolite but also the synthesis of PTH.

## Actions of PTH

PTH acts on osteoblasts in bone and tubular cells within the kidney via G-protein-linked receptors that stimulate adenylate cyclase production of cyclic AMP (*Box 5.13*). In bone, within 1 or 2 hours, PTH stimulates a process, known as osteolysis, in which calcium in the minute fluid-filled channels (canaliculi/lacunae) is taken up by syncytial processes of osteocytes and transferred to the external surface of the bone and, thence, into the extracellular fluid (*Box 5.33*). Some hours later, it also stimulates resorption of mineralized bone, a process that releases both $Ca^{2+}$ and $P_i$ into the extracellular fluid. The $P_i$ is rapidly removed from the circulation because the most dramatic effect of PTH on the kidney is to inhibit reabsorption of $P_i$ in

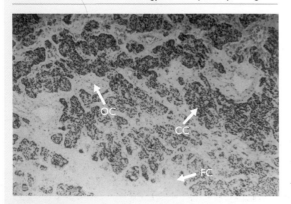

The gland has a connective tissue capsule and contains numerous chief cells (CC) and fewer oxyphil (OC) cells. The latter are larger with more cytoplasm. With age fat cells (FC) become more numerous.

This image is available in color on the website.

**Structural features of the Ca²⁺ receptor**

P   Protein kinase C phosphorylation sites
x   Location of inactivating mutations of the receptor
*   Location of activating mutations of the receptor
⋎   Glycosylation sites

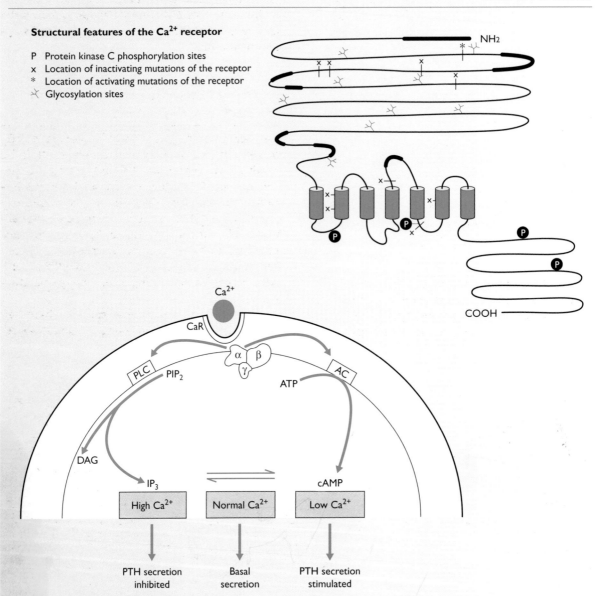

The circulating concentration of Ca²⁺ is detected by a unique G-protein-linked calcium receptor (CaR) on the cell surface of the chief cells. When the Ca²⁺ concentration is high the α-subunit of the G-protein preferentially stimulates phospholipase C (PLC) with the hydrolysis of phosphatidyl inositol 4, 5-bisphosphate (PIP₂) IP₂ to diacylglycerol (DAG) and inositol 1, 4, 5-trisphosphate (IP₃). Adenylate cyclase (AC)-induced cAMP generation is inhibited and so is PTH secretion. The reverse occurs when the Ca² concentration is low and thus PTH secretion is stimulated. When calcium concentrations are within their normal limits the two second messenger pathways are balanced and basal secretions of PTH are maintained.

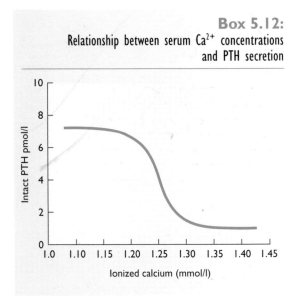

**Box 5.12:**
Relationship between serum $Ca^{2+}$ concentrations and PTH secretion

the proximal tubule and markedly increase its excretion. At the same time, PTH also enhances $Ca^{2+}$ reabsorption in the ascending loop of Henlé and the distal convoluted tubule by increasing the

active uptake of calcium by $Ca^{2+}$-ATPase and a $Na^+$-$Ca^{2+}$ antiporter. Calcium excretion rate is reduced. As noted previously, PTH also stimulates the C-1 hydroxylation of 25-hydroxy-vitamin D within the kidney, thus indirectly stimulating $Ca^{2+}$ reabsorption by the gut.

## Hypercalcemia and primary hyperparathyroidism

It is clear from the foregoing that an excess of PTH or vitamin D leads to hypercalcemia and that the resulting symptoms will be multiple (*Box 5.14*). *Clinical Case 5.1* underwent radiological investigation of the bones in which she suffered aches and pains (*Box 5.15*). This showed marked abnormalities in her humerus and also her hands. At the time her serum $Ca^{2+}$ was 4.1 mmol/l her serum PTH concentration was inappropriately elevated (35 pmol/l, NR 1–6 pmol/l), indicating primary hyperparathyroidism.

This is the most common cause of hypercalcemia with an annual incidence of about 45 per

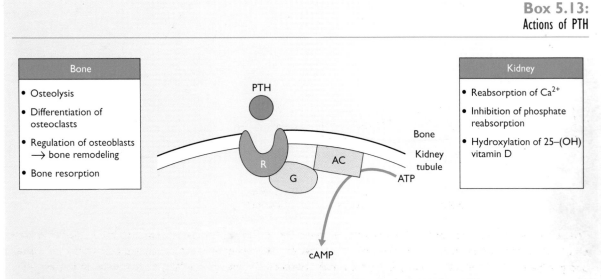

**Box 5.13:**
Actions of PTH

Parathyroid hormone (PTH) acts via a G-protein (G) linked receptor (R) to activate adenyl cyclase (AC) which converts ATP to cAMP. This second messenger stimulates signal transduction processes that activate various functions on bone cells (see also *Box 5.18*) and kidney tubular cells.

**Box 5.14:**
Clinical features of hypercalcemia

| **Symptoms**† | | **Signs**† |
|---|---|---|
| | **None*** (~60%) | |
| | **Cardiovascular** | |
| | | Hypertension (~50%) |
| | **Neurological and ophthalmological** | |
| Malaise and fatigue (~30%) | | Mental obtundation (~5%) |
| Depression (~30%) | | Dementia (~5%) |
| Muscle weakness (~10%) | | Band keratopathy+ (~<1%) |
| | | Cognitive impairment (~5%) |
| | | Coma (~<1%) |
| | **Gastrointestinal** | |
| Constipation (~30%) | | Epigastric tenderness (~5%) |
| Anorexia (~30%) | | |
| Nausea and vomiting (~10%) | | |
| | **Renal** | |
| Polydipsia (~30%) | | |
| Polyuria (~30%) | | |
| Renal colic (~10%) | | |
| | **Rheumatological** | |
| Joint pains (~10%) | | Joint swelling (~1%) |
| Bone pains (~10%) | | Bone deformity (~<1%) |
| | | Fractures (~<1%) |

*Most patients with hypercalcemia are now picked up on routine testing with few symptoms and even fewer signs.
†The frequency of symptoms and signs is dependent on the degree of hypercalcemia and its cause, so the percentage frequencies are very approximate.
+An ophthalmological sign seen only in very severe cases

100 000 (*Box 5.16*). It occurs approximately 2.5 times more frequently in women than in men and its incidence increases with age. Unlike that of *Clinical Case 5.1*, many cases are asymptomatic. In about 80% of the cases it results from a benign parathyroid adenoma and in about 15% a primary hypertrophy of the gland. Parathyroid carcinoma is rare (<0.5%).

The ability to measure total serum $Ca^{2+}$ routinely, simply and cheaply in blood samples means

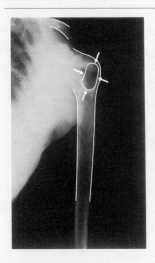

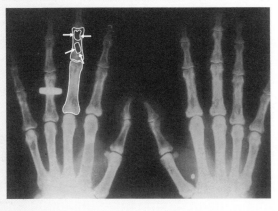

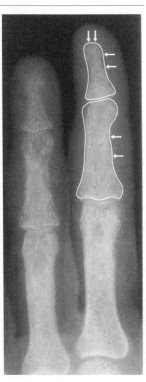

**Left humerus.** The arrows delineate a large osteolytic area. The most common cause of this appearance is metastatic tumor. In this case it is due to a 'brown' tumor or collection of osteoclasts.

**Hands.** The arrows show the position of additional osteoclast activity causing local cyst formation and subperiosteal erosion.

These images are available on the website.

that cases such as *Clinical Case 5.1* with severe hypercalcemia and marked symptoms are now rarely seen in the clinic. In this patient, radiological studies showed a large osteolytic lesion in the head of the humerus and marked erosion of the terminal phalanges, together with cyst formation. Such appearances are due to PTH-induced resorption of bone. The osteolytic lesion is caused by the PTH-induced localized accumulation of osteoclasts within the bone, termed a brown tumor because of the color when seen by the naked eye.

## Hyperparathyroidism and multiple endocrine neoplasia (MEN)

The finding of hyperparathyroidism should always suggest the possibility of multiple endocrine neoplasia because of the implications for affected families. Detailed enquiry into the family history of patients is, therefore, important. Hyperparathyroidism is the most common feature of MEN-1, being present in virtually all gene carriers by the age of 40 years, and is usually the first manifestation of the disease process. MEN-1 is due to loss of function mutations in the putative tumor suppressor gene *menin* and is characterized by tumors of the parathyroids (in ~90%), pituitary gland (~60%) and the pancreas (~70%). Hyperparathyroidism is also seen in approximately 10–30% of families with MEN-2a that is due to loss of function mutations in the putative tumor suppressor gene *ret*. Since MEN-2a is associated with the development of pheochromocytoma, such patients should undergo measurements of urinary or serum catecholamines (see *Clinical Cases 5.8 and 4.7*). Families with MEN

## Hypercalcemia and vitamin D excess

Vitamin D excess is usually due to an excessive intake of the vitamin. As the C-1 hydroxylation is tightly regulated, it is more often seen as a result of accidental therapeutic overdose with hydroxylated pharmaceutical products rather than as a result of vitamin supplementation with non-hydroxylated prohormones; unless, of course, the prohormones are taken in very large doses (>50 000 U/d). It is also seen in about 10% of patients with sarcoidosis, tuberculosis and other granulomatous disorders. This is due to extra-renal conversion of 25-hydroxyvitamin D to the active 1,25-dihydroxyvitamin D by the granulomata, a process that is not regulated by PTH. The characteristic clinical feature of such hypercalcemia is that it responds to high doses of immunosuppressant glucocorticoid steroid such as prednisolone.

**Common**

Primary hyperparathyroidism (~99% of ambulant patients)

> Single adenoma (~80%)
> Hyperplasia (~15%)
> Double adenoma (~2%)
> Carcinoma (~ <1%)

Malignant disease (~99% of ill patients)

> Metastases and myeloma – secreting osteoclast activating factors
> PTHrp secreting
> Lymphoma – cells containing C-1 hydroxylase
> PTH secreting (exceptionally rare)

**Uncommon (~ <1%)**

Vitamin D excess

> Exogenous (therapeutic use of 1,25-dihydroxy-vitamin D)
> Endogenous (e.g. sarcoidosis, tuberculosis)

Tertiary hyperparathyroidism[+]

Hyperthyroidism – usually mild and due to a direct action of thyroid hormone on osteoclasts

**Rare[*] (~ <0.01%)**

Familial hypocalciuric hypercalcemia

Jansen-type metaphyseal chondrodysplasia

[+]Tertiary hyperparathyroidism arises when hypocalcemia (e.g. in vitamin D deficiency) causes a compensatory secondary hyperparathyroidism. The drive to parathyroid hyperplasia results in parathyroid autonomy.

[*]Immobilization, milk-alkali syndrome, vitamin A intoxication and adrenal failure are all quoted in large texts on the parathyroid gland but are exceedingly rare in modern medical practice. Thiazide diuretics are also quoted but are only implicated in the presence of concomitant hyperparathyroidism.

## Hypercalcemia and malignancy

### Clinical Case 5.2:

A 63-year-old male factory worker was referred to the clinic with weight loss, general malaise and a cough. He drank four pints of beer and smoked 20 cigarettes a day. There was no history of excessive intake of vitamin supplements and he took no regular medication. Blood tests revealed normal renal and liver function but a serum $Ca^{2+}$ of 3.8 mmol/l (NR 2.2–2.6 mmol/l) with an albumin of 37g/l (NR 38–48 g/l). The serum PTH concentration was below the assay detection limits. In view of his cough and smoking history, a chest X-ray was performed (*Box 5.17*). X-rays of his skeleton were normal.

*Clinical Case 5.2* clearly differs from *Clinical Case 5.1* in having appropriately suppressed PTH concentrations and there was no history of excess vitamin D intake. His smoking history and the chest X-ray appearances clearly suggested an underlying malignant neoplasm, probably lung cancer.

should be followed in specialized multi-disciplinary clinics with regular, structured screening programs.

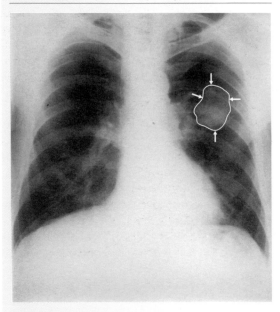

**Box 5.17:**
Chest X-ray of *Clinical Case 5.2*

The arrows delineate a mass in the left lung that in the presence of a strong history of cigarette smoking is very suggestive of a lung cancer.

This image is available on the website.

Malignancy is the second most common cause of hypercalcemia overall, but in hospitalized patients it is the most common cause. Malignancy causes hypercalcemia via two main mechanisms. Hematological malignancies (e.g. myeloma) and those that metastasize to bone (e.g. breast or prostate cancer) produce local factors that act in a paracrine manner to activate osteoclasts (*Box 5.18*). Others, particularly squamous tumors of the lung and head and neck, produce a hormone, PTH-related peptide (PTHrp), that acts at PTH receptors. Patients with tumors secreting PTHrp, as occurred in *Clinical Case 5.2*, have appropriately suppressed PTH levels due to feedback effects of the hypercalcemia on the parathyroid glands. For the sake of completeness, note that exceptionally rarely tumors may secrete PTH itself and that some lymphomas may have increased (and unregulated) C-1 hydroxylase activity.

# Parathyroid hormone-related peptide (PTHrp)

PTHrp is synthesized in various tissues including keratinocytes, lactating mammary tissue, the placenta and fetal parathyroid glands and has actions similar to PTH. It is synthesized from a gene considered to have evolved from a common ancestor of the PTH gene. Alternate splicing of the primary transcript gives rise to three similar products that range in length from 139–173 amino acids.

The amino terminal fragments of these peptides show striking homology to the amino terminal fragment of PTH (eight of the first 13 amino acids are identical) and PTHrp binds to PTH receptors (*Box 5.19*). It was originally discovered in patients like *Clinical Case 5.2* with cancers of squamous cell origin in whom it caused hypercalcemia. However, PTHrp does not, like PTH, increase renal C-1 hydroxylase enzyme activity and, thus, patients with hypercalcemia due to PTHrp do not have the raised concentrations of 1,25-dihydroxyvitamin D seen in patients with hyperparathyroidism. The role of PTHrp in the adult is uncertain but there is evidence for its importance in regulating $Ca^{2+}$ fluxes between fetal and maternal circulations, $Ca^{2+}$ concentrations in breast milk and a role in fetal development. Recently, it has been suggested that there are secreted forms of the mid-region PTHrp viz $PTHrp_{38-94}$, $PTHrp_{38-95}$ and $PTHrp_{38-101}$ that appear to act via a separate receptor as does the carboxyl terminal peptide $PTHrp_{107-139}$.

# Treatment of hypercalcemia

### Fluids

The initial treatment of hypercalcemia is the same irrespective of its cause (*Box 5.20*). As illustrated by *Clinical Case 5.1*, the inhibitory effect of hypercalcemia on the action of arginine vasopressin leads to polyuria. Thus, the initial step is assessment of a patient's fluid balance and initiation of fluid therapy (that may need to be given intravenously). Once fluid balance has been restored, excretion of calcium may be further enhanced by a saline diuresis (because $Na^+$ and $Ca^{2+}$ reabsorption parallel each

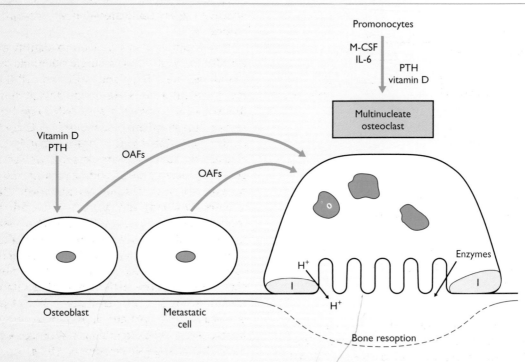

Osteoclasts arise from hematopoietic precursors of the monocyte lineage. Their differentiation is stimulated by factors such as macrophage colony-stimulating factor (M-CSF), cytokines such as IL-6 and PTH and vitamin D. A sealed space is formed by integrin (I)-mediated binding to bone surfaces, and the elaborately folded ruffled border acts, essentially, as a large lysosome secreting acid and enzymes onto the sealed bone area. This causes both demineralization and break down of the bone matrix protein. Osteoclasts do not have PTH or vitamin D receptors but their activity is regulated by osteoclast activating factors (OAFs) such as arachidonic acid derivatives and cytokines whose production can be stimulated by PTH and vitamin D. Bone metastases can also secrete OAFs and thus cause bone resorption.

other in the loop of Henle) using, for example, the loop diuretic furosemide and additional intravenous fluids.

Subsequent treatment depends on the cause (*Box 5.20*).

## Bisphosphonates

Bisphosphonates were developed in the detergent industry at Port Sunlight near Liverpool as antifoaming agents. The nucleus of the molecule contains two phosphate groups attached to a carbon and the different members of the family differ in the nature of the side chains attached to the carbon. The negative charges on the phosphate groups give the bisphosphonates their affinity for bone mineral. They are incorporated into newly formed bone. It was originally thought they reduced osteoclast action by a physicochemical action on hydroxyapatite crystals. However, it is clear that bisphosphonate absorbed to bone surface is taken up into osteoclasts and interferes with several biochemical processes. Those bisphosphonates most resembling pyrophosphate (e.g. etidronate) become incorporated into non-hydrolyzable ATP analogs

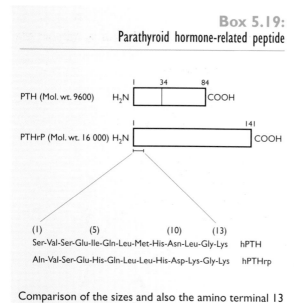

**Box 5.19:**
**Parathyroid hormone-related peptide**

PTH (Mol. wt. 9600)  H₂N  ... COOH
1   34   84

PTHrP (Mol. wt. 16 000) H₂N ... COOH
1   141

(1)    (5)    (10)    (13)
Ser-Val-Ser-Glu-Ile-Gln-Leu-Met-His-Asn-Leu-Gly-Lys   hPTH
Aln-Val-Ser-Glu-His-Gln-Leu-Leu-His-Asp-Lys-Gly-Lys   hPTHrp

Comparison of the sizes and also the amino terminal 13 amino acid sequences of PTH and PTHrp

inhibiting function and leading to cell death. Those containing nitrogen (e.g. alendronate) interfere with other reactions such as the mevalonate pathway affecting signaling functions and thus inhibiting osteoclastic bone resorption. Bisphosphonates are available for both intravenous and oral use (*Box 5.20*).

## Parathyroid surgery

The embryology of the parathyroid glands (leading to considerable anatomical variation), together with their small size, makes parathyroid surgery a specialized field. The most important question is whether a single gland has become adenomatous (the most common cause of primary hyperparathyroidism) or whether there is hyperplasia of all glands. The magnitude of the increase in serum PTH concentration does not help distinguish these possibilities, though it is said that very high concentrations of PTH are typical of the rare carcinomas. A variety of imaging techniques has been used to localize parathyroids prior to surgery, but none offers the desired degree of specificity and sensitivity most clinicians require (*Box 5.21*). Accordingly, many physicians do not use imaging

techniques, relying on the skill of experienced surgeons who generally have success rates >95%. A recent development has been the use of minimally invasive surgery using modified laparoscopic techniques.

It is incumbent on a surgeon to identify all four glands. In most cases, a single adenoma will be found and the other glands will be small (i.e. <50 mg in weight and <5 mm in greatest dimension). Biopsies of the normal glands (with rapid frozen-section histology) may be required if there is any doubt. Occasionally (i.e. approximately 1% of cases), two adenomas are present. However, the greatest problems are caused by parathyroid gland hyperplasia. In these cases, the unknown stimulus to hyperplasia may have also acted on a 5th, 6th or intrathymic gland so that the patient remains hypercalcemic despite the removal of four glands.

Furthermore, in this situation, the surgeon has to face the dilemma of whether to remove all glands (leaving the patient requiring vitamin D treatment life-long), or to remove all but part of one leaving the patient at risk of redeveloping hypercalcemia and requiring further surgery on the neck. Some surgeons remove all the glands from the neck and transplant part of one into the forearm so that only minor surgery is required if hypercalcemia returns.

The situation is different if surgery fails. It is clear that this usually arises because one or more parathyroids were not found at the first operation either because of anatomical variation or because there were more than four parathyroid glands. Selective venous catheterization of the veins in the neck and mediastinum coupled with assays of PTH has been used to localize the source of PTH prior to a second (or subsequent) operation.

## Malignancy

The treatment of malignant hypercalcemia involves the same initial generic therapy followed by bisphosphonates and treatment of the malignancy. The specific treatments for the latter are under constant review and are not covered here. The most common tumors metastasizing to bone are prostate, breast and lung. The tumors most likely to secrete PTHrp are squamous cancers of the

**General**

Fluid replacement that may need to be given intravenously ± a diuretic active on the loop of Henle such as furosemide

**Medical**

| Drug* | Use | Advantages | Disadvantages/side effects |
|---|---|---|---|
| Bisphosphonate e.g. pamidronate, alendronate | Any form of hypercalcemia in which there is osteoclast hyperactivity especially PTH or PTHrp excess | Rapidly acting and effective | Pamidronate given intravenously. Others orally active but poor gut absorption. Temporary effects |
| Glucocorticoid steroid e.g. prednisolone | Hypercalcemia due to excess 1,25 dihydroxyvitamin D especially sarcoidosis or lymphoma | Effective in specific circumstances and cheap | Iatrogenic Cushing's syndrome |
| Calcimimetic e.g. calcium receptor agonist NPS R-568 | Hyperparathyroidism of any type | Orally active | Experimental |

*Large texts on the parathyroid gland also include calcitonin, gallium nitrate, plicamycin and phosphate. Given the effectiveness of bisphosphonates and glucocorticoids, they are virtually never needed.

**Surgical**

| Procedure | Use | Advantages | Disadvantages/side effects |
|---|---|---|---|
| Parathyroidectomy† | Patients with hyper-parathyroidism | 'Definitive' (~95%) | Expensive and scarring. Recurrent laryngeal nerve palsy (~ 0.5%) Persistent hyperparathyroidism (~2%) Carotid/jugular damage and hemorrhage (~0.5%) |

†Procedures for parathyroid hyperplasia differ according to surgeon. Some advocate total parathyroidectomy, others removal of $3^{1}/_{2}$ glands whilst still others transplant part of a gland into the forearm.

**Adjunctive**

This includes other radiotherapeutic and pharmacological treatments for malignancy

lung, head and neck and esophagus although breast, renal and bladder cancers may also do so. Hypercalcemia resulting from an excess of PTHrp secreted by malignant tumors is best treated with bisphosphonates. Metastases to bone may be treated by local radiotherapy.

## Hypervitaminosis D

When this has resulted from an excess oral intake, treatment after initial generic treatment of hypercalcemia is simply to withhold the source of the excess, though glucocorticoid steroids such as prednisolone may also be used. As noted above, vitamin

| Technique | Advantages | Disadvantages |
|---|---|---|
| CT scan | Non-invasive<br>Sensitivity 50–70%<br>Widely available | Ionizing radiation |
| MR scan | Non-invasive<br>Sensitivity 50–70%<br>No ionizing radiation exposure | Less widely available than CT |
| Ultrasound | No ionizing radiation exposure<br>Cheap, widely available<br>Non-invasive | |
| Angiogram | Quoted as 'gold standard' | Invasive |
| Venous sampling<br>(with PTH assays) | Helpful for ectopic glands | Invasive and expensive<br>Only localizes the vein draining the parathyroid |
| Radionuclide scans†<br>⁹⁹ᵐTc- ²⁰¹Tl<br>subtraction<br>⁹⁹ᵐTc-sestamibi | Non-invasive<br>Sensitivity 50%<br>May detect metastases<br>Sensitivity 50%<br>May detect metastases | Radioisotope exposure |

*Note that techniques are constantly improving and are subject to major differences in local expertise. As a result, for example, sensitivities quoted for CT scans may not apply to spiral CT or multi-slice techniques.
†Radionuclide images of the parathyroids together with details of the technique are on the Website.

D excess associated with sarcoidosis and tuberculosis is treated with steroids and additional therapy according to the underlying diagnosis.

## Mutations of the Ca²⁺ or PTH receptors

It is apparent that the normal function of the parathyroid gland Ca²⁺ receptor (*Box 5.11*) is crucial to the regulation of serum Ca²⁺ concentration. Situations in which its function is decreased (loss of function mutations) falsely signal to the parathyroid gland chief cells a low serum concentration and hyperparathyroidism will result, leading to hypercalcemia. This is seen in two clinical conditions, familial benign hypercalcemia and neonatal severe hyperparathyroidism (*Box 5.22*).

To some extent these vary in severity according to whether the patients are heterozygous or homozygous and, therefore, have one or two copies of the mutation.

Similarly, if the PTH receptor were to contain mutations leading to increased biological activity (gain of function mutations) that are independent of serum PTH concentrations then hypercalcemia would also result. This occurs in the very rare, dominantly inherited condition Jansen-type metaphyseal chondrodysplasia. This is characterized clinically by short-limbed dwarfism, hypercalcemia and hypercalciuria. Whilst PTH secretion is suppressed by the hypercalcemia and, hence, serum concentrations of PTH are low, there is evidence of increased bone resorption. In both cases, the 'set points' for the control of PTH secretion have been shifted.

Box 5.22:
## Clinical conditions associated with mutations of the Ca²⁺ receptor

**Loss of function mutation of the Ca²⁺ receptor**
- Familial hypocalciuric hypercalcemia (FHH)
  - Autosomal dominant
  - Persistant relatively asymptomatic hypercalcemia due to generalized resistance to Ca²⁺
  - Unresponsive to parathyroidectomy
- Neonatal severe hyperparathyroidism
  - Severe hypercalcemia, may be associated with fractures that may be multiple
  - May be children of two parents with FHH
  - Recently also described in offspring of single parent with FHH and thought to result from a dominant negative effect of the aberrant Ca²⁺ receptor on normal receptor function

**Gain of function mutation of the Ca²⁺ receptor**
- Familial hypercalciuric hypocalcemia
  - Autosomal dominant
  - May be asymptomatic but many have seizures or carpopedal spasm
  - Treatment should be reserved for symptomatic individuals because complications are common with oral vitamin D

# Hypocalcemia and its treatment

Hypocalcemia, as judged by routine analysis of serum (i.e. total) calcium concentrations, is quite common, particularly in a hospitalized population in which a low serum albumin concentration is frequently seen. A low serum ionized (i.e. Ca²⁺) concentration is much less common. It is clear from the foregoing that hypocalcemia arises because of the inability of the body to respond to low serum calcium concentrations. Thus, chronic hypocalcemia is likely to be the result of a deficiency of PTH or vitamin D or a resistance to one or other hormone. It is important to note, however, that in the presence of normal parathyroid glands, low vitamin D concentrations (of whatever cause) will result in compensatory secondary hyperpara-

thyroidism; *severe* hypocalcemia is likely, therefore, to be due to hypoparathyroidism. The causes of hypocalcemia (and to some extent the clinical symptoms and signs) differ according to the age of the patient. The next clinical case illustrates the presentation in early life.

## Clinical Case 5.3:

A 3-week-old girl of Indian parents had been noted by her mother (who had brought her to the Emergency Room) to have intermittent twitching of her left-hand-side limbs over the previous 4 days. The girl had been born normally at 39 weeks of gestation and was being breast-fed. Examination revealed nothing abnormal. Investigations were performed into the cause of these symptoms. As a result of these, the baby was found to have a low total serum calcium concentration of 1.39 mmol/l (NR 2.2–2.75 mmol/l) a high serum phosphate of 2.87 mmol/l (NR (1.55–2.0 mmol/l) and normal albumin of 38 g/l (NR 38–48 g/l).

For the reasons given above, hypoparathyroidism is the most common cause of hypocalcemia (*Box 5.23*). In adults, this is usually caused by the surgeon's scalpel related to the fact that thyroid disease is common. *Clinical Case 5.3* presented very soon after birth suggesting that she had congenital hypoparathyroidism. As might be expected from the embryology of parathyroid gland development (see *Box 3.21*), congenital absence of the parathyroid glands is likely to be associated with maldevelopment of the 3rd, 4th and 5th branchial arches giving rise to defective thymus and cardiac development (known as Di George syndrome). Familial congenital hypoparathyroidism may also be inherited as an X-linked or recessive condition. These are, however, exceedingly rare and *Clinical Case 5.3* was phenotypically normal.

To understand fully the neonatal presentation, it is important to appreciate fetal–maternal calcium balance outlined in *Box 5.24*. It is clear that maternal hyperparathyroidism leading to hypercalcemia

**Common** (~99%)

**Neonatal**

- Maternal disorder e.g. pre-eclampsia, diabetes, placental insufficiency, hyperparathyroidism
- Prematurity

**Adulthood**

- Post-surgical damage

**Rare** (~<1%)

**Neonatal**

- DiGeorge syndrome
- X-linked or autosomal inherited hypoparathyroidism
- Activating mutations of the parathyroid gland $Ca^{2+}$ receptor (see *Box 5.22*)
- PTH gene mutations (usually in the signal or intronic sequences leading to loss of function)

**Childhood**

- Autoimmune (in polyglandular syndrome type I with mucocutaneous candidiasis)

**Adulthood**

- Iron (hemochromatosis) or copper deposition (Wilson's disease) or metastases

*See also the causes of vitamin D deficiency. For the reasons given in the text this rarely gives rise to *symptomatic* hypocalcemia.

**Box 5.24:**
Materno–fetal calcium balance

- The average neonate contains ~20 g of calcium, most of which is accumulated during the 3rd trimester (weeks 28–40)
- Maternal serum $Ca^{2+}$, $P_i$ and PTH concentrations are within the non-pregnant normal range throughout pregnancy.
- Maternal vitamin D concentrations rise early in pregnancy to about twice the normal non-pregnant values as a result of increased renal and placental $1\alpha$-hydroxylation. This leads to a doubling of gut $Ca^{2+}$ absorption.
- Maternal serum calcitonin concentrations also increase probably as a result of synthesis in the placenta and breast.
- Bone turnover in the mother increases in the 3rd trimester.
- The fetus maintains a relative hypercalcemia irrespective of ambient maternal serum $Ca^{2+}$ concentration. The physiological significance of this is unknown.
- The fetus is capable of secreting PTH from early gestation (e.g. 10–12 weeks). PTH does not cross the placenta.
- Evidence from animal studies suggests that 1,25-dihydroxyvitamin D deficiency has no effect on fetal skeletal formation and calcification or maintenance of normal serum $Ca^{2+}$ concentration.
- PTHrp is produced by many fetal tissues, circulates at higher concentrations than in the mother and regulates fetal serum $Ca^{2+}$ concentration and also fetal–placental transport of the ion. The active transplacental transport of $Ca^{2+}$ is essentially one-way, mother to fetus.

may be translated by the placenta into fetal hypercalcemia suppressing PTH secretion by the fetal parathyroid glands. In the extrauterine environment, the fetal (now neonatal) system (essentially the kidneys) clears the hypercalcemia but the parathyroid glands, having been suppressed fetally, take time to recover. Thus, a neonate subjected to fetal life in a hypercalcemic environment may present with symptoms and signs of hypocalcemia (*Box 5.23*). Noteworthy is the high serum phosphate measured in the infant. This is because in hypoparathyroidism the effect of PTH on $P_i$ excretion by the kidney is lost and thus hyperphosphatemia develops.

The serum calcium in the mother of *Clinical Case 5.3* was measured and found to be high (2.9 mmol/l, NR 2.2–2.6 mmol/l) with an albumin of 39 g/l (NR 38–48 g/l) and phosphate of 1.11 mmol/l. The mother's serum PTH was reported to be 23.9 pmol/l (NR 1–6 pmol/l) whilst that of the baby was 5.7 pmol/l. These values were inappropriately high and low respectively for the serum calcium concentrations. The daughter's serum calcium corrected spontaneously over a number of weeks; the mother underwent removal of a single parathyroid adenoma prior to undertaking a second pregnancy.

Hypoparathyroidism also occurs in rare syndromes that have associated features suggesting an autoimmune etiology (*Box 5.25*). The targets of the autoimmunity are as yet unknown; autoantibodies blocking functions have been suggested in some studies.

Whilst endocrine deficiencies are usually treated with replacement therapy of the deficient hormone (e.g. insulin, $T_4$, glucocorticoids), PTH deficiency is treated with vitamin D because it is cheap and orally active (see *Box 5.29*). PTH produced by recombinant DNA technology is currently being developed for use in osteoporosis (see below). In acute situations, as occurred in the patient in *Clinical Case 5.3*, intravenous $Ca^{2+}$ can be used.

## Pseudohypoparathyroidism

The first hormonal resistance syndrome to be described was that of PTH resistance. In 1942, Fuller Albright and his colleagues described patients who were hypocalcemic and hyperphosphatemic with a typical phenotype of short stature, short neck, brachydactyly (short fingers especially affecting the 4th and 5th metacarpals), obesity, and subcutaneous calcification. When injected with PTH they did not show the normal responses of increased serum $Ca^{2+}$ concentrations and increased $P_i$ and cAMP concentrations in the urine. As would

be expected of a resistance syndrome, such patients have high serum concentrations of PTH.

The disease was termed pseudohypoparathyroidism, a cumbersome term that remains in widespread use. A better term would, perhaps, be PTH resistance. Since that time pseudohypoparathyroidism has been divided into several types depending on the stage at which PTH signal transduction is affected. In some, the typical phenotypic features described (now known as Albright's hereditary osteodystrophy, AHO) are not present even though there is resistance to PTH.

In type Ia pseudohypoparathyroidism, there is an approximately 50% reduction in the activity of the stimulatory G-protein linked to the PTH receptor and typical features of AHO. Different mutations of the $G_s$ protein are seen in different families and these are inherited in an autosomal dominant manner. Some family members of patients with type Ia pseudohypoparathyroidism show features of AHO and reduced $G_s$ activity although they show a normal urinary phosphate and cAMP response to PTH administration. This abnormality has been termed pseudo-pseudohypoparathyroidism (an inelegant term) and is paternally transmitted. However, when the abnormal $G_s$ gene is maternally transmitted, patients tend to exhibit PTH resistance (no kidney response) as well. This suggests that other factors/genes are involved in PTH resistance other than mutations in the $G_s$ gene.

Other types of pseudohypoparathyroidism, classified as type Ib, show features of tissue-specific resistance to PTH with hypocalcemia, hyperphosphatemia and secondary hyperparathyroidism, yet they lack features of AHO or abnormal $G_s$ activity. These cases tend to occur sporadically and it is thought that the resistance is caused by an abnormal receptor or an abnormality in the transduction of the signal after activation of the G-protein.

## Vitamin D deficiency

As has been emphasized, lack of vitamin D rarely leads to symptomatic hypocalcemia because the secondary increase in PTH compensates. Vitamin D deficiency has marked effects on bone as illustrated

---

**Box 5.25:**
**Autoimmunity and the parathyroid gland**

**Polyglandular autoimmune syndrome type I**
Characterized by the triad of clinical features:
- Mucocutaneous candidiasis (~100%)
- Hypoparathyroidism (~80%)
- Addison's disease (~70%)

Also associated with:
- Gonadal failure (~50% of women, ~15% of men)
- Dental enamel hypoplasia (~70%)
- Alopecia (~30%)
- Pernicious anemia (~15%)
- Hypothyroidism (~5%)

in *Clinical Case 5.4*, chosen for its particularly eloquent additional demonstration of the non-classical actions of the hormone.

## Clinical Case 5.4:

A 28-year-old Asian woman from East Africa was admitted for investigation of suspected aplastic anemia. She was barely able to walk and was brought by wheel chair to the ward. A history revealed that she had delivered a normal baby a few months previously. She was thought to have aplastic anemia and had been treated with repeated blood transfusions. She complained of aches in her hips and was noted to have a severe proximal myopathy (weakness of the muscles around her hips). Her serum calcium was 1.96 mmol/l (NR 2.2–2.6 mmol/l), serum phosphate 0.66 mmol/l (NR 0.8–1.4 mmol/l) and albumin of 37 g/l (NR 38–48 g/l). Her serum creatinine was normal but she was noted to have a marked hyperchloremic acidosis (serum chloride 114 mmol/l (NR 99–109 mmol/l), serum bicarbonate 19

mmol/l)). The serum concentration of the bone isoform of the enzyme alkaline phosphatase (that is involved in mineralization) was markedly elevated at 1239 IU/l (NR 30–120 IU/l). X-rays of her hips showed marked deformation of the hip joint sockets on both sides and those of the lumbar spine osteopenia and osteoporosis. Detailed history taking revealed that she had become so weak during pregnancy that she had been unable to leave the house. Her only other symptom was of recurrent loose bowel motions that had become more marked during pregnancy.

The clinical features were dominated by the weakness due to a proximal myopathy and aches and pains in bones. The anemia was severe and bone marrow examination showed a marked lack of blood-forming cells (*Box 5.26*). The hypocalcemia was mild and the serum biochemistry dominated by the hypophosphatemia and hyperchloremic acidosis. The latter resulted from PTH-mediated inhibition of renal reabsorption of

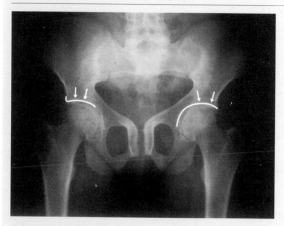

The pelvis X-ray shows the molding of the hip joint (arrows) that has occurred as a result of the loss of the tensile strength of bone.

These images are available on the website.

**Box 5.26:**
**The bone marrow appearances of Clinical Case 5.4**

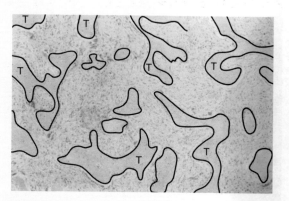

The low power photomicrograph of the bone marrow trephine shows the sparse cells of the trabeculae of bone (T). The cells between these trabeculae are not those forming the cellular elements of blood but fibroblasts.

phosphate, bicarbonate and sodium thereby increasing their urinary excretion.

*Clinical Case 5.4* had a serum 25-hydroxy vitamin D concentration of 6 nmol/l (NR 20–100 nmol/l) and a diagnosis of osteomalacia (loss of bone mineralization) due to vitamin D deficiency was made. The causes of vitamin D deficiency are given in *Box 5.27* and the clinical features in *Box 5.28*. The diagnostic question in this patient was the cause of the vitamin D deficiency. In the UK (with substantially less sun than East Africa), lack of sun exposure and poor dietary intake (or absorption) lead to a much higher prevalence in high risk populations including Asians and the elderly. In this case dietary intake was regarded as adequate.

The only symptom to give a clue to the cause came from the gut, suggesting the failure to absorb dietary vitamin D. The patient had symptoms of diarrhea without those such as loss of blood or mucus to suggest large bowel involvement. This suggested the possibility of a small bowel disease such as celiac disease. This is an immune-mediated condition leading to loss of intestinal villi and, therefore, impaired absorption of a number of important dietary materials. Duodenal biopsy was performed and confirmed the diagnosis of celiac

disease. This, together with her lack of exposure to sunlight, had caused her vitamin D deficiency.

The treatment of vitamin D deficiency is, naturally, hormone replacement. The principles of oral replacement are given *Box 5.29*. In *Clinical Case 5.4*, it was recognized that oral vitamin D may not be absorbed and intramuscular vitamin D was given. At the same time, she was given dietary advice to avoid foods containing wheat that contains the protein gluten to which there is hypersensitivity in celiac disease. Once this was done and a repeat duodenal biopsy showed recovery, she was treated with oral vitamin D. The bone marrow showed marked recovery (see Website).

## Non-classical actions of vitamin D

The widespread distribution of vitamin D receptors (VDRs) in the body suggests functions for the hormone far beyond that of the regulation of $Ca^{2+}$ and $P_i$ (*Box 5.30*). VDRs have been located in at least 30 different tissues and over 70 genes are regulated by the VDR. These include genes associated with mineral homeostasis, cell differentiation and proliferation, oncogenes, metabolism and signal transduction proteins. The antiproliferative and maturational effects of vitamin D on keratinocytes have been put to clinical use; vitamin D is used to treat psoriasis, a proliferative skin disorder. In the bone marrow, vitamin D acts to suppress the production of cytokines by megakaryocytes (the precursors to platelets) and, in the absence of the hormone, the cytokines produced inhibit normal marrow function (as seen in *Clinical case 5.4*).

Vitamin D is also involved in immunomodulation. It stimulates the differentiation of promonocytes to monocytes and macrophages (believed to be precursors of osteoclasts that resorb bone), reduces the production of cytokines by immune cells and decreases the proliferation of T and B lymphocytes. Thus, vitamin D increases non-specific immunity but suppresses antigen-specific immunity. No major immune defect, however, is notable in individuals who lack vitamin D receptors. In contrast, life-long alopecia (hair loss) is frequently associated with loss of VDRs indicating that the

---

### Box 5.27:
### Causes of vitamin D deficiency

**Common (~95%)**
- Deficient intake or cutaneous synthesis e.g. dietary deficiency or reduced sunlight (particularly seen in the UK in the elderly and Indian subcontinent Asian populations)

**Less common (~5%)**
- Deficient absorption e.g. celiac disease or pancreatic insufficiency
- Increased metabolism e.g. hepatic P450 enzyme induction during anticonvulsant medication

**Rare (~<1%)**
- Impaired C-25 hydroxylation e.g. liver disease
- Impaired C-1 hydroxylation e.g. renal failure or type I vitamin D resistance
- Target organ resistance e.g. type 2 vitamin D resistance

## Childhood
Rickets
- Bony deformity e.g. bowing of long bones ①, widening of cartilage at growth plate ②
- Bone pain
- Weakness

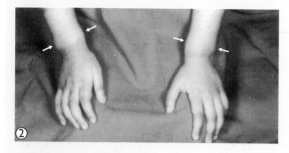

Epiphyseal widening at wrists

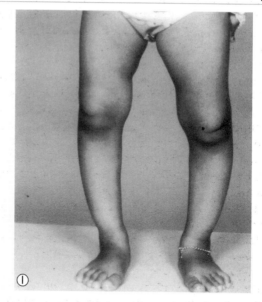

Marked bowing of legs

## Adulthood
Osteomalacia
- Bone pains
- Proximal myopathy
- Fractures e.g. through Looser's zones ③

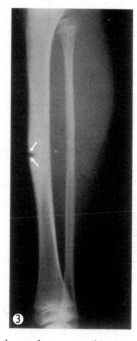

Arrows show Looser's zone on tibia

These images are available on the website.

## Box 5.29:
### Principles of the treatment of hypocalcemia

- In the acute situation with severe symptoms (e.g. neuromuscular irritability), intravenous calcium will usually be required.
- Oral calcium (1–3 g daily) supplementation is usual. In clinical situations associated with magnesium deficiency, replacement of this element in addition is essential.
- In hypoparathyroidism, deficiency of PTH results in reduced C-1 hydroxylation of vitamin D so treatment with 1α-hydroxyvitamin D is used.
- In vitamin D deficiency, the metabolite, dose and method of administration chosen depend on the underlying cause and also factors such as absorption and patient compliance. Thus:
  - In situations associated with reduced C-1 hydroxylation e.g. renal failure or type 2 resistance, the 1α-hydroxyvitamin D is used
  - When absorption is poor, parenteral (intramuscular) vitamin D may be given
  - Rapid replenishment of body stores may be achieved by intramuscular non-hydroxylated vitamin D (that is taken up into fat stores)
  - Higher doses are required in patients with increased vitamin D metabolism e.g. those taking anticonvulsants
- Treatment may need to be life-long and doses titrated to keep the serum $Ca^{2+}$ in the normal range. Hypercalcemia should be avoided and regular assays of serum $Ca^{2+}$ are required. Patient education is important.

## Box 5.30:
### Genomic actions of vitamin D

**Classical**
- Increased calcium binding proteins
- Increased calcium pumps in basolateral surface of intestinal villus and crypt cells
- Stimulated production of paracrine signals on osteoblasts which recruit and activate ostoclasts
- Increased alkaline phosphatase and osteocalcin for bone mineralization
- Increased 24-hydroxylase activity

**Non-classical**[*]
- Decreased production of interleukin-2, γ-interferon and other cytokines in monocytes and activated T lymphocytes
- Inhibition of the cell cycle (antiproliferative, prodifferentiating effects) of, for example
  - proliferating T and B lymphocytes
  - proliferating keratinocytes
  - smooth muscle cells, cardiac myocytes
  - myometrium and endometrium of uterus

[*]Vitamin D receptors are also found in pancreatic islets, anterior pituitary gland, hypothalamus, placenta, ovary, aortic endothelium and could account for a variety of other actions of vitamin D that are not involved in calcium regulation.

vitamin is important in the maturation of the hair follicle.

# Vitamin D resistance and rickets

As with other hormones, resistance to vitamin D also occurs, but it is rare. As inherited defects, they present in childhood with clinical features of the bone disease rickets. There are two forms of resistance. Type 1, also known as pseudovitamin D deficiency, is not actually a true resistance but is caused by a defect in its C-1 hydroxylation. Hence, the active form of the hormone is not produced and bone formation is impaired. It is easily treated by oral administration of the active 1,25-dihydroxylated hormone.

Type 2 vitamin D resistance, otherwise known as hereditary vitamin D resistant rickets (VDRR), is due to a true end-organ resistance and is inherited in an autosomal recessive manner. Several different mutations in the vitamin D receptor have been documented. Some decrease the binding affinity for the hormone whilst others affect the subsequent processes involved in the transcription of genes normally controlled by the hormone receptor complex. Rickets is discussed further in the context of *Clinical Case 5.5*, a rare case chosen to introduce bone disease.

## Clinical Case 5.5:

An 18-month-old child first walked at 14 months of age. She was noted to have an odd gait and deformity of the legs. Dietary vitamin D deficiency rickets was diagnosed at another hospital and she was treated with vitamin D2. By the age of 2 years her deformity was more marked (*Box 5.31*). She was reinvestigated. When taking her vitamin D2, her serum calcium was 2.32 mmol/l (NR 2.2–2.6 mmol/l) with a phosphate of 0.58 mmol/l (NR 1.16–1.91 mmol/l). The serum PTH concentration was 12 pmol/l (NR 1–6 pmol/l).

The child was diagnosed as having dietary vitamin D deficiency but the clinical features deteriorated while taking apparently adequate treatment; either the family had not been administering the treatment or the diagnosis was incorrect (or both). Family frictions made it difficult to obtain a full family history but, after lengthy discussions, the child's mother later admitted to having been treated for rickets in childhood and blamed her own mother for her childhood difficulties associated with this disease.

A diagnosis of X-linked dominant hypophosphatemic rickets was made and the child was treated with 4-hourly oral phosphate supplements and 1,25-dihyydroxyvitamin D. The dramatic radiological and clinical benefits of treatment can be seen (*Box 5.31*). Hypophosphatemic rickets remains to be fully understood. It is characterized by a defect in proximal renal tubule function resulting in phosphate wasting plus low or inappropriately normal concentrations of serum 1,25-dihydroxyvitamin D and defective bone mineralization. Studies in *hyp* mice, a model of the disease, have shown defects in the C-1 hydroxylation of 25-hydroxyvitamin D in the same cells that have a defect in phosphate absorption. It appears to be

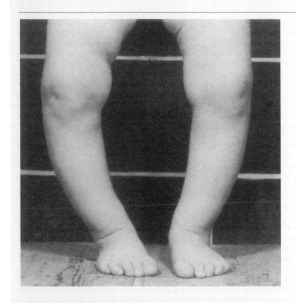

Clinical photograph of the lower legs at presentation. Note the marked bowing.

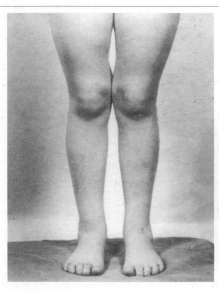

Clinical photograph of the lower legs after 7 years treatment with regular oral phosphate and vitamin D. A vivid demonstration of the ability of bone to remodel.

due to a mutation in the PHEX gene – a *PH*osphate-regulating gene with homologies to *E*ndopeptidases located on the *X*-chromosome. It has been suggested that PHEX codes for a membrane enzyme that cleaves the putative hormone phosphatonin that is involved in regulating $P_i$ absorption. Inadequate cleavage of phosphatonin leads to increased circulating concentrations of the protein, decreased expression of renal $Na^+/PO_4^{3-}$ co-transporters and, thus, $P_i$ wasting.

## Hormones and the skeleton

*Clinical Case 5.5* (*Box 5.31*) shows the spectacular ability of bone to remodel and correct deformities and the requirement of vitamin D for bone mineralization. *Clinical Cases 5.1* and *5.3* have demonstrated the importance of vitamin D and PTH in regulating $Ca^{2+}$ and $P_i$ concentrations. There are, in addition, several endocrine conditions that can give rise to skeletal abnormalities in the absence of changes in serum calcium concentration, and without alterations in vitamin D or PTH status. Since many hormones can affect bone formation and remodeling (*Box 5.32*) and so give rise to skeletal abnormalities it is appropriate to discuss these processes in more detail.

## Structure, formation and function of bone

Bone is composed of an organic matrix (primarily collagen) impregnated with hydroxyapatite crystals $(Ca_{10}[PO_4]_6[OH]_2)$. Other minerals are also present (e.g. magnesium) and bone is an important store of these. There are two types of bone, cortical and trabecular, the former constituting approximately 80% of the total bone mass. In the long bones of the skeleton, cortical or compact bone predominates and is characterized by an outer layer of circumferential rings of bone surrounding columns of concentric rings of bone (*Box 5.33*). Each column surrounds a Haversian canal that contains blood and lymph vessels and nerves. Inside this thick hard shell is the trabecular bone that is made up of spicules of bone or trabeculae arranged in lamellae. Between these spicules lie the bone marrow ele-ments and connective tissue cells, as well as blood and lymphatic vessels. In the axial skeleton (skull, ribs, vertebrae etc.) there is only a relatively thin layer of circumferential cortical bone with a much greater mass of trabecular or spongy bone. Since trabecular bone has five times as much surface area as compact bone – i.e. the surfaces within bones exposed to the ECF – it is far more important than compact bone in phosphate and calcium homeostasis.

Bone formation and resorption (remodeling) occurs on bone surfaces of microscopic units called osteons (*Box 5.32*). Formation is carried out by active osteoblasts that extrude collagen into the extracellular space. Subsequently (about 10 days later), calcium and phosphate are deposited in this osteoid and mature hydroxyapatite crystals are slowly formed. Alkaline phosphatase is required for this mineralization process as well as adequate concentrations of calcium and phosphate. Vitamin D is essential and this is why lack of, or resistance to, this hormone leads to impaired mineralization as seen in *Clinical Case 5.5*.

As the osteoblasts become surrounded by mineralized bone these cells lose their activity and become interior osteocytes. However, they remain in contact with the bone surfaces, and hence the ECF, through long cytoplasmic processes (syncytial processes) that extend through the fluid-filled lacunae traversing the bone lamellae. The syncytial processes form gap junctions with surface osteoblasts. It is through these connections that calcium can be released from bone – a process termed osteocytic osteolysis and under the control of PTH (*Box 5.33*).

Bone resorption also occurs on bone surfaces and is carried out by giant multinucleate cells (up to 100 μm diameter) formed by the fusion of several progenitor cells (*Box 5.18*). These osteoclasts literally tunnel their way into mineralized bone. The actions of numerous enzymes break down the hydroxyapatite crystals and destroy the osteoid leaving craters on the bone surface. These pits are subsequently filled in with new bone by osteoblasts so bone resorption and formation are coupled.

Under normal circumstances, bone formation and resorption are co-ordinated processes occurring in osteons and responsible for the continual remodeling of bone. In any one year, it is estimated

### Bone remodeling and hormonal control of bone resorption

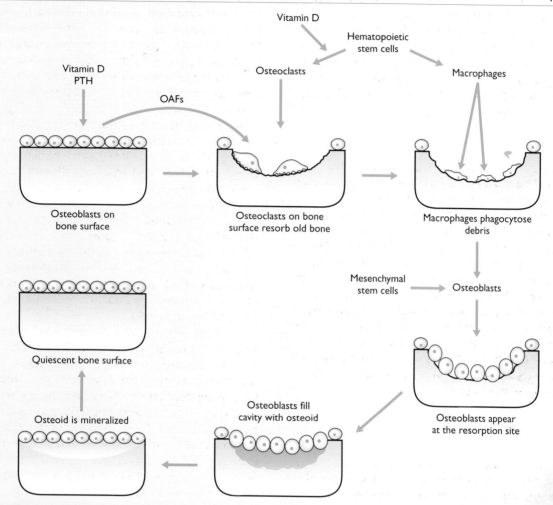

On bone surfaces osteoblasts secrete collagen into the extracellular space and subsequently calcium and phosphate are deposited in this osteoid. Eventually the osteoblasts become surrounded by the newly formed bone and become osteocytes remaining in contact with the bone surfaces by syncytial processes. Osteoclasts are multinuclear cells that resorb bone. PTH and vitamin D are thought to induce bone resorption by stimulating osteoblasts to produce osteoclast activating factors (OAFs). These are paracrine signals (e.g. cytokines and prostaglandins) that attract and activate osteoclasts.

that there is a turnover of approximately 25% of trabecular and 3% of cortical bone. It should be noted that peak bone mass is considered to be reached at about the age of 30 years and studies in twins have indicated that approximately 80% of the variation in bone mineral density is due to genetic factors. It is clear that up to this age bone formation must exceed resorption and both bone formation and its remodeling are controlled by a vast array of hormones. These include growth fac-

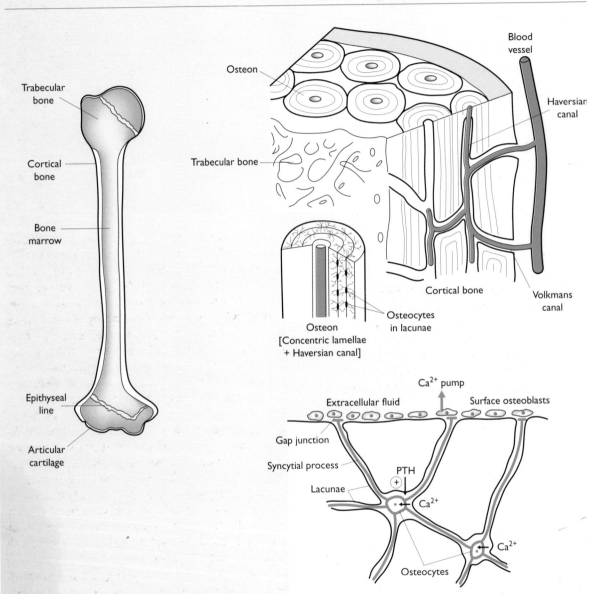

A schematic diagram of cortical and trabecular bone is shown in the upper figure together with the osteons where bone remodeling occurs. Surface osteoblasts become osteocytes as they become surrounded by mineralized bone but they remain in contact with the bone surface through long synctial (cytoplasmic) processes which run in the fluid filled lacunae. They are connected to the surface osteoblasts through gap junctions. $Ca^{2+}$ in the lacunae is in equilibrium with plasma $Ca^{2+}$ but, under the action of parathyroid hormone (PTH), $Ca^{2+}$ is taken up by the osteocytes, transported to the surface osteoblasts which pump the $Ca^{2+}$ into the extracellular fluid, thus raising plasma $Ca^{2+}$ concentrations.

tors and cytokines (many better known for roles played in the immune system), some of which stimulate bone formation or resorption, others inhibiting these processes.

# Osteoporosis

Osteoporosis is one of the most common endocrine diseases. It differs from osteomalacia (in vitamin D deficiency) in that collagen as well as mineral is lost from bone. It occurs when bone resorption exceeds formation. Normally these bone remodeling processes are tightly co-ordinated by a wide variety of hormones and growth factors, allowing compensation for any change. If, for example, the primary action of a hormone is to stimulate bone resorption, this can be partially balanced by a secondary increase in formation. Thus, the net effect of any endocrine abnormality depends on the degree of compensatory coupling.

The most common form of osteoporosis is age related and there is a gradual loss of bone from the age of 30–40 years onwards. In women, bone loss is accelerated in the postmenopausal years due to the loss of estrogens and this occurs in both men and women at any age when there is a deficiency of sex hormones or other defined diseases. Osteoporosis is also a major problem in patients confined to chronic bed rest because immobilization increases bone resorption as does space flight owing to the loss of gravity.

Osteoporosis may occur as a result of a reduced peak bone mass or a mismatch between bone formation and resorption. It has been calculated that lifetime risk of osteoporotic fracture over the age of 50 years is 40% for females and 13% for males. These fractures cost the Health Service many hundreds of millions of pounds per year. To emphasize that the disease is not restricted to elderly women, *Clinical Case 5.6* is an unusual example of a young man with severe osteoporosis.

## Clinical Case 5.6:

A 26-year-old man had been under long-term follow up for hypopituitarism as a result of the treatment of a very large 3rd ventricular brain tumor presenting at the age of 15 years. He had been treated by the insertion of a ventricular–peritoneal shunt to reduce hydrocephalus and 5500 cGy of craniospinal irradiation. Over the course of his 26th year, it was noted that his standing height decreased by 6 cm. His serum biochemistry was normal. In particular, the serum calcium was 2.45 mmol/l (NR 2.2–2.6 mmol/l), the $P_i$ 1.1 mmol/l (NR 0.8–1.4 mmol/l) and the albumin 38 g/l (NR 38–48 g/l) and his replacement endocrine medication of hydrocortisone, thyroxine and mixed testosterone esters was unchanged. X-rays of his spine reveal marked osteoporosis (*Box 5.34*) that was confirmed on bone biopsy. Bone mineral density by dual X-ray absorptiometry was markedly reduced.

Osteoporosis arises when bone resorption exceeds its formation and its major causes are given in *Box 5.35*. In *Clinical Case 5.6* there is a number of possible etiologies. Whilst hypogonadism is well recognized to cause osteoporosis, he was being treated with intramuscular androgens and there was no evidence of a past or present deficiency. Osteoporosis is also a feature of Cushing's syndrome and high doses of exogenous glucocorticoids. Again, in this case, there was no evidence that his glucocorticoid replacement was instrumental in its development. Radiotherapy also gives rise to osteoporosis but in this case bones in non-irradiated areas were also affected. It seems likely that a deficiency of pituitary somatotrophin (growth hormone) played a role in causing the bone disease.

Somatotrophin provides a constant stimulus to bone formation and this stimulus can be promoted by insulin-like growth factors and other local growth factors. Cortisol inhibits bone formation and stimulates resorption, whilst the sex steroids have opposite effects. Cytokines generally stimulate bone resorption. Thus, the osteoporosis seen in *Clinical Case 5.6* was likely to be caused by the loss of somatotrophin stimulation on bone formation and that this loss could not be compensated for by other bone-promoting hormones and growth factors. The syndrome of adult somatotrophin deficiency and its treatment is discussed in more detail on the website. The treatments for osteoporosis are given in *Box 5.36*.

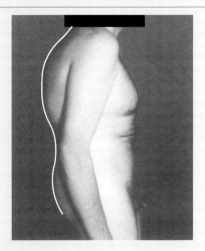

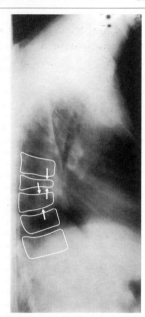

Clinical photographs of *Clinical case 5.6* age 26 years. Note the shortening and marked antero-posterior curvature (termed kyphosis) of the spine, particularly noticeable in the thoracic region. This arises as a result of the combination of a reduction in the vertical height of vertebrae and also the tendency for this to be greatest in the anterior part of the vertebral bodies resulting in a wedge shape.

This is well seen in the lateral X-ray of the spine of *Clinical Case 5.6* (arrowed).

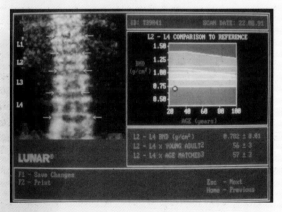

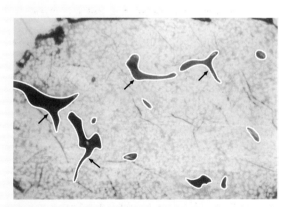

Quantification of bone mineral density in the lumbar spine using dual X-ray absorptiometry (DEXA) shows that *Clinical Case 5.6* has only approximately 56% the expected bone density for a man of his age.

These images are available in color on the website.

Bone biopsy showing sparse bony spicules (arrowed) compared with broad expanse of fat-filled marrow cavity. Compare with the bone marrow trephine in Box 5.26.

**Definition:** A disease characterized by low bone mass and microarchitectural deterioration of bone tissue leading to enhanced bone fragility and a consequent increase in fracture risk.

**Diagnostic categories:** Non-invasive diagnosis is made using bone densitometry. Osteoporosis is defined as a bone mineral density more than 2.5 standard deviations (SD) below the mean for young adults. Osteopenia is defined as a bone mineral density 1–2.5 SD below the young adult mean. Severe or established osteoporosis is defined as being present when the above bone density criterion is met and there are one or more fragility fractures.

**Causes***
**Primary**
**Secondary**
• Endocrine
  Hypogonadism of any cause
  Glucocorticoid excess of any cause (most commonly iatrogenic)
  Hyperthyroidism
  Pregnancy (rare)
• Hematopoietic diseases e.g. multiple myeloma, leukemia, sickle cell disease
• Connective tissue disease e.g. osteogenesis imperfecta, Marfan's syndrome (all rare)
• Drug induced e.g. heparin, anticonvulsants, methotrexate
• Renal disease e.g. chronic renal failure
• Nutritional e.g. malabsorption

*The division into primary and secondary osteoporosis is somewhat arbitrary since epidemiologically the 'primary' disease is clearly related (and, thus, secondary) to ageing and to the hypogonadal state of the menopause in women.

# Paget's disease (osteitis deformans)

## Clinical Case 5.7:

A 78-year-old widow presented to the Rheumatology clinic with a several year history of deformity and discomfort in the lower right leg (Box 5.37). Her serum $Ca^{2+}$ was 2.76 mmol/l (NR 2.2–2.6 mmol/l) with a $P_i$ of 1.03 mmol/l (NR 0.8–1.4 mmol/l) and an alkaline phosphatase of 335 IU/l (NR 30–100 IU/l). She was treated with an oral bisphosphonate. Nine years later she tripped on a pavement fracturing her right tibia (Box 5.37). At that time the serum $Ca^{2+}$ was 2.57 mmol/l with a $P_i$ of 1.00 mmol/l and an alkaline phosphatase of 684 IU/l. She was treated with a plaster of Paris cast and the fracture healed over the subsequent 6 months. Seventeen years after presentation, she complained of deteriorating hearing and was referred to the audiology department. At the age of 95 years her serum $Ca^{2+}$ was 2.42 mmol/l with a $P_i$ of 0.92 mmol/l and an alkaline phosphatase of 513 IU/l.

*Clinical Case 5.7* vividly illustrates the origin of the name of the condition osteitis deformans and it is clear that Paget's disease is a disorder of bone remodeling. It is prevalent in Northern Europe, affecting up to 4% of people over the age of 40 and up to 10% over the age of 60. It is not known why large, somewhat bizarre-looking osteoclasts, with up to a hundred nuclei, stimulate bone metabolism and initiate bone remodeling in a disorganized way. An infectious etiology has been implicated (e.g. paramyxovirus or canine distemper) and other studies have suggested a genetic trait. The result of the disorganized remodeling is focal areas of highly vascular and cellular bone, with either a mosaic pattern of lamellar bone or woven bone. The disease can affect any bone but the most common sites are the sacrum and spine, femur, skull and the pelvis.

**General**

A number of recommendations have been made to reduce the risk of the development of osteoporosis. These include adequate calcium and vitamin D intake, regular weight-bearing exercise, moderate alcohol intake and not smoking.

**Specific**

| Drug[*] | Use | Advantages | Disadvantages/side effects |
|---|---|---|---|
| Bisphosphonate e.g. alendronate, etidronate | Decreases bone resorption | Effective in the treatment of established osteoporosis. Used orally. May be added to estrogen. May be used to prevent glucocorticoid associated osteoporosis | Used long-term. Some specific side effects e.g. gastrointestinal |
| Estrogen | Prevention or treatment of established osteoporosis | Effective. Also has other benefits e.g. on cardiovascular risk | Used long-term some increase in risk of breast cancer and venous thromboembolism |
| PTH | Stimulates bone deposition. Treatment of established osteoporosis | Effective in short term studies | Expensive. Given by injection. Currently experimental. Not currently licensed |
| PTH secretagogue e.g. NPS2143 | Promotes PTH secretion by inhibiting the parathyroid $Ca^{2+}$ receptor | Effective when used in conjunction with an inhibitor of bone resorption (estrogen) | Currently experimental |
| Proton pump inhibitor e.g. SB242784 | Prevents acidification of the osteoclast space and thus inhibits bone resorption | Effective in animal models of hypogonadal osteoporosis | Experimental |

[*]Note that experimental agents have been included.

In the initial stages of the disease, osteoclastic activity usually predominates so that bones become soft and deformed and may fracture as vividly illustrated by *Clinical Case 5.7*. Later, increased osteoblastic activity results in thickened deformed bone. This can trap nerves or leave abnormal bone in the joint areas. Thus, neurological (such as deafness as in *Clinical Case 5.7*) and rheumatological symptoms are associated with Paget's disease. The worst complication is the progression to bone sarcoma, but this occurs rarely (<1%). In the main, this disorder is asymptomatic and diagnosed coincidentally from radiological investigation performed for another purpose.

Biochemical investigations of this disease show that serum calcium is usually in the normal range whilst serum alkaline phosphatase is raised. This is a useful marker of disease activity and for assessing the response to bisphosphonate therapy used to inhibit bone resorption. Indications for treatment with bisphosphonates include deformity, pain and the involvement of bones that are prone to lead to complications (e.g. weight bearing or the base of the skull).

*Clinical Case 5.7* was used to illustrate the presentation of Paget's disease and some of its complications but also because she demonstrates the chronic course of hyperparathyroidism in many patients. At

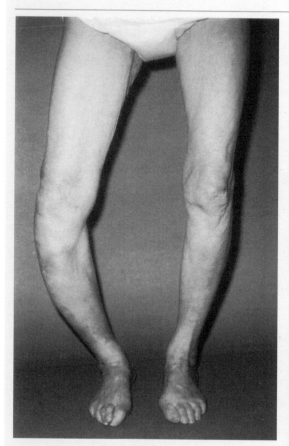

Clinical photograph of the patient's right tibia on presentation.

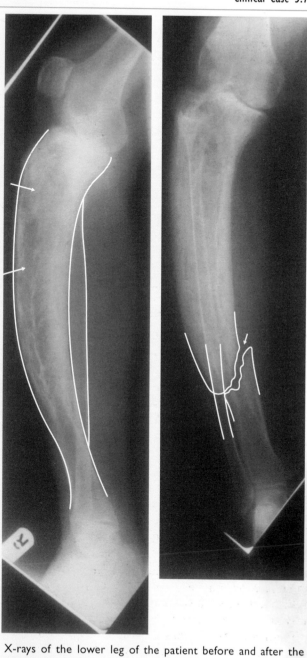

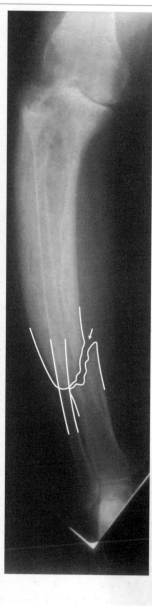

X-rays of the lower leg of the patient before and after the fracture. Note the bowing and marked irregularity of the cortex of the bone of the tibia (arrowed) compared with that of the neighboring fibula. The fracture demonstrates the weakness of the disorganized bone. Note that the much smaller fibula is intact.

These images are available on the website.

presentation, when the serum $Ca^{2+}$ was 2.76 mmol/l, she was noted to have a serum PTH concentration of 8.2 pmol/l (NR 1–6 pmol/l). It has been suggested that patients with Paget's disease have an increased prevalence of primary hyperparathyroidism and it may be these patients that are particularly prone to develop marked hypercalcemia when immobilized after, for example, a fracture. As she had normal renal function, no kidney stones and no evidence of parathyroid bone disease, parathyroid surgery was not considered appropriate.

## Calcitonin and calcitonin gene-related peptide

At the beginning of this chapter, it was noted that $Ca^{2+}$ homeostasis was unaffected by the absence of calcitonin from the thyroid gland. Thus, its physiological role (at least in man) remains problematic even though circulating concentrations rise when serum $Ca^{2+}$ concentrations increase. However, there are some important clinical and physiological aspects of this hormone and calcitonin gene-related peptide (CGRP). Both these hormones are synthesized from the same gene and different post-transcriptional processing of exons and introns give rise to two different hormones (*Box 5.38*). This contrasts with the synthesis of PTH and PTHrp which are coded from different genes evolved from a common ancestral gene.

Diseases in which calcitonin features are much less common than those in which PTH plays a major role and the next clinical case exemplifies the lack of effect of calcitonin on $Ca^{2+}$ homeostasis in the human.

### Clinical Case 5.8:

A 27-year-old woman was seen in the clinic complaining of a lump in her neck that had increased in size over the previous year. She was clinically and biochemically euthyroid and the lump had not caused any problems from its size or position. Her serum calcium was normal. She had been adopted and no family history of thyroid disease was available. There were no abnormal findings on examination apart from a 1 x 2 cm mass in the left lobe of the thyroid gland.

To diagnose the cause of the lump in her neck, she underwent a fine needle aspiration cytological investigation (see *Box 3.33*) and the diagnosis of medullary cell carcinoma was made (*Box 5.39*). This is a tumor of calcitonin-secreting interstitial C-cells in the thyroid gland and it usually presents as a thyroid mass. Additional symptoms such as diarrhea are unusual and suggest metastatic disease and large tumor bulk. Treatment of this carcinoma is total thyroidectomy and lymph node dissection and therapeutic success can be monitored using serum calcitonin assays (two-site IRMA) with or without stimulation with a calcium infusion or pentagastrin.

A diagnosis of medullary cell carcinoma should, like that of hyperparathyroidism, always suggest the possibility of multiple endocrine neoplasia (MEN, *Box 5.40*). Whilst hyperparathyroidism is usually present in MEN type 1 syndrome, it only occurs in about 30% cases of MEN-2a. Evidently the *ret* oncogene is less important for parathyroid growth than for interstitial C-cells of the thyroid gland. Thus, although the serum calcium concentration was normal in *Clinical Case 5.8* this does not exclude MEN type 2a. It later transpired that this patient's biological mother had died suddenly aged 45, suggesting the possibility of a pheochromocytoma. Since she had recently married and was planning to have children she underwent genetic investigation for the *ret* oncogene.

## Structure and synthesis of calcitonin and calcitonin gene related peptide

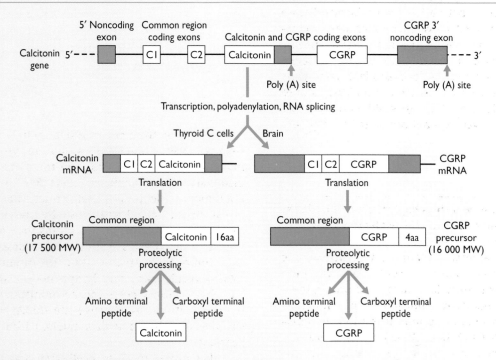

Human calcitonin

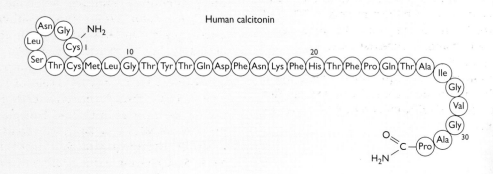

## Box 5.39:
### Medullary cell carcinoma of the thyroid gland

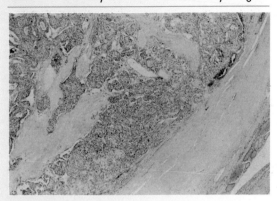

Color image available on website.

- This is a multicentric neoplasm of the C cells of the thyroid gland.
- The earliest abnormality is hyperplasia of the C cells followed by progression to nodular hyperplasia and then carcinoma.
- Lymph node metastases are common as size of tumor increases above I cm diameter.
- Treatment is *total* thyroidectomy with regional lymph node dissection where appropriate.
- Tumor monitoring is by measurements of serum calcitonin (usually following stimulation by the peptide pentagastrin). Other tumor markers such as CGRP have also been used.
- Members of families with MEN carrying loss of function mutations in the *ret* gene may undergo prophylactic thyroidectomy when the serum calcitonin rises above the normal range.

## Box 5.40:
### Multiple endocrine neoplasia

**Type I**
- Autosomal dominant with incomplete penetrance.
- Loss of function mutations in the menin gene on chromosome 11.
- Affects parathyroid glands (~100%), pituitary gland (~60%) and the pancreas (~60%).
- Screening with serum $Ca^{2+}$ and PTH (± gastrin and prolactin) measurements combined with MR imaging of the pituitary and pancreas.

**Type 2**
- Associated with loss of function mutations in *ret* gene coding for a tyrosine kinase receptor for an as yet unknown ligand.
- Autosomal dominant with incomplete penetrance.
- Type 2a associated with medullary cell carcinoma of the thyroid (~100%), unilateral or bilateral pheochromo-cytoma (~50%), parathyroid abnormalities (~35%). There are some rare variants of MEN-2a.
- Type 2b associated with medullary cell carcinoma, pheochromocytoma and mucosal neuromas. Other features include tall, slim appearance and concavity of the chest (pectus excavatum).

# CLINICAL CASE QUESTIONS

The following are examples of applied pathophysiology and these clinically based questions can be answered with the information provided in this chapter. Answers and additional material are available on the website.

---

## Clinical Case Study Q5.1

A 6-yearold boy was seen in the Emergency Room with 18 h severe nausea and vomiting associated with a decrease in conscious level. He was seen initially by the Duty Surgical team who referred him to the Duty Medical Team. In the past, there was a poorly documented history of recurrent abdominal pain and polyuria. There was no history of therapeutic or 'over-the-counter' medication or vitamin supplementation. When admitted, he had a serum $Na^+$ of 143 mmol/l (NR 135–145 mmol/l), $K^+$ 3.6 mmol/l (NR 3.5–4.5 mmol/l), urea 16.6 mmol/l (NR 2.5–8.0 mmol/l), creatinine 51 µmol/l (NR 60–110 µmol/l). The serum $Ca^{2+}$ was 5.14 mmol/l (NR 2.2–2.6 mmol/l) with a $P_i$ of 1.75 mmol/l (NR 0.8–1.4 mmol/l) and an albumin of 49 g/l (NR 38–48 g/l) and an alkaline phosphatase of 231 IU/l (NR 30–100 IU/l).

---

**Question 1:** List the possible causes of hyper-calcemia and outline what investigations you would perform.

**Question 2:** How should he be treated?

## Clinical Case Study Q5.2

A 53-year-old woman was seen in the Outpatient Clinic complaining of muscle weakness and, in particular, of difficulty going upstairs. Her past medical history was noteworthy for the fact that she had undergone jejuno-ileal bypass surgery 25 years previously for morbid obesity (*Box Q5.2*). Over the previous 3 years, she had suffered from several episodes of renal colic due to kidney stones that on analysis were shown to be predominantly of calcium oxalate. She was 1.63 m tall and prior to the bypass operation she had weighed 125 kg. At the time of her regular outpatient clinic visit, she weighed 78 kg. Direct questioning revealed that she had tripped over several times recently and that she had stopped driving her car at night. Serum biochemical tests revealed normal serum concentrations of $Na^+$, $K^+$, urea and creatinine. The serum $Ca^{2+}$ was 2.03 mmol/l (NR 2.2–2.6 mmol/l) with a $P_i$ of 0.8 mmol/l (NR 0.8–1.4 mmol/l), albumin of 38 g/l (NR 38–48 g/l), alkaline phosphatase of 143 IU/l (NR 30–100 IU/l).

**Jejuno-ileal bypass surgery for severe obesity**

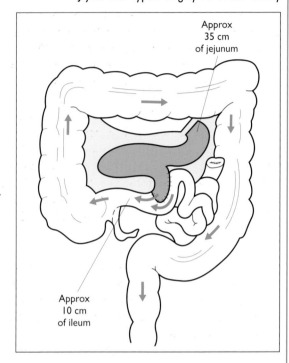

Approx 35 cm of jejunum

Approx 10 cm of ileum

Box Q5.2: In this operation, the amount of small intestine available for digestion and absorption is markedly reduced. Fat malabsorption is nearly universal.

**Question 1:** Outline the synthesis and metabolism of vitamin D. How are her current symptoms related to her previous surgery?

**Question 2:** What other investigations would you perform?

**Question 3:** How would you treat her?

## Clinical Case Study Q5.3

A 56-year-old previously well pub owner was seen in the Emergency Room with a 5 h history of central ominal pain and vomiting. He smoked 20 cigarettes and drank half a bottle of whisky a day during the course of his duties. He was placed 'nil by mouth', admitted under the surgeons and treated with intravenous fluids and nasogastric tube drainage of the stomach. The serum $Na^+$ was 138 mmol/l (NR 135–145 mmol/l), the $K^+$ 3.9 mmol/l (NR 3.5–4.5 mmol/l), the urea 11.0 mmol/l (NR 2.5–8 mmol/l) and creatinine 110 μmol/l (NR 50–110 μmol/l). The serum amylase was 1098 (NR<200 IU/l), the $Ca^{2+}$ 2.43 mmol/l (NR 2.2–2.6 mmol/l), the $P_i$ 1.1 mmol/l (NR 0.8–1.4 mmol/l) and the albumin 40 g/l (NR 38–48 g/l). A diagnosis of acute pancreatitis, probably secondary to alcohol, was made. Ultrasound examination of the abdomen revealed no signs of gall stones but evidence of pancreatic inflammation. Three days after admission, he complained of paresthesiae ('tingling') in his extremities accompanied by painful cramps in his hands. Trousseau's sign was positive (Box Q5.3). The serum $Ca^{2+}$ was 1.45 mmol/l and the albumin 29 g/l.

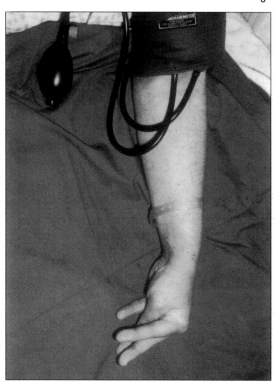

Box Q5.3: In this test the sphygmomanometer cuff is inflated to 300 mmHg for 3 minutes. The carpopedal spasm is painful.

**Question 1:** List the causes of hypocalcemia. What process occurred over the first 3 days of the patient's admission to cause the precipitous fall in serum $Ca^{2+}$ concentration?

**Question 2:** Which further investigations would you perform and how would you treat this patient?

## CHAPTER 6

# The gonad

## Chapter objectives

*Knowledge of*

1. Anatomy and embryology of sexual differentiation and its abnormalities
2. Physiological regulation of the testis and ovary
3. Normal processes of puberty and their abnormalities
4. Menstrual cycle
5. Causes of hypogonadism and infertility, their investigation and treatment
6. Causes of erectile dysfunction and their treatment
7. Endocrine therapies for contraception and the menopause

*'Can either sex assume, or both: so soft*
*And uncompounded is their essence pure…*
*in what shape they choose,*
*Dilated or condensed, bright or obscure'*
*Paradise Lost, John Milton*

It is self-evident that the sexual dimorphism of human external genitalia is so marked that sex assignment at birth can usually be done at a cursory glance. More than 2000 years ago Aristotle thought that the sex of children was determined by the temperature of sperm at the time of copulation. Sex in some reptilian species is, indeed, determined by the temperature at which fertilized eggs are incubated. This is not the case in the human in which sex is determined by a complex (and still incompletely understood) interplay of genes and hormones.

The ovary and the testis, like the adrenal gland, secrete cholesterol-derived steroid hormones under the control of the secretions of the hypothalamo-pituitary axis. The two major functions of the gonads in the adult are steroid hormone production and gametogenesis. Reproductive hormones are also pivotal in sexual differentiation, fetal development, growth and sexual maturation. The major hormones that control the development and maintenance of the male and female phenotype are the androgens and estrogens and progestagens, respectively. These are regulated by gonadotrophin releasing hormone (GnRH) from the hypothalamus and the gonadotrophins, luteinizing hormone (LH) and follicle stimulating hormone (FSH) from the anterior pituitary gland. The complexity of the determination of the external genitalia is illustrated by *Clinical Case 6.1.*

## Clinical Case 6.1:

A 26-year-old West African man was referred to the Endocrine Clinic by the Urology team. In his teens, he had had bilateral breast development (termed gynecomastia) and at the age of 14 years he vividly remembered having an operation in Africa on a kitchen table in which both testes were removed from his groins under local anesthesia. Surgery was also performed to remove the breast tissue. He had had no further treatment since that time. His sexual identity had been unequivocally male. On examination, the absence of testes was noted and he had a small penis with a hypospadias (urethra opening at the base of the penis *Box 6.1*). Serum testosterone concentration was unmeasurably low (<0.5 nmol/l,

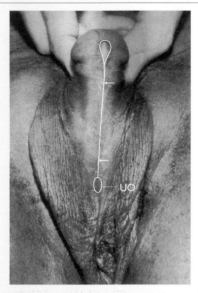

The photograph of the genitalia shows the small penis with empty scrotum. The urethral opening is at the base of the penis (UO) and the line of the urethral groove ending in a pit at the end of the penis is clearly shown (arrows).

This image is available on the website.

NR 9.5–25 nmol/l). Chromosomal analysis revealed that he was genetically female (46XX).

An understanding of this case clearly requires information on the genetic regulation of the external genitalia.

## Genetic determination of sexual differentiation

Each mature ovum contains 22 autosomal chromosomes and one X sex chromosome. A mature sperm contains 22 autosomal chromosomes and either one Y or one X sex chromosome. A fertilized egg, therefore, contains 22 pairs of autosomal chromosomes and one pair of sex chromosomes, either 46XX (female) or 46XY (male). At least 100 autosomal genes are present on the X chromosome and mutations of these genes cause a variety of sex-linked disorders including color blindness, hemophilia and Duchenne muscular dystrophy. In contrast, the Y chromosome has very few autosomal genes. One of the X chromosomes in females is inactivated, producing the Barr body. The inactivated chromosome must be reactivated when cells replicate and divide.

In the human, the default pattern of genital development is female. There are three important steps in sexual differentiation and the development of the normal male phenotype. The first is the differentiation of bipotential gonad primordia (identical in both XX and XY fetuses) into testes that secrete testosterone. The second is the development of the internal reproductive tract. In male fetuses, this requires the presence of anti-Müllerian hormone (AMH, see *Box 6.47*) that causes involution of the Müllerian ducts, the anlagen for the female type reproductive tract. The third is the development of the external genitalia that requires testosterone and, in some target tissues, its more potent metabolite 5α-dihydrotestosterone (DHT). Female differentiation occurs by default in the absence of these hormones. It is evident that the gonads are paired bilateral structures; in very rare circumstances the developmental processes may be different on either side.

The genes involved in gonadal differentiation have been summarized in *Box 6.2*. To date, three genes have been identified in the formation of the bipotential gonad. *WT1* and *LIM1* code for zinc-finger DNA binding proteins and are expressed early in gonadal development. *FTZ-F1* codes for an orphan nuclear hormone receptor, steroidogenic factor-1 (SF-1). Several functions have been ascribed to SF-1 including differentiation and maintenance of both gonadal and adrenal tissue, increasing the synthesis of testosterone and reducing its conversion to estradiol via the transcriptional regulation of the hydroxylases and P450 aromatase, respectively. It may also regulate transcription of the AMH gene.

The importance of the Y chromosome in male development is that its short arm possesses a *sex-*

**Box 6.2:**

Summary of the genes that code for transcription factors that induce differentiation of a bipotential gonad into either a testis or an ovary and subsequent differentiation of the internal reproductive tracts as described in the text

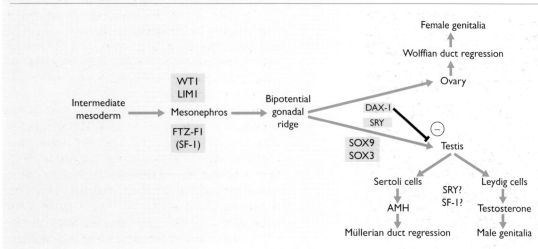

determining region on the *Y* gene (SRY) that codes for a DNA-binding protein termed the 'testis-determining factor' (TDF). This protein is a transcription factor that regulates the expression of other genes or interacts with other transcription factors. Whilst the majority of XX males carry the *SRY* gene, only 15–20% human XY females have loss of function mutations in the *SRY* gene. This implies the involvement of other genes in sexual differentiation. Experimental studies have shown that SRY regulates the expression of genes coding for P450 aromatase and AMH, but a direct interaction between SRY protein and the *AMH* gene is not yet proven. Two other genes, also implicated in gonadal differentiation, are *SOX9* and *SOX3*, so called because they have sequence homologies to a specific region (the HMG box) of the SRY gene – hence SRY-*box*-related.

The identification of genes that control male differentiation has progressed because mutations in such genes lead to the development of a female phenotype. This is not true for female differentiation that occurs by default. This is reflected in the fact that only one gene has so far been identified that appears to be required for ovarian, but not testicular, development. *DAX-1* was originally identi-

fied on the short arm of the X chromosome and known as the *do*sage-sensitive *s*ex (DSS) reversal locus. This was because duplications in this part of the chromosome were present in some XY females. The DAX-1 protein has been found to be a repressor of StAR expression. StAR transports cholesterol to the inner mitochondrial membrane where the first step in steroid synthesis occurs (see *Box 4.4*). Mutations of *DAX-1* may lead to hypogonadism and adrenal hypoplasia although the precise action of *DAX-1* in this respect is not known. Dosage-sensitive models have been proposed. For example, SRY protein could suppress *DAX-1* expression but in duplication there may be insufficient SRY protein. Alternatively, SRY could out-compete *DAX-1* binding to the StAR promoter leading to autorepression of *DAX-1* and, hence, testis formation.

The male determining region of the Y chromosome is so powerful that individuals with 47 XXY or even 49 XXXXY are unequivocally male at birth. The inheritance of only one X chromosome (45 XO, termed Turner's syndrome) still leads to the development of a female phenotype even though there are additional phenotypic features (see *Box 6.49*). *Clinical Case 6.1* is important because further detailed genetic analysis demonstrated the complete absence of the *SRY* gene, thus indicating the involvement of other genes in governing (albeit incomplete) male sexual differentiation. *Clinical Case 6.2* demonstrates that, despite the importance of the Y chromosome, there are circumstances in which its defining actions are abrogated.

# Sexual differentiation of the gonads and internal reproductive tracts

## Clinical Case 6.2:

A 16-year-old girl was referred to the endocrine clinic because of primary amenorrhea. When seen, she had a normal female post-pubertal appearance with good breast development but very little axillary and pubic hair. She was 1.65 m tall and weighed 60 kg. A mass was palpable in the inguinal canal of each groin. Endocrine investigation revealed that she had very low circulating concentration of estradiol (60 pmol/l, NR 70–500 pmol/l), normal gonadotrophin concentrations and serum prolactin and normal male concentration of testosterone (19.5 nmol/l, male NR 9–25 nmol/l). Ultrasound scan confirmed the presence of inguinal masses and a scan of the pelvis showed that the uterus was absent.

An understanding of this case requires further knowledge of the development of the Wolffian and Müllerian duct systems. The gonadal ridges originate from the intermediate mesoderm which gives rise to the mesonephros, the medial aspects of which form the gonadal ridges (see *Boxes 4.7* and *6.3*). Around the 5th week of gestation, germ cells migrate from the yolk sac into the gonadal ridges, and this process is complete by about the 6th week. At this stage, the gonadal primordia look the same histologically in either genetic sex (*Box 6.3*). They consist of three cell types: the germ cells that develop into oogonia (primitive eggs) or spermatogonia (stem cell precursors of sperm); the supporting somatic cells that become either the Sertoli cells or the granulosa cells; and the stromal or interstitial

cells. Considerable experimental work has shown that a number of autosomal genes is involved in the development of the primordial gonad.

Differentiation of the testes begins around the 7th week of gestation when the somatic cells form sex cords (the future Sertoli cells) that incorporate the primitive germ cells. At this stage, the human fetus has both Müllerian (paramesonephric) and Wolffian (mesonephric) ducts that are the respective anlagen of the female and male reproductive tracts (*Box 6.3*). Sertoli cells begin to secrete AMH, a dimeric glycoprotein (molecular weight 70 000) that causes involution of the Müllerian ducts.

By the 8th fetal week, Leydig cells appear in the differentiating testis and begin to secrete androgens, the actions of which are essential to the masculinization of the fetus. With the regression of the Müllerian ducts and under the influence of testosterone, the Wolffian ducts develop into the epididymis, the vas deferens and the seminal vesicles (*Box 6.3*).

Testicular descent during sexual development occurs in two phases. The first is relative to development rather than actual movement and it reaches the internal inguinal ring by week 24. The second phase occurs in the last 2 months of fetal life with the testis passing through the inguinal canal to reach the scrotum. Androgens are an absolute requirement for this migration and in 97% of normal newborns the testes are in a scrotal position.

In the absence of AMH, the Müllerian ducts develop to form the Fallopian tubes, uterus, cervix and upper part of the vagina (*Box 6.3*). This differentiation begins around the 10th week of gestation and the Wolffian ducts begin to degenerate. Around the same time, the germ cells, that are now destined to become oogonia, enter their first meiotic division and are subsequently surrounded by a layer of granulosa cells to form primordial follicles. Such follicular development does not begin until about 15 weeks gestation (some 8 weeks later than the differentiation of the testes). At birth, each ovary contains about 2 million primordial follicles though this declines to about 200 000 primordial follicles by menarche. Each primordial follicle contains a primary oocyte half way through its first

Schematic overview of the differentiation of the internal male and female reproductive tracts from the Wolffian and Müllerian ducts

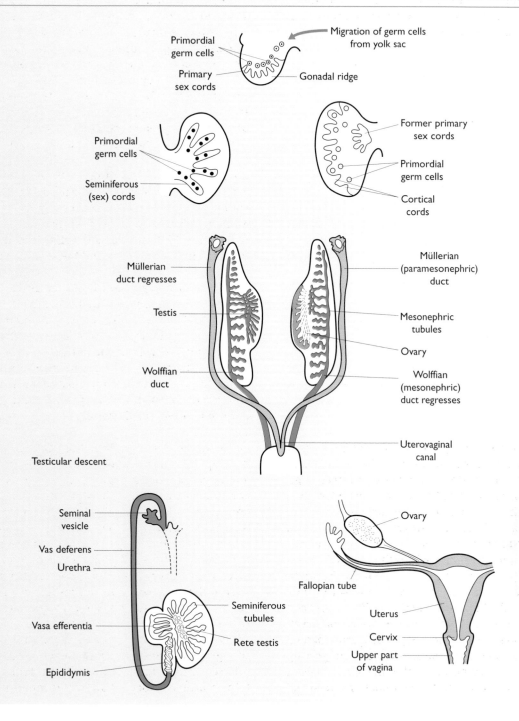

meiotic division. There is a vast over provision of potential oocytes and many become atretic well before the menopause. Thus, females are born with all the eggs they will ever have. This contrasts with the male germ cells or spermatogonia that, from puberty and throughout life, continue their ability to divide and to produce sperm.

Imaging performed by ultrasound on the patient in *Clinical Case 6.2* showed that she had no Fallopian tubes or uterus and only the lower two-thirds of her vagina. She had male concentrations of circulating testosterone synthesized by the testes in her inguinal canals, and yet she showed no signs of masculinization. Her external genitalia were female and completely normal. Thus, during fetal development the Müllerian ducts regressed under the influence of *SRY* and other genes encoding for transcription factors that stimulated AMH production. Loss of Wolffian duct development was due to her complete insensitivity to the masculinizing actions of fetal testosterone and its metabolites. This also explains the lack of pubic and axillary hair, additional manifestations of androgen action, in her teens.

Surgical removal of her undescended testes was undertaken because of the high risk of malignant transformation. The diagnosis of androgen-insensitivity syndrome was confirmed by laboratory studies on cells obtained from a biopsy of genital skin taken at the same time. Fibroblasts grown from the biopsy demonstrated very low binding of radiolabeled testosterone, confirming an abnormality in the androgen receptor. Androgen insensitivity may not be complete and the phenotype depends crucially on the extent to which testosterone signaling is handicapped. In some cases, radiolabelled testosterone binding studies are normal because the loss of function mutation in the testosterone receptor affects DNA binding, not hormone binding.

## Sexual differentiation of the external genitalia

Sexual differentiation of the male external genitalia is critically dependent on androgens and, as the next clinical case illustrates, defects in androgen signaling can result in ambiguous genitalia at birth.

### Clinical Case 6.3:

A man in his 50s was referred to the Endocrine Clinic from the Urology Clinic where he had attended for stress incontinence. He had been noted to have no palpable prostate gland and a wide bladder neck leading to the problems of incontinence, particularly when he coughed. This had been exacerbated by his asthma. The past medical history was noteworthy. He had been brought up as a girl until the age of 5 years and he remembered playing with dolls (and tea-sets) and had had no inkling of being a boy. At the age of 5 years, his hair had been cut short for his first term at school and he had been dressed in shorts. He vividly remembered the first time he tried to urinate in the standing position like other boys, an event that led to the soaking of his trousers and socks. A series of plastic surgical operations had been undertaken in his teens allowing the correction of the hypospadias, closure of the urogenital sinus and construction of a penis (*Box 6.4*). At the age of 16 years, his birth certificate had been changed from female to male. He was well aware of the implications of his anatomy. He found that sexual intercourse required 'some innovation' but had never been in any doubt that he was male. He had married but had no children. Examination in the Urology clinic revealed a small penis and two normal sized testes in a small scrotum (*Box 6.4*).

Like the gonads, but unlike the internal reproductive tracts, the structures that develop into the external genitalia are initially identical in males and females. They develop from the same anlagen: the genital or labioscrotal swelling; the genital or urethral folds; the genital tubercle and the urogenital sinus (*Box 6.5*). The development of the external male phenotype requires the actions of testosterone. This, however, requires the conversion of testosterone to its active metabolite, 5α-dihydrotestosterone (DHT) within the cells of the anlagen for normal differentiation (*Box 6.6*).

Clinical photographs of the external genitalia of *Clinical Case 6.3* before and after surgery

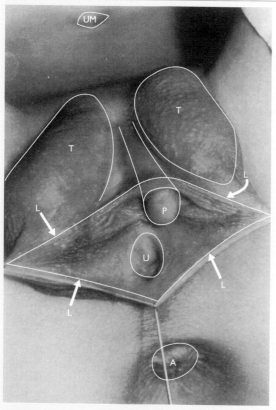

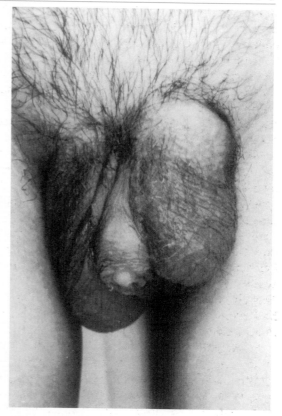

Prior to surgery. Pubic hair has been removed. The folds forming the labia minora have been retracted to show the urogenital sinus. A = anus; L = labial folds (retracted); P = penis/large clitoris; T = testes; U = urogenital sinus; Um = umbilicus.

After surgery. Note the female pattern pubic hair.

These images are available on the Website.

In a male fetus, between 7 and 13 weeks gestation: the genital swellings migrate and become the scrotum; the urogenital folds enlarge and enclose the penile urethra and corpus spongiosa; the genital tubercle becomes the glans penis; and the urogenital sinus forms the prostate gland (*Box 6.5*). Hypospadias arises when the urethra is not completely enclosed by the urogenital or urethral folds. At 15 weeks gestation, the size of the external genitalia is roughly the same in males and females and it is not until the latter two-thirds of pregnancy that growth of the male external genitalia takes place and descent of the testes into the scrotal sac is completed.

Female differentiation begins later and, in the absence of testosterone: the genital swellings form the labia majora; the genital folds remain unfused and form the labia minora; the genital tubercle forms the clitoris and the urogenital sinus the lower part of the vagina (*Box 6.5*). This is the 'standard' or default pattern of differentiation and appears to be independent of gonadal steroids.

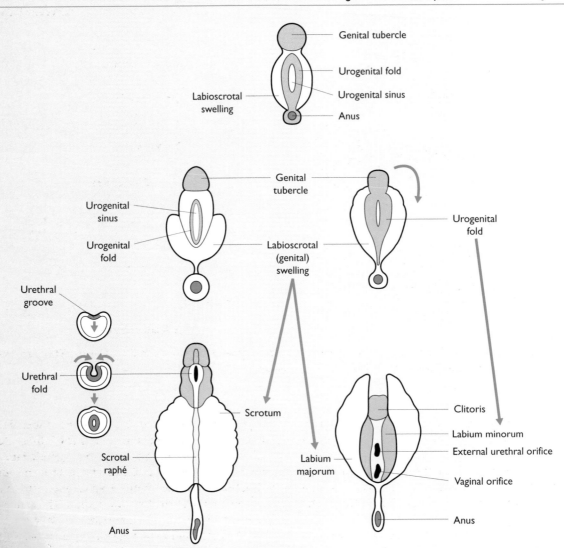

The genital tubercle elongates and forms the shaft and glans of the penis. The urogenital sinus becomes continuous with a groove that develops on the caudal face of the genital tubercle and this groove closes to become the penile part of the urethra while the fused urogenital folds enclosing the sinus becomes the prostate part of the urethra. In the most distal part of the penis, invagination of a cord of epithelial cells covering the glans meets the penile urethra and when this cord canalizes the formation of the urethra is complete. The line of fusion along the urethra and scrotum is called the raphé. The labioscrotal folds form the scrotum.

In females, the genital tubercle bends inferiorly to form the clitoris, the urogenital folds, that do not fuse, form the labia minora and the genital swellings develop into the labia majora. The vagina and the urethra open into the vestibule of the urogenital sinus.

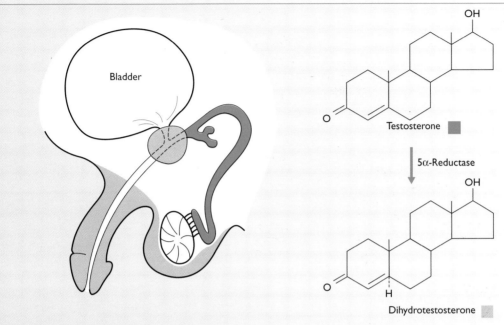

The roles of testosterone (T) and 5α-dihydrotestosterone (DHT) in the development of the male internal and external reproductive tract

The reduction of T to DHT is performed by the enzyme 5α-reductase expressed in the tissues shown. There are two isoforms (type 1 and 2) that differ in tissue distribution and kinetics.

The patient in *Clinical Case 6.2* was completely insensitive to testosterone and DHT (androgen insensitivity) due to a receptor defect and, thus, had normal female external genitalia including a blind ending vagina. She was, thus, capable of a sexually active life as a female but without the ability to be fertile.

In contrast, *Clinical Case 6.3* showed clear evidence of masculinization of the external genitalia and, hence, of androgen actions, but this was incomplete. The patient had normal circulating blood concentrations of testosterone but low levels of its metabolite, DHT. A defect in 5α-reductase results in complete or partial failure in the masculinization of the external genitalia (depending on the degree of enzyme deficiency). The lack of the full effect of DHT during the fetal life of *Clinical Case 6.3* led to his designation at birth as female.

It is, thus, clear that abnormalities of sexual differentiation occur when there is one of three situations. There may be virilization of a genetic female, incomplete virilization of a genetic male or the rarest situation of all when both testicular and ovarian tissue are present (true hermaphrodite). The causes of these abnormalities are summarized in *Box 6.7*.

The presentation of ambiguous genitalia at birth is a medical emergency. Since ambiguous sex is surrounded by a maelstrom of emotion and misunderstanding, its management requires the logical application of these embryological principles so that the situation can be resolved rapidly and with the minimum of investigations (*Box 6.8*). A clinically based approach is given in *Box 6.9* and treatment will require appropriate endocrine induction of puberty, maintenance of adult sex steroid replacement and reconstructive surgery as dictated by the individual anatomy.

**Virilization of a genetic female with ovaries**
- Fetal androgens – e.g. congenital adrenal hyperplasia, adrenal adenoma or hyperplasia
- Maternal androgens – e.g. ovarian or adrenal tumors
- Iatrogenic – exogenous androgens or progestagens with androgenic activity

**Incomplete virilization of a genetic male with testes**
- Defect of testis development (termed gonadal dysgenesis leading to impaired AMH and testosterone production) – e.g. loss of SRY (Y-linked XY dysgenesis), additional DSS (X-linked dysgenesis), loss of SOX9 (autosomal-linked dysgenesis). Dysgenetic testes are at increased risk of malignant transformation and, therefore, removal is recommended
- Leydig cell hypoplasia – e.g. loss of function mutation of the LH receptor. AMH is still produced so the phenotype is female with no Müllerian duct system
- Impaired testosterone production – e.g. defects in synthetic enzymes including 3β-hydroxysteroid dehydrogenase or 17α-hydroxylase
- Androgen insensitivity syndrome – (see *Clinical Case 6.2*), may be variable severity
- 5α-reductase deficiency – (see *Clinical Case 6.3*).

**True hermaphroditism** – both external and internal structures show gradations between normal male and female. The initial presentation is with genital ambiguity but more rarely isolated cliteromegaly or penile hypospadias. Virtually all have a urogenital sinus and uterus. Most are raised as males

*These are all rare.
†Classification is based on gonadal morphology. A true hermaphrodite possesses both testicular and ovarian tissue. A male pseudo-hermaphrodite possesses differentiated testes but is incompletely virilized whilst a female pseudo-hermaphrodite has ovaries but is virilized.

## Control of steroid production in the fetal gonads

The major control of steroid synthesis in the fetal and adult gonad is through the actions of the

1. Elicit family history and any consanguinity
2. Examine for dysmorphic features
3. Take blood for karyotype (chromosome analysis)
4. Palpate gonads:
- If none palpable, patient is likely to be female with virilization, most likely due to congenital adrenal hyperplasia. Measure blood 17α-hydroxyprogesterone and 11-deoxycortisol concentrations
- If two palpable, patient is likely to be male with incomplete virilization, most likely due to impaired testosterone biosynthesis, androgen insensitivity or 5α-reductase deficiency. Perform a 3 day hCG test (1000 U daily for 3 consecutive days) with blood taken on days 0 and 4 for testosterone, dihydrotestosterone, dehydroepiandrosterone and androstendione analysis. Consider androgen binding studies, molecular studies and pelvic ultrasound
- If one palpable, patient is likely to have a form of gonadal dysgenesis or true hermaphroditism. Perform an hCG test and gonadal biopsy. Consider pelvic ultrasound and laparoscopy to define anatomy

*Usually involves a multidisciplinary team including endocrinologist, geneticist, pediatric gynecologist/urologist.

gonadotrophins, LH and FSH, secreted by the pituitary gland (see *Box 6.13*). In the fetus, the hypothalamo-hypophyseal vascular connections responsible for LH release by hypothalamic GnRH are only established between 11 and 12 weeks after conception. This is some 3 weeks after the onset of testosterone production in the Leydig cells of the testis. Early sexual differentiation depends, therefore, on human chorionic gonadotrophin (hCG) secreted from the placenta in high concentrations during the first trimester of pregnancy. This hormone, the detection of which forms the basis of the commonly used pregnancy test, is homologous to LH and acts on the same G-protein linked receptor. There is a good correlation between the circulating concentrations of hCG and testosterone and it is clear that hCG is also important for the proliferation and differentiation of Leydig cells.

## Box 6.9:
### Ambiguous genitalia — principles of management and treatment

- Avoid the use of gender-specific pronouns or the term intersex (that promulgates the idea of the neonate being of neither sex) and simply make reference to 'your baby'
- Avoid an early provisional opinion prior to a complete assessment
- The sex of rearing is independent of the genetic sex (or karyotype)
- Decision on sex of rearing should be taken jointly by a multidisciplinary team including endocrinologist, gynecologist or urologist and the parents. Anatomy and biochemical test results must be considered
- Virilized females with congenital adrenal hyperplasia should in general be raised as females. Long-term outcomes for these patients (in terms of a full female role) may be less than ideal
- Genetic males with severe genital abnormalities and testosterone insensitivity should also be raised as females. Low radio-labeled androgen binding or poor clinical reponse to administered testosterone (e.g. 50 mg monthly for 3 months) would support this decision
- Cultural, ethical and social issues or the special case of puberty in patients with $5\alpha$-reductase deficiency may affect the final decision (see Website)

Estrogen formation in the fetal ovaries also begins early in development even though primordial follicles do not start to develop until the second trimester of pregnancy. At this early stage, the ovary does not contain all the enzymes required for the synthesis of estrogen and it may be produced from conversion of androgens. Its physiological role is uncertain.

Gradually, gonadotrophin secretion from the fetal pituitary takes over the role of hCG and peripheral blood concentrations of fetal pituitary LH and FSH peak around mid-gestation falling to low levels by the time of birth. This later reduction is thought to result from the maturation of the negative feedback effects of steroids on the hypothalamo-pituitary axis. During the latter two thirds of pregnancy, these steroids are required for further virilization (e.g. growth of the penis) and the final shaping and growth of the female external genitalia. A second, but smaller peak, of LH and FSH secretion occurs post-partum stimulating increased steroid secretion. This post-natal peak is thought to be due to the loss of the negative feedback effects of steroids from the feto–placental unit.

The post-natal period of relatively high steroid concentrations gives rise to an interesting phenomenon and two clinically important sequelae. The phenomenon is 'witches' milk' that occurs as a result of estrogen effects on the neonatal breast leading to milk production. The first clinical sequela is that it allows the investigation of the hypothalamo-pituitary-gonad axis. If this opportunity is missed it does not occur again for about a decade, at the onset of puberty. It also allows a therapeutic window of opportunity for male children born with small penis (micropenis) or undescended testes, both processes being dependent on testosterone. Depot injections of testosterone (e.g. 50 mg intramuscularly each month for 3 months) can be used to increase penis size or to encourage testicular descent. At this time, there is relatively little adverse effect of such therapy on bone development.

In the post-natal period, a new equilibrium is soon established and circulating androgen and estrogen concentrations decrease over several months to the very low levels that characterize childhood (when serum testosterone and estradiol are unmeasurable in the usual clinical assays). Then follows the organized mayhem of puberty.

# Puberty

Puberty marks the transition from a non-reproductive state into a reproductive state and its name is derived from the Latin word *pubes* meaning hair. It is a time of widespread endocrine changes including the adolescent growth spurt, skeletal changes (e.g. increase in hip width, in females), increase in muscle and fat tissue and profound psychological changes. Other physical changes associated with puberty are development of pubic and axillary hair (pubarche) and development of breasts (thelarche).

The age at which puberty occurs has decreased dramatically during the last century and this is thought to be due to better nutrition and health. The ages at which pubertal changes occur, however, vary greatly among individuals and there are ethnic differences. In order to assess the speed and extent of development, Tanner and co-workers developed a set of stages for axillary and pubic hair development, and breast and male genital development. They are widely used and referred to as Tanner stages (*Box 6.10*) although it must be remembered that there is nothing stepwise about normal puberty. Unlike males, who have no noteworthy event by which its passage may be timed, females usually remember the year of the onset of menstruation (termed menarche). It is to be emphasized that normal puberty consists of a smooth ordered progression of processes often termed consonance.

In terms of the endocrinology of human puberty this consists of two processes, adrenarche and gonadarche that are independently regulated. Adrenarche refers to the increase in androgen secretions from the zona reticularis of the adrenal cortex that occurs between the ages of about 6 and 8 years whilst gonadarche, occurring several years later, refers to the activation of gonadal sex steroid production. Disorders of sex steroid action cause the major clinical problems at puberty.

The onset of puberty is characterized by increasing secretions of LH and FSH that stimulate gonadal activity. These are induced by an increasing drive from the hypothalamic GnRH neurons. Thus, it is pertinent to discuss the hormones of the hypothalamo-pituitary-gonadal axis before embarking on the hormonal changes that occur in puberty and the endocrine disorders that can cause abnormal pubertal development.

## GnRH and the control of gonadotrophin synthesis and secretion

GnRH is synthesized in about 1000–3000 neurons diffusely situated in the arcuate nucleus and other nuclei of the hypothalamus. Most of their axons terminate on the hypophyseal portal capillaries in the median eminence through which the GnRH is transported to the gonadotrophs of the anterior pituitary gland (see *Box 7.3*). Some axons project to other brain areas and animal studies suggest these may play a role in sexual behavior. GnRH is also synthesized in the placenta, gonad, breast, lymphocyte and pituitary gland where its exact physiological roles remain uncertain.

It is synthesized as a large pre-prohormone (*Box 6.11*) consisting of a 23-amino-acid signal sequence at the N-terminal, the 10 amino acids which form GnRH, a 3-amino-acid sequence used for molecular processing and a 56-amino-acid sequence at the carboxy-terminus known as GnRH associated peptide (GAP). GnRH and GAP are cleaved before secretion. In the adult, GnRH is secreted in a pulsatile manner with a single pulse occurring approximately hourly. Different patterns are seen in infants, and during puberty a diurnal rhythm of pulsatile GnRH secretion is seen. GnRH acts on the pituitary gonadotroph via typical G-protein-linked receptors that predominantly activate phospholipase C with the resulting hydrolysis of $PIP_2$ to $IP_3$ and increased intracellular calcium and generation of diacylglycerol and activation of protein kinase C (*Box 6.11*).

GnRH stimulates both the synthesis and release of LH and FSH and it is the pattern (amplitude and frequency) of GnRH secretory pulses that is thought to regulate these functions. Thus, low-amplitude, high frequency pulses, as seen in women in the follicular phase of the menstrual cycle, may preferentially stimulate synthesis and secretion of the FSH β-subunit. High-amplitude, low-frequency pulses typical of the luteal phase of the menstrual cycle may preferentially stimulate synthesis of the LH β-subunit.

The LH and FSH responses to a given pulse of GnRH are governed by two further factors, the feedback action of gonadal steroids on the pituitary gonadotrophs and the regulation on GnRH receptors on these cells. In the absence of regular GnRH pulses, pituitary gonadotrophs lose GnRH receptors and become less and less sensitive. As will be seen in *Clinical Case 6.6*, patients with hypothalamic hypogonadism have a small gonadotrophin response to an intravenous injection of synthetic GnRH.

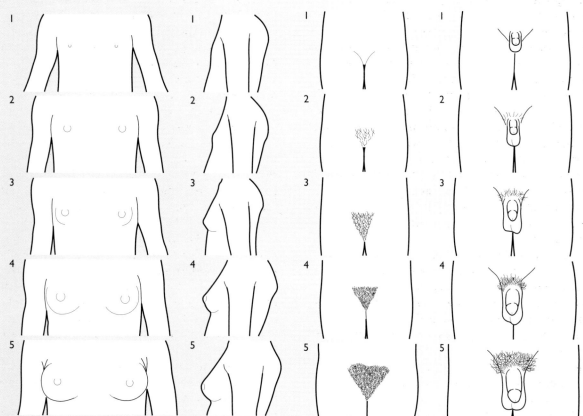

**Female**

| Stage | Breast development |
|---|---|
| 1 | Prepubertal. No breast tissue |
| 2 | Areolar enlargement with breast bud |
| 3 | Enlargement of breast and areola as single mound |
| 4 | Projection of areola above breast as double mound |
| 5 | Adult; papilla projects out of areola that is part of breast contour |

**Male**

| Stage | Genital development |
|---|---|
| 1 | Prepubertal |
| 2 | Testes enlarge (4 ml); scrotum larger, reddened and skin coarser |
| 3 | Penis enlarges, initially in length. Continued growth of testes and scrotum |
| 4 | Penis grows in length and breadth; continued growth of testes and scrotum that becomes pigmented |
| 5 | Testes, scrotum and penis adult size |

**Both sexes**

| Stage | Pubic hair development | Stage | Pubic hair development |
|---|---|---|---|
| 1 | None | 4 | Small adult configuration |
| 2 | Few darker hairs along labia or at base of penis | 5 | Adult configuration with spread onto inner thighs |
| 3 | Curly pigmented hairs across pubes | 6 | Adult configuration with spread to linea alba |

## Synthesis of GnRH and its actions on pituitary gonadotrophs

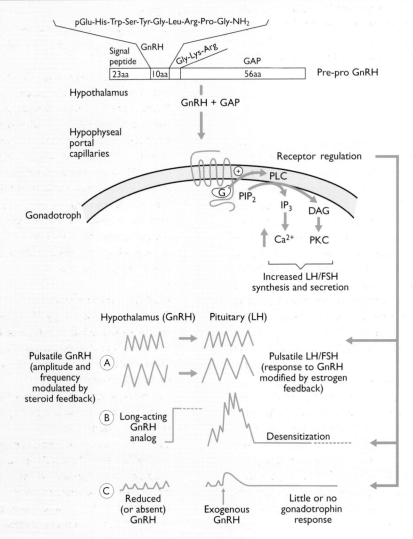

GnRH is synthesized as a large prohormone and released with gonadotrophin associated peptide (GAP). It acts on the gonadotroph via a G-protein (G) linked receptor that activates phospholipase C (PLC) that stimulates the inositol signaling pathway (see *Box 1.10*).

Ⓐ  GnRH is secreted in a pulsatile manner with one pulse occurring approximately each hour and a half.

Ⓑ  Administration of long-acting agonist analogs induces an initial stimulation of LH (and FSH) but over a few days causes complete desensitization of the pituitary gonadotroph.

Ⓒ  Loss of endogenous GnRH secretion induces loss of GnRH receptors and the LH response to a bolus injection of GnRH is very low.

Abbreviations: $PIP_2$, phosphatidylinositol 4, 5-bisphosphate; $IP_3$, inositol 1,4,5-trisphosphate; DAG, diacylglycerol; PKC, protein kinase C.

Repeated pulses of GnRH approximately 90 min apart up-regulate its receptors and the gonadotrophin response. In contrast, continuous (non-pulsatile) infusions of GnRH cause an initial stimulus to gonadotrophin secretion followed by a down-regulation of GnRH receptors and loss of responsiveness. This has important clinical consequences (*Box 6.12*).

## The gonadotrophins – LH and FSH – and their actions

The gonadotrophins, like TSH and hCG, are glycoproteins (molecular weights approximately 30 000) made up of a species-specific common α-subunit and a β-subunit that confers biological specificity to each hormone. LH and FSH are important regulators of steroidogenesis in the gonads and, like GnRH, their receptors are also typical G-linked proteins. Receptor activation by gonadotrophin binding stimulates adenylate cyclase and a consequent rise in cAMP. There is also evidence that LH/hCG can signal via the activation of phospholipase C and phosphoinositide hydrolysis (*Box 6.13*).

Just like the action of ACTH on adrenal cortical cells, LH and FSH increase intracellular concentrations of free cholesterol, its transport to the mitochondria and the transport of cholesterol to the inner mitochondrial membrane by the StAR protein. Here, cholesterol is converted to pregnenolone by side chain cleavage enzyme (*CYP11A1*, see *Box 4.5*) and subsequent synthetic processes depend on the target cell. The rate-limiting step in gonadotrophin-induced steroid synthesis is the regulation of StAR and cholesterol side-chain cleavage activity.

These mechanisms are common to both male and female but divergence arises in regard to the target cells and actions of gonadotrophins in the gonads. In the testis, LH is the exclusive steroidogenic hormone acting only on the interstitial or Leydig cells whilst FSH acts exclusively on the Sertoli cells. In the ovary, both LH and FSH are involved in the control of steroidogenesis and each acts on more than one cell type. There are numerous isoforms of circulating LH and FSH and biological potency depends on the degree and sites of

---

**Box 6.12:**
**Clinical uses of GnRH and its analogs**

**Principles:**

- GnRH is not orally active because it is rapidly broken down in the gut; it has a short half life (<15 minutes)
- Many stable, long-acting GnRH agonists and antagonists have been developed
- Agonists cause an initial stimulation of LH and FSH, but, due to the ability of GnRH to regulate its own receptors, after ~10 days treatment long-acting analogs induce loss of pituitary receptors and LH and FSH secretion is switched off. Antagonists induce an immediate inhibition of LH/FSH secretion
- Correct functioning of pituitary gonadotrophs requires a pulsatile GnRH signal that is not achievable with stable analogs
- Analogs allow clinicians to induce a 'chemical' (and reversible) gonadectomy

**Uses:**

- **Pituitary function tests**
  Single injection of 100 μg of GnRH with assays of venous serum LH and FSH concentrations before and at intervals after (see *Box 6.17*)
- **Hypothalamic hypogonadism** (with intact pituitary function)
  Pulsatile subcutaneous infusions of GnRH through a programmable infusion pump every 90 min
- **Assisted conception**
  Long-acting analogs to inhibit endogenous secretion of LH/FSH: folliculogenesis is controlled entirely using exogenous gonadotrophins
- **Endocrine dependent cancers**
  Long-acting analogs to inhibit gonadotrophin 'drive' of steroidogenesis in ovary or testis e.g. for prostate cancer
- **Endometriosis**
  Long-acting analogs used to suppress cyclical ovarian activity. Used with replacement therapy

---

glycosylation and the electrical charge of the molecule. Thus, different assays of LH and FSH concentrations may not always give a true index of biological activity (*Box 6.14*).

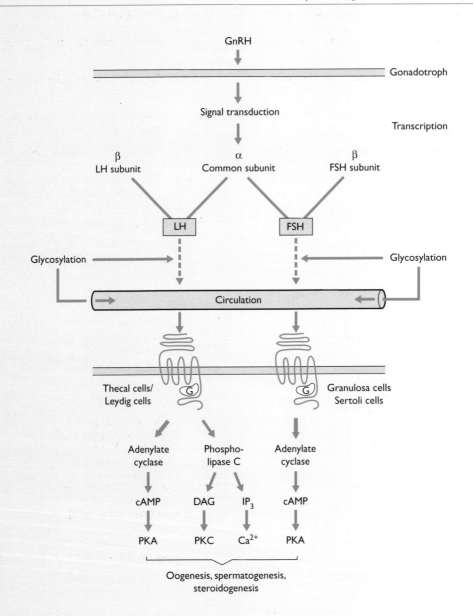

GnRH stimulates transcription of the genes coding for the common α and specific β subunits of LH and FSH. Glycosylation of the proteins occurs in the pituitary and may be modified in the circulation. Glycosylation sites and the charge of different LH and FSH isoforms alter their biological potency. They act on gonadal cells via typical G-protein linked receptors.

Abbreviations: PKA/C, protein kinase A/C; DAG, diacylglycerol; PI₃, inositol 1, 4, 5-trisphosphate.

**Box 6.14:**
Measurement of LH, FSH and hCG

| Assay method | Advantages | Disadvantages |
|---|---|---|
| Radioimmunoassays (polyclonal Abs) | Cheap, sensitive, rapid | May not reflect biological activity |
| IRMAs or ELISAs (monoclonal Abs (see *Box 3.25*) | Cheap, sensitive, rapid | May not reflect biological activity |
| Receptor binding (see *Box 3.15*) | Measures hormone binding to receptors | Detects deglycosylated hormone that is inactive |
| Bioassay (see below) | Measures bioactive hormone | Expensive, less sensitive and reproducible |

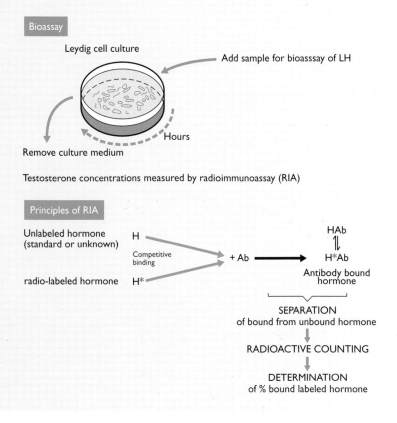

Bioassay

Leydig cell culture

Add sample for bioasssay of LH

Hours

Remove culture medium

Testosterone concentrations measured by radioimmunoassay (RIA)

Principles of RIA

Unlabeled hormone (standard or unknown) H

Competitive binding

radio-labeled hormone H*

+ Ab

HAb

H*Ab

Antibody bound hormone

SEPARATION
of bound from unbound hormone

RADIOACTIVE COUNTING

DETERMINATION
of % bound labeled hormone

The human genes coding for the LH and FSH receptors are located on chromosome 2p21 and are very large containing 10 and 11 exons, respectively. Inactivating mutations of the β-chain of the LH receptor have been described and, in males, the loss of gonadotrophin stimulation on fetal Leydig cell proliferation and development results in Leydig cell agenesis or hypoplasia. The clinical features depend on the degree of compromise in receptor function. Loss of testosterone secretion may cause an ambiguous phenotype. Other cases present as fertile males (because FSH secretion is maintained) with eunuchoidal body proportions ('fertile eunuch syndrome'). Similar inactivating mutations in females do not alter phenotype and folliculogenesis can still occur, though ovulation does not. Constitutive activating mutations of the LH receptor have been reported (see *Clinical Case 6.4*) and inactivating mutations of the FSH receptor, associated with ovarian dysgenesis and amenorrhea, have been identified.

## Endocrine changes in puberty

The next two cases are graphic demonstrations of early (precocious) sexual development and late (delayed) puberty and are used to introduce the physiological processes controlling puberty.

### Clinical Case 6.4:

A 20-month-old boy was referred to the clinic with his mother who was concerned about his abnormal development. He had been normal at birth. His mother had noted pubic hair from an early age and thought that he had always been 'much larger' than the male babies of other mothers. When seen, he was indeed tall with advanced general physical development and sexual development compatible with Tanner stage 3 but associated with small testes of 3 ml volume (Box 6.15). He had frequent erections. The rest of his development had been normal. The family history was noteworthy for the fact that two maternal cousins had been treated in Thailand for precocious sexual development, though no other information was available. The bone age (estimated from an X-ray of the left hand and wrist, see *Box 7.11*) was advanced at 4.2 years.

### Clinical Case 6.5:

A 19-year-old man was brought to the clinic by his parents because of delayed pubertal development. There was a family history of delayed development and his father remembered that he had not started shaving regularly until the age of 22 years. There was no relevant past medical history and in particular no

history of headaches or visual field problems. No family history of serious illness such as cirrhosis, diabetes mellitus or heart failure at an early age was elicited. Examination revealed him to be tall with a height of 1.85 m (his father's height was 1.74 m and his mother's height 1.60 m). His arm span was 1.92 m and his leg length was 0.98 m. He was in early puberty only, with Tanner stage 2 genitalia and 4 ml testes bilaterally.

Prior to the onset of puberty, both LH and FSH are secreted in very small amounts (with low concentrations in peripheral blood) and there is no apparent stimulation of the gonads (*Box 6.16*). However, as puberty approaches, the amplitude of LH and FSH pulsatile secretion increases (hence, mean secretion rates) and the nocturnal rise in LH secretion is amplified. It is notable that this nocturnal rhythm is specific to puberty as it disappears in adulthood. The gonad itself does not seem necessary for the changes to occur and, thus, it must be concluded that the brain is in some way programmed to produce more GnRH and, hence, LH and FSH.

Several theories have been put forward to account for this change in the secretion of GnRH. One is that there is an inherent maturation of these neurons. Another is that melatonin secretion from the pineal gland is reduced at puberty relative to increasing body mass and, thus, there is less inhibition of GnRH secretion by this hormone (see *Box 7.33*). A third idea is that the achievement of adequate body fat may be an important determinant of puberty. Finally, it has been suggested that the early pubertal rise in DHEA secretion from the adrenal cortex (adrenarche) aids maturation of the GnRH neurons. Whatever the mechanism, the increasing drive from the GnRH neurons and the increasing sensitivity of the pituitary gland to this neurohormone raises circulating concentrations of LH and FSH. This stimulates pubertal development of the gonads and, thus, an increase in the output of sex steroids. These, together with adrenal androgens, induce the physical changes that occur at this time.

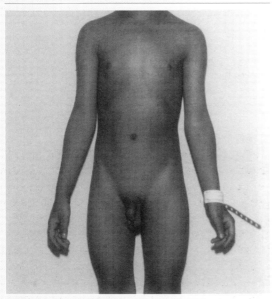

Clinical photos of *Clinical Case 6.4* demonstrate that the general body habitus is clearly much more mature than that expected from his chronological age of 20 months

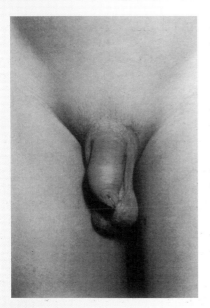

Tanner stage 3 – the penis is lengthened and broader and the scrotum larger with curly hair across the pubes. The testicular volumes are 3 ml bilaterally.

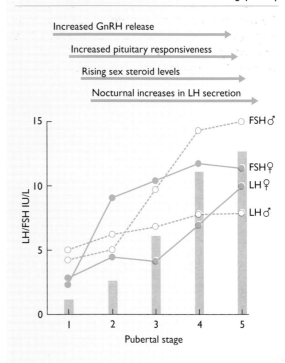

Other hormones that may play a part in puberty are the metabolic hormones, somatotrophin and leptin. The former augments the pattern of sexual maturation once a pubertal pattern of gonadotrophin secretion is established. Leptin, on the other hand, may play a part in controlling body weight (fat mass). This may be important since the onset of puberty has been associated with the body reaching a critical mass. That said, the evidence and proposed mechanisms for the relationship between body fat and leptin in regulating puberty have yet to be established.

In males, the earliest sign of increasing LH and FSH secretions is an increase in testicular volume greater than 4 ml or 2.5 cm in length. In girls, thelarche (breast development) is a sensitive indicator of LH- and FSH-stimulated ovarian steroid secretions. Prior to menarche, however, estradiol secretion fluctuates widely probably reflecting waves of follicular development that fail to reach the ovulatory stage. The estrogen stimulates growth of the uterus but menarche does not occur until the estrogens have stimulated sufficient uterine growth such that their withdrawal causes the first menstruation. The onset of menstruation is such a milestone in the development of girls that primary amenorrhea can be relied upon to indicate underlying pathology. The growth of axillary and pubic hair in both sexes is a consequence not only of increasing gonadal steroids (gonadarche) but also adrenal steroids (adrenarche).

## Precocious sexual development

Precocious sexual development results from the premature exposure of tissues to sex steroids whatever their source (*Box 6.17*). Such sexual development is not the same as precocious puberty since the latter maintains its underlying pattern or consonance. The 20-month-old boy in *Clinical Case 6.4* was tall for his age and parental heights and had Tanner stage 3 genital development and pubic hair but no signs of gonadarche; i.e. no growth of testicular volume. Thus, he had precocious sexual development not precocious puberty. This conclusion was supported by the fact that LH and FSH were unmeasurable (<0.1 IU/l) in peripheral blood. The lack of FSH explained his small testicular volume since seminiferous tubules, forming the bulk of testicular volume, are primarily stimulated by FSH.

Investigations of *Clinical Case 6.4* showed normal 17α-hydroxyprogesterone (6.2 nmol/l, NR <20 nmol/l) and androstenedione (2.1 nmol/l NR 3–8 nmol/l) and suppressed dehydroepiandrosterone sulfate (<0.5 mmol/l, NR 2.8–12 mmol/l). This indicated that the adrenal glands were not the source of androgens. Thus, his testes were producing testosterone independent of the hypothalamo-pituitary

axis. This condition, sometimes called 'testotoxicosis', is often due to an activating mutation of the LH receptor (*Box 6.13*).

The investigation and treatment of precocious sexual development follows logically from the principles outlined in the text and are summarized in *Boxes 6.17* and *6.18*. *Clinical Case 6.4* was treated with cyproterone acetate but testolactone and spironolactone were added to improve control of sexual development. There was little regression in the physical signs with which he presented to medical attention and his growth chart (see Website) indicated continued poor control in part exacerbated by poor compliance with medication. True precocious pubertal development may be arrested by treatment with a long-acting synthetic analog of GnRH (see *Box 6.12*).

## Delayed puberty

The definitions and causes of delayed puberty are given in *Box 6.19*. Just as precocious puberty prejudices final height, late puberty (in the presence of a normal GH and IGF-1 axis) leads to a final height that is above that predicted from the mid-parental value, with long legs and arms and a relatively short sitting height. This was illustrated in *Clinical Case 6.5* with markedly delayed puberty. In this young man, the serum testosterone concentration was low (1.1 nmol/l, NR 9–25 nmol/l) as were the serum gonadotrophins (LH 0.5 IU/l, FSH 1IU/l). When these results became available, the only additional piece of clinical information was that he had markedly reduced sense of smell.

The low serum gonadotrophin concentrations coupled with low testosterone and lack of testicular development indicate that he had hypogonadotrophic hypogonadism. His growth and pubic hair development, however, suggested that he had undergone normal adrenarche. This patient has Kallman's syndrome, a genetically heterogenous condition in which congenital hypogonadotrophic hypogonadism is associated with reduced sense of smell. In the X-linked form there are mutations in the *KAL* gene on the short arm of the X chromosome coding for anosmin, an adhesion molecule. The defect leads to the inability of

---

**Definition:** Development of *any* secondary sexual characteristic before the age of 8 years in girls and 9 years in boys.

**Causes** (all are rare):

- Excess GnRH secretion – idiopathic and secondary (e.g. radiotherapy, cerebral tumor) central precocious puberty, premature and variant thelarche
- Excess gonadotrophin secretion – e.g. hypothyroidism, gonadotrophin-secreting tumor of pituitary gland
- Excess adrenal androgens – e.g. premature adrenarche, congenital adrenal hyperplasia, adrenal tumor
- Excess gonadal steroids – activating mutation of the LH receptor ('testotoxicosis' – *Clinical Case 6.4*), G-protein mutation (McCune–Albright syndrome), gonadal tumor, exogenous sex steroids

**Investigations:** *All* forms of precocious sexual development associated with an increase in sex steroid concentrations demonstrate an increase in growth velocity and advancement of the bone age. Absence of these features generally indicates lack of serious pathology and no need for further investigation. It is mandatory that initial assessment should include:

- Auxology – accurate measurement of height (and comparison with parental heights)
- Pubertal staging
- Bone age estimation

Endocrine measurements:

- LH, FSH and sex steroids – single measurements are of limited value because gonadotrophins are secreted in a pulsatile manner, mainly at night, and the values are low in most patients with sexual precocity
- GnRH test – peak LH in response to 100 μg of GnRH is normal for the stage of puberty (>5 IU/l) in central precocious puberty but it is suppressed in testotoxicosis or McCune–Albright syndrome
- Adrenal steroids – may be elevated in cases with adrenal tumors; precursors such as 17α-hydroxyprogesterone are high in congenital adrenal hyperplasia

Imaging:

- MR scans of the hypothalamo-pituitary area – important in all cases of central precocious puberty
- Ultrasound scans of the pelvis – very useful in girls to determine the pubertal changes in uterine and ovarian volume and endometrial thickness (see *Box 6.25*).

---

the GnRH neurons to migrate to the hypothalamus during development.

During embryonic development nerves grow from the nasal cavity to the olfactory bulbs at the base of the cerebral hemispheres. From there the olfactory tracts project to the hypothalamus and other brain areas, a process that is complete at about 25 days gestation. The embryonic cells of the GnRH neurons also originate in the nasal cavity and normally migrate along the olfactory tracts to the hypothalamus. However, with incomplete development of olfactory nerves, the GnRH neurons have no olfactory highway to guide them in their migration and they remain in the nose, hence, the association of anosmia and one cause of hypogonadotrophic hypogonadism. *KAL* is also

expressed in other tissues and associated features of Kallman's include renal aplasia, ataxia, cleft palate. However, it is to be emphasized that the phenotype–genotype correlations are poor and, indeed, that X-linked is the least common form of inheritance. This indicates that a number of other genes or factors are operating in governing the expression of the condition.

Testicular development and normal testosterone secretion can be restored in Kallman's syndrome by treatment with pulsatile GnRH therapy (*Box 6.12*), a use that contrasts with the use of long-acting GnRH analogs to delay pubertal development. A clinical approach to the investigation and treatment based on the principles outlined in the text are given in *Boxes 6.20* and *6.21*.

| Drug | Use | Advantages | Disadvantages/side effects |
|------|-----|-----------|---------------------------|
| Cyproterone acetate | Antiandrogen (also decreases gonadotrophins) | Orally active. Effective | Some progestational and glucocorticoid actions<br>Tiredness, lethargy. Adrenal suppression. Loss of bone density |
| Flutamide | Nonsteroidal antiandrogen | Orally active. Effective | Requires contraception. Occasional but serious hepatotoxicity (<0.5%), photosensitivity (~<0.5%) |
| Ketoconozole | Inhibit testosterone synthesis | Orally active | Large doses needed. Gastrointestinal side effects and gynecomastia. Relatively toxic |
| Finasteride | 5α-reductase inhibitor | Orally active, well tolerated | Few side effects in studies |
| Testolactone | Inhibition of testosterone aromatization | Orally active, well tolerated | Few side effects in studies |
| Spironolactone | Antiandrogen (also decreases androgen production) | Orally active | Weak antiandrogen. Frequently causes polymenorrhea |
| GnRH analog e.g. leuprolide | Decrease gonadotrophin secretion in central precocious puberty | Inhibits LH and FSH secretion after initial stimulation (that may be antagonized with cyproterone). Depot injections monthly in children more useful than nasal or daily injections | Given by injection. Initial stimulatory action. Expensive |

*None may be required for situations in which there is no threat to final height and no psychological stress such as premature thelarche or normal early puberty in a psychologically adjusted family.
Treatment may prevent further advance of puberty but has little effect in causing regression of, for example, breast development. Little need be done for the signs of thelarche or adrenarche.

## Premature adrenarche

Premature adrenarche may occur between 4 and 8 years of age. Pubic hair growth in a child of, say, 5 years may cause parental concern that the child has *progressive* precocious sexual development. Most commonly, however there is no underlying medical problem and the most important evaluation is clinical assessment and careful auxology to verify that there is no progression to precocious puberty and no acceleration in growth rate. When investigations are performed, they confirm that gonadotrophin and gonadal steroid secretions are pre-pubertal and that the circulating concentrations of dehydroepiandrosterone and its sulfate (whilst elevated for age) are matched with appropriate bone age and pubic hair development. No treatment is required for premature adrenarche.

**Definitions:**

Delayed puberty: no increase in testicular volume (i.e. <4 ml) by the age of 14 years in boys and no breast development by the age of 13.5 years in girls.

Primary amenorrhea: lack of menstruation by the age of 16 years.

Pubertal arrest: no progress in puberty over 2 years.

**Causes:**

**Common** (~90%)

Constitutional delay – affecting both growth and puberty: much more common (~10 fold) in boys than girls and may be familial. By definition, investigations are normal.

**Rare** (~10%)

Hypogonadotrophic hypogonadism

- GnRH deficiency – may be isolated or associated with other features e.g. anosmia (Kallman's syndrome), cognitive impairment and dysmorphic features (Prader–Willi syndrome)
- Gonadotrophin deficiency – may be isolated (fertile eunuch resulting from LH deficiency) or more commonly associated with any form of hypopituitarism (see Box 7.9)

Hypergonadotrophic hypogonadism

- Sex chromosome abnormality – e.g. Klinefelter's syndrome in boys (47XXY and variants), Turner's syndrome in girls (45X0) – see Box 6.49
- Gonadal dysgenesis with normal karyotype
- Gonadal damage – viral (e.g. mumps orchitis), iatrogenic (surgical, chemotherapy or radiotherapy), autoimmune (often associated with Addison's disease). Gametes generally more sensitive to damage that steroid secreting cells
- Loss of function mutation in the β-LH subunit. Reduced LH bioactivity but elevated concentrations of LH in immunoassay
- Loss of function mutation in gonadotrophin receptors – resistant ovary syndrome

Temporary delay in pubertal development is very common in the presence of any serious illness e.g. renal failure, bowel or liver disease. Progress depends on the course of the underlying disease. Endocrine causes of temporary delay include hypothyroidism, GH deficiency and excess glucocorticoids of whatever cause.

# Acne, hair growth and hirsutism

Axillary and pubic hair growth are important aspects of puberty as are the problems of teenage spots. Problematical acne and excess hair growth in females (hirsutism) result from the action of androgens on pilo-sebaceous units (PSUs) of which there are four types, vellus, terminal, apo and sebaceous (Box 6.22).

It is the sebaceous PSUs that are the cause of much teenage angst. As cells of the sebaceous gland differentiate and move centrally they accumulate lipid droplets that eventually coalesce and burst the cell (it has given its all – *holo* in Greek – hence the term holocrine secretion). This sebum contains large amounts of glycerides, fatty acids and cholesterol and its production is stimulated by androgens and inhibited by estrogens. Retinoids are also involved in sebaceous gland development.

Acne is a multifactorial disorder and not simply the result of increased sebum secretion. Infection, abnormal keratinization and immune influences can all play a role. The role of adrenarche in acne, however, is supported by the fact that DHEAS concentrations are higher in pre-gonadarcheal girls with comedonal (non-scarring) or inflammatory acne than in those without. Its treatment includes antibiotics and local antiseptics to deal with the *Propionobacterium acnes* bacterial infection that occurs at puberty. Anti-androgens such as cyproterone are useful in female patients and severe disease may require 13-*cis*-retinoic acid that causes a marked reduction in sebaceous gland size.

With regard to hair growth, androgens can cause problems in two common circumstances. In females, they can cause the vellus PSUs to differentiate into terminal PSUs, though the sensitivity to androgens declines with distance from the androgen-dependent facial, pubic and axillary hairs. In the presence of excess androgens, mustache growth occurs first, followed by beard growth, extension of hair in the pubic area (e.g. up the linea alba or onto thighs) and finally terminal hair over the shoulders. The severity of this process is determined, to some extent, by family inheritance and/or ethnicity (indicating genetic factors). It can be measured by the scoring system of Ferriman and Galwey (Box 6.23).

**Clinical**
- Elicit family history of delayed puberty, anosmia, color blindness
- Examine for dysmorphic features (e.g. Prader–Willi or Turner's syndrome, see *Box 6.49*) and in a boy the genitalia for features such as micropenis (suggestive of intrauterine testosterone deficiency)
- Investigations required are greatly influenced by the sex of the child (girls more likely to have an organic cause) and simple clinical assessments that should include:
  Auxology – accurate measurement of height (including body proportions) and weight
  Pubertal staging
  Bone age (BA)

**Based on the above clinical findings endocrine investigations include:**
- Girls of normal weight
  Short, no BA delay – likely to be Turner's syndrome with primary ovarian failure: check karyotype and LH/FSH (for hypergonadotrophic hypogonadism)
  Short, marked BA delay – likely to have hypopituitarism: check LH/FSH (for hypogonadotrophic hypogonadism) then dynamic pituitary tests and MR scan of pituitary gland
  Tall/normal, some BA delay – likely to have GnRH deficiency: check LH/FSH (for hypogonadotrophic hypogonadism)
- Girls of low body weight – likely to have anorexia nervosa or systemic illness e.g. celiac disease; may be associated with marked exercise e.g. athletics
- Boys of normal weight
  Short with some BA delay – likely to have constitutional delay: may need full assessment of growth, GnRH test and MR scan of pituitary gland
  Short, marked BA delay – likely to have hypopituitarism: check LH/FSH (for hypogonadotrophic hypogonadism) then dynamic pituitary tests and MR scan of pituitary gland
  Tall/normal, some BA delay – likely to have GnRH deficiency: check LH/FSH (for hypogonadotrophic hypogonadism)
  Tall/normal with some virilization and small testes – likely to be Klinefelter's syndrome (see *Box 6.49*): check karyotype and LH/FSH (for hypergonadotrophic hypogonadism)
- Boys of low body weight - likely to have systemic illness e.g. celiac disease, rarely anorexia nervosa

Masculinization manifest as clitoral hypertrophy and breast atrophy is only seen at the very highest concentrations of androgens.

Whilst androgens cause hair growth in females, in genetically at-risk males androgen exposure causes baldness with scalp terminal hair regressing to vellus hair with a large sebaceous gland. The patient in *Clinical Case 6.3* with a deficiency of 5α-reductase had a full head of scalp hair, little beard growth, normal axillary hair and a female pattern of pubic hair. This has been seen in many patients with 5α-reductase deficiency, indicating that 5α-DHT is the active androgen in the beard and balding area and that testosterone is the active androgen in the axilla and female-distribution pubic hair.

## The breast – premature development, hypoplasia and gynecomastia

Breast development normally occurs at puberty in response to estrogen, prolactin and local hormones, although excess prolactin cannot compensate for estrogen deficiency. Premature thelarche (*Box 6.24*) is characterized by isolated breast development in young girls that either regresses or remains static. Whilst circulating estrogen concen-

| Drug | Use | Advantages | Disadvantages/side effects |
|---|---|---|---|
| Testosterone[†] | Induction of puberty in males | Effective in increasing linear growth and inducing secondary sexual characteristics. Dose and frequency varies with preparation | Oral preparations not very effective |
| Estrogens | Induction of puberty in females | Effective in increasing linear growth and inducing secondary sexual characteristics. Starting dose and age varies; may be best to start young with low dose. Orally active | Few side effects at physiological doses |
| Oxandrolone | Constitutional delay | Orally active. Effective without reducing final height. Low dose (0.05–0.1 mg/kg) | High doses associated with hepatotoxicity |

*None may be required when there is no threat to final height and no stress in a psychologically adjusted family.
†Available in oral, transdermal, intramuscular and sub-cutaneous depot preparations.

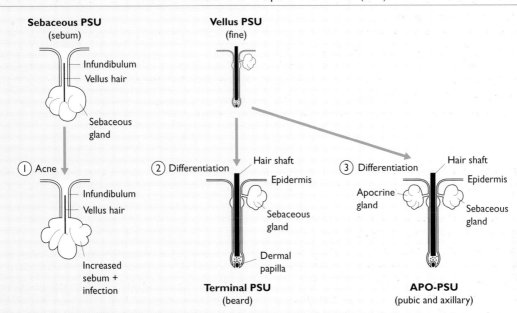

① Androgens stimulate sebum secretion and together with infection this can cause acne.
② Androgens can induce differentiation of vellus PSUs to terminal PSUs encouraging mustache and beard growth.
③ Androgens can induce differentiation of vellus hairs to apo-PSUs encouraging increased growth in areas of pubic and axillary hair.

Diagram of the Ferriman & Galwey scoring system for assessing hirsutism

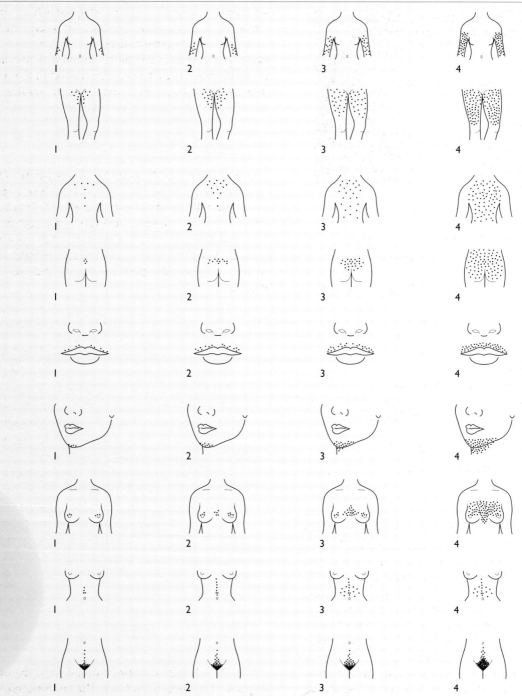

Individual scores are added to give a total.

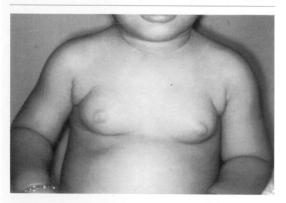

An 18-month-old child with marked breast development

**Characteristics of isolated premature thelarche**

- Breast development <2 years age, cyclical changes in size ~6 weeks
- Absence of other signs of puberty and behavioral problems
- Normal growth and bone maturation
- Predominantly FSH pulsatility in nocturnal profiles
- Lack of ovarian follicular cysts

**Thelarche variant**

- Breast development >2 years of age
- Non-cyclical or persistant breast development
- Progression to central precocious puberty may occur
- LH rather than FSH pulsatility

This image is available on the website

trations may still be low (and below the sensitivity of most radioimmunoassays), ultrasound data and cytological examination of the vaginal epithelium often indicate that estrogen concentrations are elevated relative to age-matched controls. In girls with premature thelarche, or indeed premature adrenache, the use of non-invasive pelvic ultrasound may allow discrimination from precocious puberty since the changes of puberty on the ovary and uterus have been quantified (*Box 6.25*). Lack of development of the breast (hypoplasia) is seen in delayed or arrested puberty, or when tissue is damaged e.g. local radiation (*Box 6.26*).

Gynecomastia refers to growth of mammary glands in males. This may result from changes in sex steroid production during sexual development or senescence, drugs that affect endogenous hormone production or action and genetic disorders linked with gonadal dysgenesis. Excess prolactin can also cause gynecomastia but most common is pseudo-gynecomastia due to the deposition of fat in the pectoral area. Causes of and treatment for gynecomastia are summarized in *Boxes 6.27* and *6.28*.

## Testicular function

The importance of FSH in the development and maturation of the seminiferous tubules and of LH or maternal hCG on the proliferation, differentiation and testosterone production of the Leydig cells has been defined. *Clinical Case 6.6* is the focus for discussion of their roles in controlling the adult testicular functions of spermatogenesis and steroid production.

### Clinical Case 6.6:

A 26-year-old man was seen in the long-term follow-up clinic. He had been treated for acute myeloblastic leukemia with chemotherapy at the age of 12 years. A relapse of the disease 1 year later was treated with a bone marrow transplant utilizing conditioning with busulphan and cyclophosphamide. He had been lost to follow up in the leukemia clinic for several years. He was employed as an accountant and was married. He and his wife had been trying to start a family for 2 years without success. They had sexual intercourse regularly twice a week. On examination, he had normal post-pubertal male secondary sexual characteristics but his testicular volumes were only 6 ml (normal ~ 25 ml). The serum testosterone was 9.8 nmol/l (NR 9–25 mmol/l) with a serum LH of 7 IU/l (NR 2–9 IU/l) and FSH of 34 IU/l (NR 2–9 IU/l).

The Sertoli cells and the germinal cells (the precursors of spermatocytes) are the major components of the seminiferous tubules (*Box 6.29*). These

## Box 6.25:
### Pelvic changes of puberty on ultrasound

Cheap, non-invasive and painless technique to measure bioactivity of the hypothalamo-pituitary-ovarian axis

| Tanner stage | Uterine volume (ml) | Ovarian volume (ml) |
|---|---|---|
| I | 0.5–1.5 | 0.2–0.9 |
| 2 | 1.5–3.0 | 0.9–1.5 |
| 3 | 3.0–10.0 | 1.5–2.5 |
| 4 | 10.0–30.0 | 2.5–3.0 |
| 5 | 30.0–80.0 | 3.0–10.0 |

- Uterine shape changes with age – drop shaped in infancy, tubular by age 8 years and pear-shaped in puberty
- The ratio of the lengths of uterine cervix to corpus is 2:1 pre-puberty and 1:2 post-puberty
- An angle between the corpus and cervix uteri is only seen after puberty
- Endometrial thickening is not seen pre-puberty
- Ovarian follicles may be detected from any age from early infancy. 3–4 cysts ~5 mm diameter normal at any age. Cyst number increases after the age of 8.5 years.

## Box 6.26:
### Breast hypoplasia

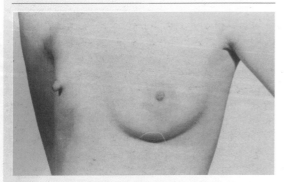

Clinical photograph of a young adult female treated in childhood with external beam radiotherapy for a tumor on the right chest wall. The radiation field included the right breast.

## Box 6.27:
### Causes of male gynecomastia

**Causes:**
**Common** (~>95%)
- Age related (non-pathological):
  Neonatal – circulating estrogen action
  Pubertal – breast aromatase activity converting testosterone to estradiol (usually disappears after 2 years)
  Old age – decreased circulating androgen concentrations
- Drugs including:
  Estrogens or estrogen precursors – e.g. testosterone
  Androgen antagonists – e.g. spironolactone, cimetidine, marijuana, progestagens
  Prolactin stimulating agents – e.g. metoclopramide, sulpiride, phenothiazines, tricyclic antidepressants

**Rare** (~<5%)
- Androgen deficiency including:
  Hypogonadism – e.g. Klinefelter's syndrome, primary testicular failure
  Androgen insensitivity (usually present with pubertal delay)
  Hypopituitarism/gonadotrophin deficiency
- Excess estrogens – e.g. tumor of adrenal or testis
- Other hormone – e.g. hypothyroidism, hyperprolactinemia, hCG-producing tumor
- Systemic disease – e.g. liver disease (increase in SHBG concentrations leads to relative increase in free estrogens over androgens)

tubules, that are surrounded by a basement membrane and form the bulk of the testis, drain into the vas deferens. Sertoli cells span the thickness of the tubule wall and at their base they are connected to adjacent Sertoli cells through tight junctions. These tight junctions form a blood–testis barrier (somewhat analogous to the blood–brain barrier) that enables the Sertoli cells to maintain an extracellular environment within the tubule that is different from normal extracellular fluid. The blood–testis barrier also helps to protect maturing sperm from potential toxins and immune assault and leakage of sperm out of the tubule. Sertoli cells organize and nurture waves of spermatogenesis.

**Box 6.28:**
Treatment of gynecomastia in men

**Medical**

| Drug | Use | Advantages | Disadvantages/side effects |
|------|-----|------------|----------------------------|
| Tamoxifen[†] | Antiestrogen[*] | Orally active. Effective[#] (~80%) | Loss of libido, erectile dysfunction |
| Clomiphene[†] | Antiestrogen | Orally active. Effective (~40%) | Hepatitis, psychiatric changes |
| Testolactone[†] | Aromatase inhibitor | Orally active. Effective (~70%) | Few side effects in reported studies |
| Danazol[†] | Antiandrogen[*] | Orally active. Effective (~30%) | Hepatic dysfunction, gastrointestinal upset, CNS effects |

**Surgical**

| Procedure | Use | Advantages | Disadvantages/side effects |
|-----------|-----|------------|----------------------------|
| Breast removal | Reduce gynecomastia | 'Definitive'. Also reduces risk of breast cancer | Complications include scarring (100%) and infection (~<5%) |

[*]Not strictly true as these agents have both agonist and antagonist actions depending on tissue.

[#]Effectiveness and in particular relative effectiveness is difficult to judge since comparative trial data is only now becoming available and the condition has a natural tendency to remit. The values given are very approximate.

[†]Not a licensed indication.

Leydig cells lie between the tubules (hence the term interstitial cells) and comprise less than 5% of the total testicular volume. Their prime function is to synthesize and release androgens including androstenedione, dehydroepiandrosterone and testosterone, the latter being the most important in potency and quantity (*Box 6.30*) Testosterone diffuses into the seminiferous tubules where it is essential for maintaining spermatogenesis. Some binds to an androgen-binding protein (ABP) that is produced by the Sertoli cells and is homologous to the sex-hormone binding globulin that transports testosterone in the general circulation. The ABP carries testosterone in the testicular fluid where it maintains the activity of the accessory sex glands and may also help to retain testosterone within the tubule and bind excess 'free' hormone. Some testosterone is converted to estradiol by Sertoli cell-derived aromatase enzyme.

## Control of testicular function

Leydig cell steroidogenesis is controlled primarily by LH with negative feedback of testosterone on the hypothalamic-pituitary axis (*Box 6.31*). FSH acts on Sertoli cells to stimulate protein synthesis, mobilization of energy resources, production of testicular fluid, and the output of Sertoli cell proteins such as inhibin and ABP. The actions of testosterone and FSH on Sertoli cells is synergistic allowing spermatogenesis to be completed. FSH stimulates production of an androgen receptor that makes the Sertoli cell responsive to androgens. Androgens stimulate the synthesis of FSH receptors.

In the human, the feedback control of FSH secretion is less clearly defined than that of LH. Administration of testosterone reduces LH secretion but has little, if any, effect on FSH secretion. Inhibin, secreted by Sertoli cells (see *Box 6.47*),

Diagram of the structural organization of the human seminiferous tubule Ⓐ and the stages of spermatogenesis Ⓑ

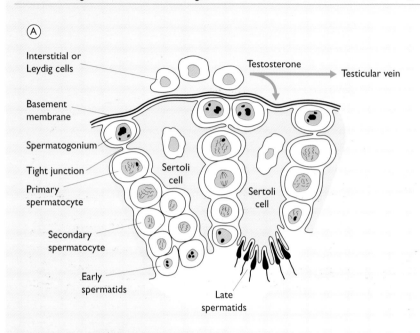

Ⓐ

Interstitial or Leydig cells

Testosterone → Testicular vein

Basement membrane

Spermatogonium

Tight junction

Primary spermatocyte

Sertoli cell

Sertoli cell

Secondary spermatocyte

Early spermatids

Late spermatids

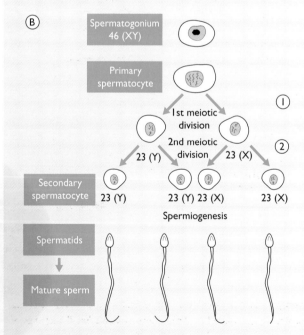

Ⓑ

Spermatogonium 46 (XY)

Primary spermatocyte

1st meiotic division

2nd meiotic division

Ⓘ

Ⓐ

23 (Y)    23 (X)

②

Secondary spermatocyte

23 (Y)    23 (Y) 23 (X)    23 (X)

Spermiogenesis

Spermatids

↓

Mature sperm

Spermatogonia push their way through the tight junctions between adjacent Sertoli cells and become primary spermatocytes. In the first meiotic division Ⓘ each of the 46 chromosomes doubles up and then forms a pair with another doubled up chromosome during which time there is exchange of genetic material (crossing over). The cell divides and each daughter cell contains one of the pairs of chromosomes. In the second meiotic division ② each double chromosome simply separates producing genetically identical secondary spermatocytes. (The ovum, XX, undergoes the same meiotic divisions although completion of the first meiotic division and initiation of the second only occurs after the LH surge and completion of the second does not occur until after fertilization.)

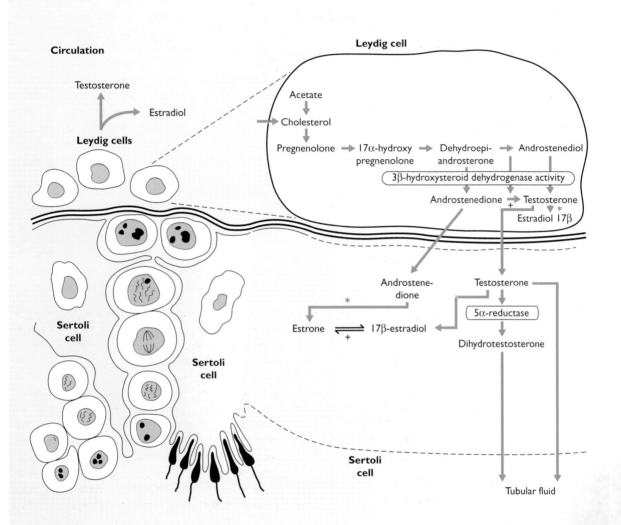

Testosterone and smaller amounts of androstenedione not only enter the circulation but diffuse into the seminiferous tubules where they may bind directly to androgen receptors or first be converted to dihydrotestosterone. Small amounts of estradiol are also formed in both cell types, perferentially in the Sertoli cells prepubertally and in the Leydig cells postpubertally.

+, conversions by 17β-hydroxysteroid dehydrogenase; *, conversions by aromatase.

binds to target cells in the anterior pituitary gland and has a selective negative feedback action on FSH secretion (*Box 6.31*). There is also evidence that the small amount of estrogen that is formed from the peripheral aromatization of testosterone can inhibit both FSH and LH secretion.

It is clear that testicular damage may result in loss of testosterone production or the loss of spermatogenesis or both. Loss of androgen production results in hypogonadism, the symptoms of which (*Box 6.32*) reflect the functions of testosterone and the causes of which will be essentially those discussed previously causing delayed male puberty (see *Box 6.19*).

The requirement of spermatogenesis for high local concentrations of testosterone means that loss of androgen production is likely to be accompanied by loss of spermatogenesis. Indeed, if testicular androgen production is inhibited by the administration of exogenous androgens then spermatogenesis ceases. This is the basis of using exogenous testosterone as a male contraceptive. The patient in *Clinical Case 6.6* had normal adult male secondary sexual characteristics and libido and his peripheral venous testosterone concentration was as expected in the normal range as was the serum LH concentration. His small testicular volume and high serum FSH concentration (a result of reduced inhibin secretion from the Sertoli cells) indicated that his Sertoli cells had been damaged resulting in loss of spermatogenesis and infertility.

## Transport, metabolism and actions of androgens

The testis secretes 4–10 mg testosterone daily, over 95% of the circulating testosterone. The rest is derived from peripheral conversion of adrenal androgens (*Box 6.33*). The testis also secretes small amounts of the more potent DHT, the weak androgens DHEA and androstenedione and estradiol and progestagens. Most of the DHT and estradiol circulating in men is derived from peripheral conversion of testosterone.

Only about 2% of circulating testosterone is in the free form and able to enter cells. The rest is either bound to albumin (approximately 40%) or to sex-hormone-binding globulin (SHBG) and is in equilibrium with the free form. SHBG is synthesized in the liver and its circulating concentration is increased by estrogen or excess thyroid hormones and decreased by exogenous androgens, glucocorticoids or growth hormone and by hypothyroidism, acromegaly and obesity.

Most circulating testosterone is converted in the liver to metabolites such as androsterone and etiocholanolone that, after conjugation with glucuronide or sulfate are excreted in the form of 17-ketosteroids (*Box 6.34*). Note that the majority of urinary ketosteroids are of adrenal origin and, thus, determinations of ketosteroids do not reliably reflect testicular secretion.

In many target tissues, testosterone is rapidly converted to DHT by the 5α-reductase enzyme before it interacts with the androgen receptor, a protein that is encoded by a gene on the X chromosome. The binding of either testosterone or DHT with the receptor induces release of a heat shock protein, dimerization of two receptors and translocation to the nucleus where the dimer binds to an estrogen-like hormone response element (see *Box 6.35*) on DNA. Other transcription factors may be involved in modulating transcription of a number of genes. As with other steroid hormones there is evidence that testosterone may exert nongenomic effects on certain cells via cell surface molecules and also that SHBG may mediate some of these actions.

## Spermatogenesis

Spermatogenesis begins at puberty and involves mitotic proliferation, meiotic division and extensive cell modeling (*Box 6.29*). It starts with the spermatogonia or germinal cells dividing mitotically to produce a small clone of diploid (46XY) cells termed spermatocytes. The spermatocytes migrate through the tight junctions at the base of the Sertoli cells and, in their new environment cradled by the Sertoli cells, undergo two meiotic divisions. In the first division, pairs of chromosomes come together and exchange DNA (crossing over) and separate into two haploid cells (23X or 23Y) known

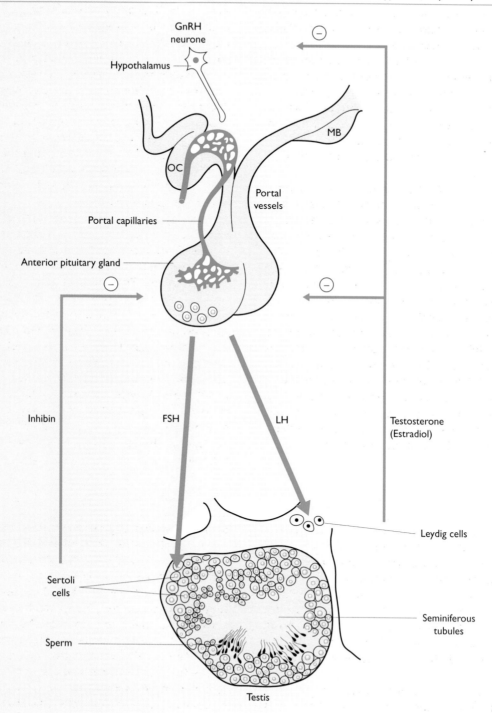

GnRH neurone

Hypothalamus

MB

OC

Portal vessels

Portal capillaries

Anterior pituitary gland

Inhibin

FSH

LH

Testosterone (Estradiol)

Leydig cells

Sertoli cells

Seminiferous tubules

Sperm

Testis

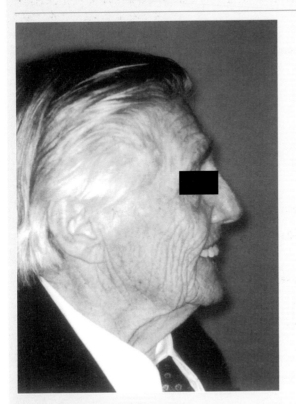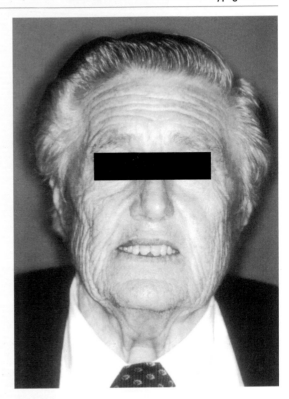

Finely wrinkled facial skin may be the only obvious feature of adult male hypogonadism

**Symptoms**

Decreased libido

Decreased erections

Decreased stamina/muscle strength

Hot flushes

(usually only with acute hypogonadism)

**Signs**

Decreased secondary sexual hair

Smooth (finely wrinkled) skin around eyes

Decreased muscle bulk

Decreased testis size

*These are the result of lack of testosterone. Failure to produce sperm is symptomless and only apparent (apart from changes in the appearance of ejaculate) as a result of infertility. Determining the frequency of the signs and symptoms is extremely difficult, not least because androgens appear to play a major role in initiation of certain processes (e.g. beard growth) but are not absolutely required for their continuation.

as secondary spermatocytes. Almost immediately, a second meiotic division takes place in which the two chromatids that make up a single chromosome separate. These haploid cells, thus, contain 23 single half chromosomes and are called spermatids.

At this stage, they are still simple round cells but, before they leave the nurturing of the Sertoli cells, an acrosome (essential for fertilization) is formed at the head of the sperm and a tail develops. They are extruded from the Sertoli cells into the lumen of the seminiferous tubule. This whole

Box 6.33:

Gonadal versus adrenal androgen production or peripheral conversion as a percentage contribution to total circulating androgens in males and females

| Male | Testis | Adrenal | Peripheral conversion |
|---|---|---|---|
| Testosterone | 95 | <1 | <5 |
| 5α-DHT | 20 | <1 | 80 |
| Androstenedione | 20 | <1 | 90 |
| DHEA | 2 | <1 | 98 |
| DHEA-S | <10 | 90 | – |

| Female | Ovary | Adrenal | Peripheral conversion |
|---|---|---|---|
| Testosterone | 5–25 | 5–25 | 50–70 |
| 5α-DHT | – | – | 100 |
| Androstenedione | 45–60 | 30–45 | 10 |
| DHEA | 20 | 80 | – |
| DHEA-S | <5 | >95 | – |

Total serum concentrations of testosterone — male: 9–25 nmol/l
— female: 0.5–2.5 nmol/l

Abbreviations: DHT, dihydrotestosterone; DHEA(-S), dihydroepiandrosterone (-sulfate).

process of spermatogenesis takes approximately 74 days and about 300–600 sperm/gram of testis are produced each second. Not all survive.

From the seminiferous tubules, the sperm are washed towards the rete testis which drains into the vasa efferentia and from there into the epididymis, a highly convoluted tube that finally drains into the vas deferens (Boxes 6.39 and 6.45). During the 12 day passage from the testis to the vas deferens, the sperm become motile and mature to reach full fertilizing ability. As a result of fluid absorption in the epididymis, sperm also become highly concentrated.

Whilst spermatogenesis is dependent on the hormonal drive from the gonadotrophins and testosterone, temperature also plays a critical factor in this process. Normal spermatogenesis is impaired if the testis is maintained at normal body 'core' temperature (as occurs in cryptorchidism or through tight clothing). The temperature of the testes is normally maintained about 2°C lower than core body temperature because they lie outside the body, moving freely in the scrotal sac. Three layers of membranes enclose each testis and extensions of the fibrous tunica albuginea form septa that divide the gland into 200–300 lobes. In appearance, the testes are white with an oval shape (approximately 4 × 2 × 3 cm with a volume of about 25 ml and weighing between 10–14 g). Seminiferous tubules constitute 70–80% of this mass and each testis has approximately 200 m of seminiferous tubule. The blood supply comes from the testicular arteries that are branches of the internal spermatic arteries.

A fully functioning testis normally achieved by the age of 16 years has the capacity to produce over 200 million sperm each day. Only one is required for fertilization, but each tiny sperm (a few thousandths of a millimeter in length) must travel some

**Box 6.34:**
Major metabolic pathways of the three principal steroids secreted by the gonads

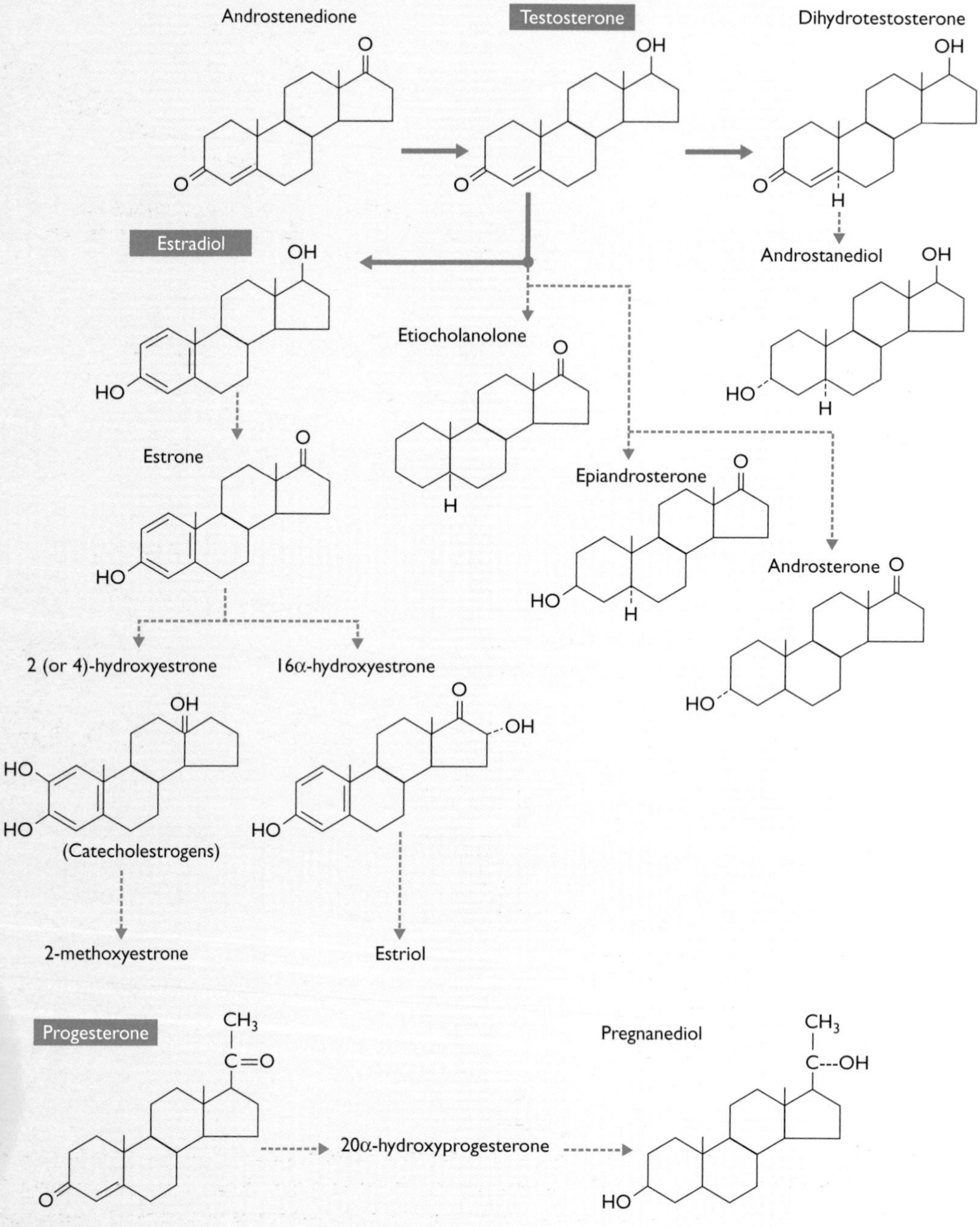

Androstenedione    Testosterone    Dihydrotestosterone

Estradiol

Etiocholanolone

Androstanediol

Estrone

Epiandrosterone

Androsterone

2 (or 4)-hydroxyestrone    16α-hydroxyestrone

(Catecholestrogens)

2-methoxyestrone    Estriol

Progesterone    Pregnanediol

CH₃
C=O

20α-hydroxyprogesterone

CH₃
C---OH

Most steroids are converted ( ----- ) in the liver to various metabolites and then conjugated with glucuronide or sulfate before being excreted in the urine

## Box 6.35: Intracellular receptor mechanisms for the three major gonadal steroids

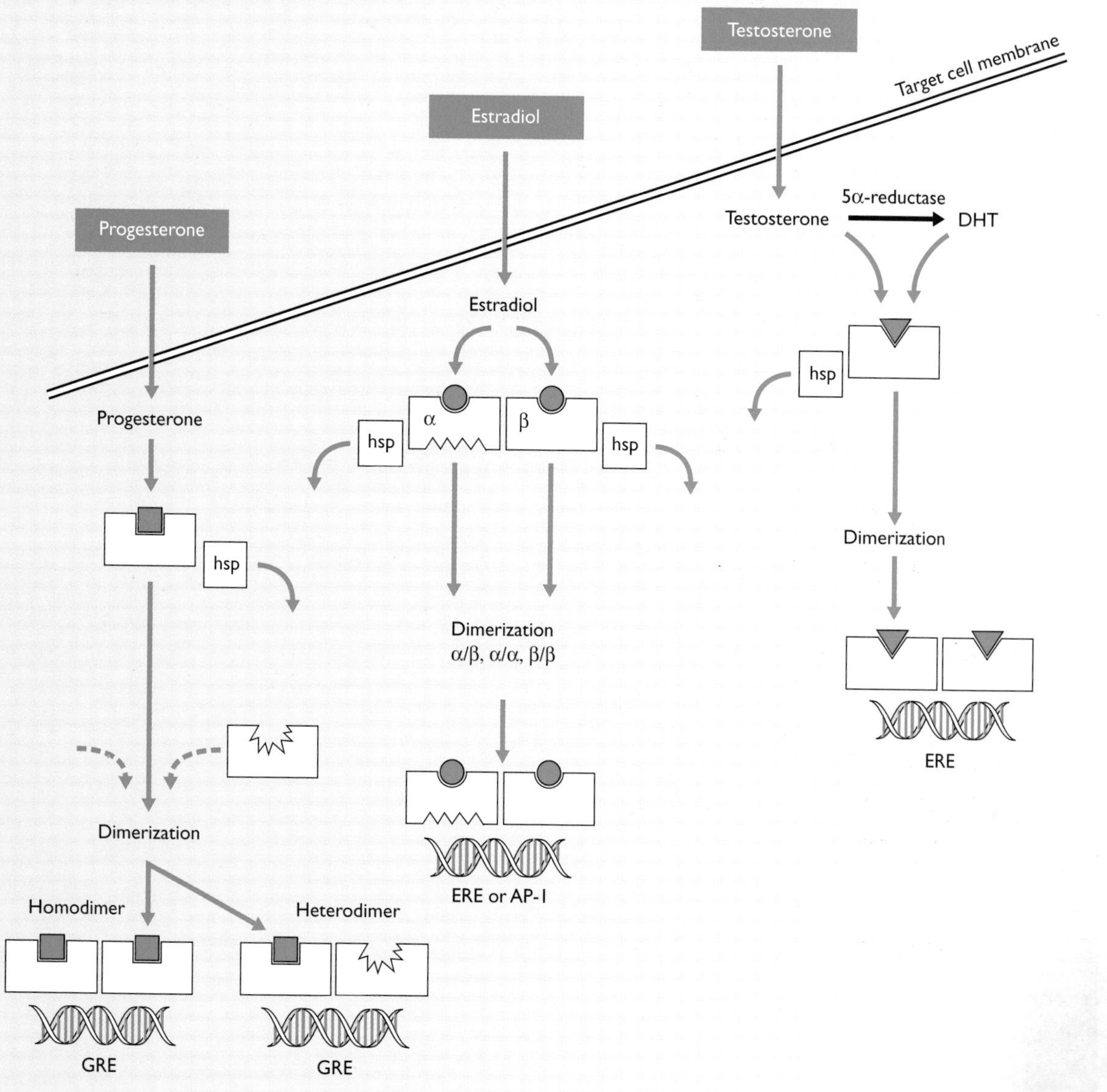

Receptors are mainly located in the cytoplasm attached to heat shock proteins (hsp). Upon ligand binding the hsp are released, receptors dimerize and are translocated to the nucleus. In some target tissues testosterone must first be converted to dihydrotestosterone (DHT) before it interacts with its receptor. Two forms of estradiol receptor have been identified, α and β which form different dimers as indicated. Progesterone can form homo- and heterodimers and interacts with a GRE concensus sequence on DNA.

Abbreviations: ERE, estrogen response element; GRE, glucocorticoid response element (see *Box 1.12*)

30–40 cm (100 000 times its own length) of the male and female reproductive tract before it reaches its final destination in the Fallopian tube. Less than 1 in a million ever completes this journey, though they are helped by the process of ejaculation.

Clinical Case 6.6 had normal Leydig cell function but clear evidence that his Sertoli cells had been damaged resulting in loss of spermatogenesis and infertility. There are a number of causes of this (Box 6.36) but it is highly likely given his past medical history that the cytotoxic drug cyclophosphamide was the cause. Clinical Case 6.6 underwent testing of his seminal fluid and it was found that he had azoospermia (Box 6.37). Treatment is possible in a number of causes of male infertility (Box 6.38) but currently there is none available for cyclophosphamide-induced azoospermia. Cryopreservation of ovary and testis of patients prior to undergoing such therapies is under active consideration (see Website).

## Erection and ejaculation

Sperm can be stored up to 5 weeks in the tail of the epididymis and vas deferens before they are released at ejaculation. In the absence of ejaculation sperm dribble into the urethra and are washed away in the urine. In men who have undergone a vasectomy (ligation of the vas deferens) sperm build up behind the ligation and are either removed by phagocytosis in the epididymis or leak through the epididymal wall.

The ejaculatory response is evoked by a complex series of reflexes and the physiological phases of this response have been defined as erection, emission and ejaculation. Failure to achieve penile erections has been termed impotence, but the word conjures up such images of functional incapacity that the term erectile dysfunction is recommended.

### Clinical Case 6.7:

A 56-year-old man was seen in the diabetic clinic. He had had diabetes mellitus type 2 for 15 years and was complaining of inability to achieve erections. He had had treatment with laser photocoagulation for diabetic retinopathy and mild renal failure with a serum creatinine of 130 µmol/l (NR 60–110 µmol/l).

---

**Box 6.36:**
Causes of male infertility*

**Testicular disease** (50% of total)
- Unknown (~50%)
- Maldescent (~20%)
- Torsion/trauma (~5%)
- Klinefelter's (~20%)
- Orchitis (~5%)
- Chemotherapy (~5%)

**Duct obstruction** (~15% of total) – may occur in rete testis or the result of too tight coiling of the seminiferous tubules: most commonly in the epididymal duct (as a result of infection, trauma, congenital abnormality). Obstruction of the vas deferens is usually surgical but may be congenital particularly in patients heterozygous for the ΔF508 mutation causing cystic fibrosis.

**Endocrine** (~2% of total) – any cause of hypopituitarism (see Box 7.9)

**Autoimmune** (~5% of total)

**Sperm abnormalities** (~25% of total)

**Ejaculatory problems** (~5% of total)

*It is difficult to establish the exact frequencies of the causes of infertility. The exact roles of, for example, varicocele or autoimmunity continue to be debated.

---

**Box 6.37:**
Tests evaluating male fertility

**Descriptive tests** – these include:
- Sperm number
- Sperm motility
- Sperm morphology
- Sperm antibodies
- Seminal fluid ATP

**Tests of sperm function** – these include:
- Penetration of cervical mucus
- Binding of mannose
- Penetration of hamster oocytes
- Zona pellucida binding

- The majority of male infertility is untreatable because of irremediable damage to the germ cells
- Endocrine therapies are highly successful (e.g. GnRH pump or gonadotrophins) but are only applicable to a very small number of men
- *Intracytoplasmic sperm injection* (ICSI) has revolutionized therapy for those men with either duct obstruction or sperm abnormalities. Pregnancy rates in excess of 50% have been achieved. However, concerns continue to be expressed over the issue of quality of the material injected and the reproductive future of the adult product of the fertilized ovum.

Erection is induced by tactile stimulation of the genital region, particularly the glans penis, or from visual cues or emotions that can stimulate descending pathways from the brain (*Box 6.39*). Such sensory stimulation induces dilatation of arterioles in the penis and the sinuses of the corpus spongiosum and cavernosa become engorged with blood. As these erectile bodies are surrounded by a strong fibrous coat the penis becomes rigid, elongated and increases in girth. This compresses venous outflow so that while inflow increases out-flow does not. At the same time, parasympathetic nerves stimulate the bulbo-urethral glands to produce a mucoid-like substance to aid lubrication.

Emission involves contractions of the smooth muscle in the walls of the vas deferens and genital ducts that push sperm into the upper part of the urethra. At the same time, the seminal vesicles and prostate gland (accessory sex glands) contract and seminal fluid is released into the urethra. At ejaculation, the semen (sperm plus seminal fluid) is expelled from the posterior urethra by contractions of the bulbo-cavernous and urethral muscles. The passage of semen from the upper part of the urethra back into the bladder is normally prevented by sympathetic contraction of the urethral sphincter. Failure of this sphincter can cause retrograde ejaculation.

In the resolution phase, all the physiological changes of sexual arousal (e.g. erection of the nipples, increased heart rate and blood pressure, flushing on the face neck and chest) are reversed. A man becomes refractive to any further sexual stimulation for a period from a few minutes to several hours.

Any interference with spinal reflexes or blood supply can cause erectile dysfunction although libido will be unaffected. Over 50% of cases of erectile dysfunction have a physical basis (*Box 6.40*). The complications of diabetes mellitus include both neuropathy and vascular damage and the disease is one of the most common causes of erectile dysfunction. Doppler blood flow studies of *Clinical Case 6.7* showed normal vascular supply but tests of autonomic nerve function showed a marked dysfunction indicating a neurological cause. He was treated with oral sildenafil (better known as Viagra, *Box 6.41*) with some improvement.

The possible role of testosterone in male sexual behavior is clouded by the variance between individuals and is also markedly influenced by learning. Thus, loss of androgens before puberty reduces the normal pubertal sex drive, but when androgens are deficient after puberty there is a gradual loss of sex interest and an increasing incidence of erectile dysfunction.

The sexual response may also be suppressed by the central nervous system either consciously or subconsciously leading to erectile dysfunction, loss of sexual interest, premature ejaculation, ejaculatory failure or a loss of generalized orgasm at erection. These are all common defects of this complex reflex response and may have a psychogenic basis in some patients. They are often amenable to behavioral therapy.

Given what is known of the embryology and anatomy of the male and female external genitalia, it could be asked whether there is a female equivalent of male erectile dysfunction. The recent experience with the drug sildenafil suggests that this drug is not only effective in treating erectile dysfunction in men but it can also help women to achieve orgasm. It seems highly likely that is works by improving clitoral erection and, thus, sensory sexual stimulation.

## Ovarian control and the menstrual cycle

The ovary shows cyclical activity, unlike the testis that is maintained in a more or less constant state

Diagram of mid-sagittal section through the male pelvis and a testis and the major nervous pathways involved in penile erection

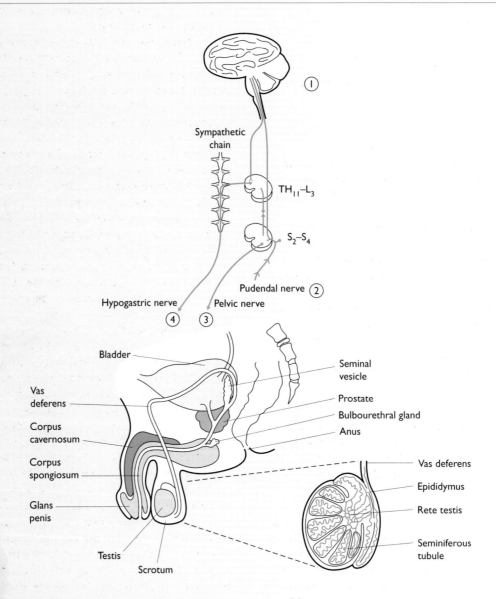

Psychogenic stimuli from the brain ① or from tactile receptors on the penis (via the pudendal nerve) ② activate efferent parasympathetic fibers of the pelvic nerve ③. This stimulates vasodilatation increasing blood flow into the corpora cavernosa and to a lesser extent in the corpus spongiosum. This involves the neurotransmitters, acetylcholine and vasoactive polypeptide and increased nitric oxide production. The sympathetic outflow of the hypogastric nerve ④ normally maintains myogenic tone in the flaccid penis but this is counteracted by the parasympathetic activity during sexual arousal. Prostaglandin $E_1$ or a synthetic analog or $\alpha$-adrenergic blockers can reduce tone and cause tumescence.

Box 6.40:
Causes of erectile dysfunction

**Psychogenic** – this includes
- performance anxiety
- depression
- schizophrenia

**Neurogenic** – this includes:
- cerebral lesions – such as stroke or Alzheimer's disease
- spinal cord lesions
- pelvic injury
- neuropathy – e.g. diabetes mellitus

**Endocrine** – e.g. hyperprolactinemia or hypogonadism

**Vascular** – this includes problems of arterial supply due to atherosclerosis and also venous failure due to trauma

**Drug-induced** – many drugs have been implicated, including:
- centrally acting agents affecting neurotransmitter pathways such as antipsychotics, antihypertensives, antidepressants
- antihypertensive agents including β-adrenergic blocking agents and thiazide diuretics
- antiandrogens such as spironolactone, cimetidine, cyproterone or estrogens

**Other diseases** – e.g. renal, heart or hepatic failure

of activity. Hormone secretions vary according to the phase of the menstrual cycle (*Box 6.42*) and gonadal steroids have both negative and positive feedback effects on the control of gonadotrophin secretion (*Box 6.43*).

The first day of the menstrual cycle is defined as the first day of menstruation when estrogen and progesterone secretions from the ovary are low and FSH secretion has increased as a result of the loss of negative feedback effects. The increased FSH stimulates the growth and differentiation of cohorts of preantral or antral follicles that are at different stages of development (see *Box 6.46*). As a consequence steroid production in the ovary increases.

The ovary requires both LH and FSH to produce sex steroids (*Box 6.44*). LH stimulates the thecal cells surrounding the follicle to produce proges-

terone and androgens. The androgens diffuse across the basement membrane to the granulosa cell layer, where, under the action of FSH, they are aromatized to estrogens, mainly estradiol. The developing follicle selected to become dominant (see *Box 6.46*) progresses to full maturity.

Ovulation requires that the follicle rises to the surface of the ovary and the granulosa cells develop LH receptors. At this stage, circulating concentrations of estradiol have reached a critical concentration (>750 pmol/l) and, 24–48 hours after peak production, its negative feedback effect on gonadotrophin secretion is switched to a positive feedback. Such positive feedback is a rare biological phenomenon and is thought to be the result of estrogen increasing the amplitude and frequency of GnRH pulses and a consequent up-regulation of GnRH receptors. Estrogen also increases the responsiveness of the pituitary gonadotrophs. Together, these effects induce a preovulatory peak of LH secretion and a smaller increase in FSH secretion. Ovulation occurs 9–12 hours after the LH surge and involves local paracrine mechanisms and induction of proteolytic enzymes.

After ovulation, the empty follicle is remodelled and plays an important role in the second half or luteal phase of the menstrual cycle. The granulosa and thecal cells remaining in the ruptured follicle proliferate rapidly and form the corpus luteum (from Latin, 'yellow body'). This phase is dominated by progesterone and, to a lesser extent, 17β-estradiol secretion by the corpus luteum. Significant quantities of 17α-hydroxyprogesterone and inhibin are also secreted and these, together with other steroids, may help to modulate the actions of gonadotrophs in luteal development and maintenance. Small amounts of gonadotrophins, particularly LH, are required to maintain the function of the corpus luteum and in the luteal stage, high-amplitude, low-frequency LH pulses are observed compared to the high-frequency, low-amplitude pulses seen in the follicular stage of the cycle (*Box 6.42*).

In the absence of fertilization the corpus luteum breaks down by a process known as luteolysis. The precise mechanisms that induce this degeneration are unknown (although in some species it involves

**Box 6.41:**
Treatment of erectile dysfunction

**Medical**

| **Drug** | **Use** | **Advantages*** | **Disadvantages/side effects** |
|---|---|---|---|
| Sildenafil | Phosphodiesterase 5 inhibitor Potentiates NO action (see *Box 8.7*) | Effective (~50–80%), orally active | Absolutely contraindicated with nitrate therapy. Headache (~15%), flushing (~10%), colored vision (~3%) |
| Phentolamine | $\alpha_2$-receptor antagonist | Effective (~40%), orally active | Headache (~15%), flushing (~5%), nasal congestion (~30%) |
| Yohimbine | $\alpha_2$-receptor antagonist | Most effective in non-organic erectile dysfunction (~20–30%). Orally active | Palpitation (~10%), tremor (~10%), anxiety (~5%), elevation of blood pressure (~5%) |
| Alprostadil (transurethral) | Prostaglandin $E_1$ | Effective (~40%) | Administration route. Penile pain (~30%), urethral pain (~15%), hypotension (~5%) |
| Alprostadil‡ (intracavernosal) | Prostaglandin $E_1$ | Effective (~70%) | Administration route. Penile pain (~30%), fibrosis (~5%), priapism (~<1%) |
| Papaverine‡ (intracavernosal) | Phosphodiesterase inhibitor | Effective (~40–70%). Low cost | Priapism (~20%), fibrosis (~30%) |
| Phentolamine‡ (intracavernosal) | $\alpha_2$-receptor antagonist | Effective when combined with papaverine (~70%) | Hypotension (~10%), palpitations (~15%) |

**Surgical**

| **Procedure** | **Use** | **Advantages** | **Disadvantages/side effects** |
|---|---|---|---|
| Vacuum device | Increase tumescence and rigidity | Non-invasive, cheap. No systemic side-effects | Unnatural erection, petechiae, numbness (~20%) Trapped ejaculate |
| Prosthesis | Implanted device (various types) | Effective | Unnatural erection, expensive, infection. Requires replacement after 5–10 years |

*The nature of the condition makes accurate assessment of efficacy difficult.
†Trazodone, a serotonin reuptake inhibitor, is sometimes used in combination with yohimbine.
‡These intracavernosal agents are often used together in lower doses than those used singly.

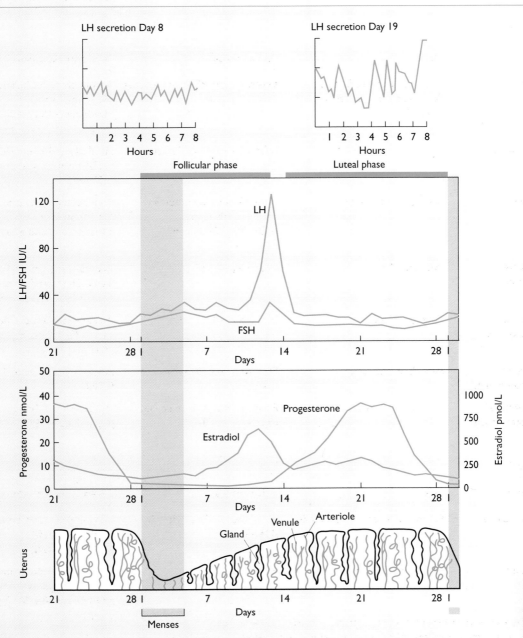

The graph shows average serum concentrations of hormones during a typical 28 day menstrual cycle along with changes in the uterine endometrium. LH, FSH and GnRH, are secreted in a pulsatile pattern with the frequency and amplitude changing according to the stage of the menstrual cycle as shown for LH (top). The pulsatile pattern of GnRH may determine the preferential synthesis and secretion of either LH or FSH. Positive feedback effects of peak concentrations of estradiol induces the pre-ovulatory LH surge.

**Box 6.43:**
**Feedback control of the hypothalamo-pituitary-ovarian axis**

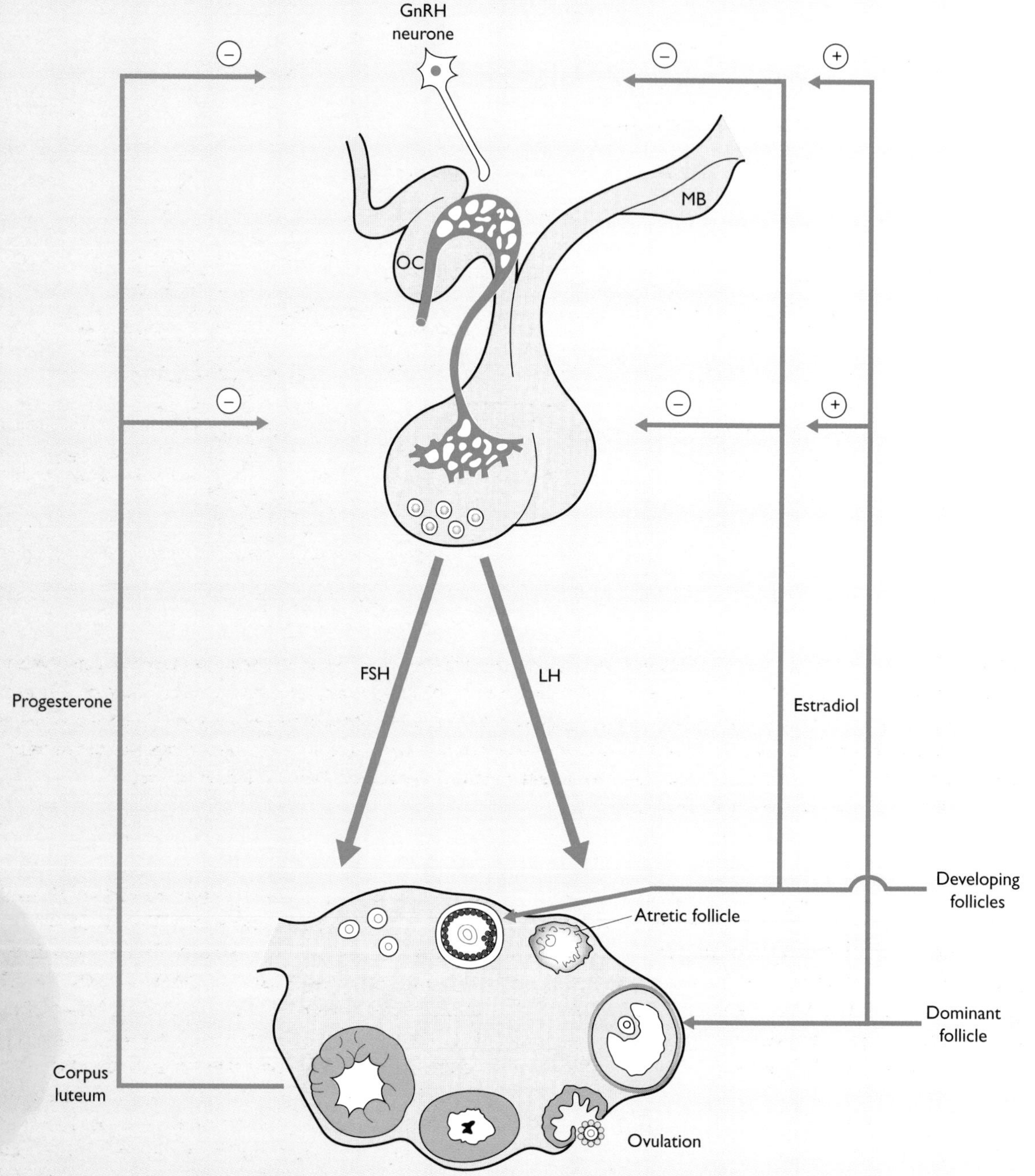
GnRH
neurone
MB
OC
FSH
LH
Progesterone
Estradiol
Developing
follicles
Atretic follicle
Dominant
follicle
Corpus
luteum
Ovulation

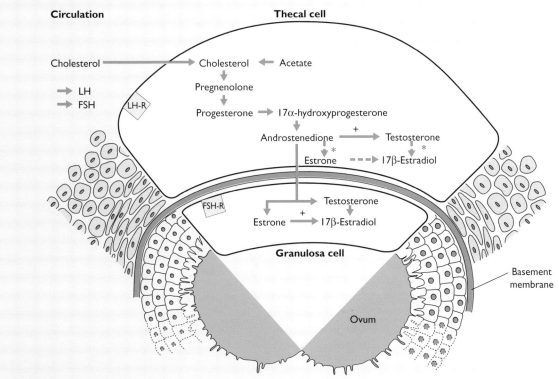

Androstenedione, formed in thecal cells under the stimulatory effects of LH, diffuses across the basement membrane where, under the action of FSH, it is converted to estradiol. In the developing follicle, LH receptors (LH-R) are only located on the thecal cells and FSH receptors (FSHR) on the granulosa cells. The 'dominant' pre-ovulatory follicle develops LH-Rs on the granulosa cells prior to the LH surge. Thecal cells of the preovulatory follicle also develop the capacity to synthesize estradiol (dotted lines) and this persists when the thecal cells become incorporated into the corpus luteum.
*Aromatase; +, 17β-hydroxysteroid dehydrogenase type I

prostaglandins) but it may be that there is simply insufficient LH to maintain the corpus luteum. The consequences are that progesterone and estrogen secretions from the corpus luteum decline. The loss of the negative feedback of the steroids induces a selective rise in FSH secretion, more follicles are recruited and a new cycle begins.

## Transport, metabolism and actions of ovarian steroids

Estradiol, the most important steroid secreted by the ovary because of its biologic potency and diverse actions, is transported bound to albumin (approximately 60%) and about 30% to SHBG. It is rapidly converted to estrone by 17β-hydroxysteroid dehydrogenase in the liver and, whilst some estrone re-enters the circulation, most of it is further metabolized to estriol via 16α-hydroxyestrone or to 2- or 4-hydroxyestrone (catechol estrogens) by the action of catecho-O-methyltransferase. The latter metabolites can be formed in the brain and may compete with receptors for catecholamines. Metabolites are conjugated with sulfate or glucuronide before excretion by the kidney (Box 6.34).

Progesterone is mainly bound to albumin in the circulation and, to a lesser extent, *cortisol-binding globulin*. It is rapidly cleared from the circulation, being converted to pregnanediol and conjugated with glucuronic acid in the liver in which form it can be excreted. The ovaries also produce small amounts of testosterone, DHT, androstenedione and DHEAS and these are metabolized like the testicular hormones.

Estrogen and progesterone, like testosterone, also have multiple target cells and their actions are mediated by intracellular receptors which, upon ligand binding, release a heat shock protein, dimerize with another receptor and bind to a hormone response element or an AP-1 promoter region on DNA (*Box 6.35*). Within the last few years two forms of the estrogen receptor have been identified – α and β. They have different distributions in estrogen target tissues and can form different dimers – α/β, α/α and β/β. The different dimers may have different biological effects. The progesterone receptor, unlike the estrogen receptor, can form heterodimers and, instead of binding with an estrogen response element on DNA, as does testosterone (see *Box 1.12*), progesterone-bound receptors bind to a response element similar to that of glucocorticoids. The specificity of the response is determined by which receptor is present in the cell as well as other cell-specific transcription factors.

## The ovary – folliculogenesis and oogenesis

Each ovary nestles in a small depression of the posterior wall of the broad ligament on each side of the peritoneal cavity and just above the pelvic brim. They are connected to the fimbriated ends of the Fallopian tubes (*Box 6.45*). The ovaries are dull white in color, oval in shape ($3 \times 2 \times 1$ cm) and weigh about 5–8 g. They are enclosed in a tough fibrous capsule, the tunica albuginea, and consist of an outer cortex and an inner medulla. The cortex contains all the follicles and remains of ruptured follicles embedded in vascular fibrous tissue. The inner medulla is where the blood vessels, lymphatics and nerves enter the ovary. The appearance of the ovary varies with the age of the woman.

Before puberty, the glands are smooth and rather solid in consistency and contain many primordial follicles. Between puberty and the menopause, their surfaces become more corrugated in appearance due to the activity of the gland during each ovarian cycle. After the menopause, they shrink and are covered with scar tissue, the result of monthly follicular rupture.

At birth, the cortex of the immature ovary contains about half a million primordial follicles consisting of flattened cells surrounding a primary oocyte that is halfway through its first meiotic division. At the time of puberty, the total number has been reduced to around 300–400 000 and <1.0% ever reach full maturity and ovulate. When primordial follicles enter their growth phase, granulosa cells begin to divide, the oocyte enlarges and becomes surrounded by a zona pellucida. Gradually the follicles become secondary follicles and, when fibroblast cells in the inner thecal layer differentiate, the secondary follicle is defined as a preantral follicle (*Box 6.46*). The early growth phase is considered to be independent of gonadotrophin stimulation despite the evidence for FSH receptors on these immature follicles. It is not known why a few primordial follicles begin to grow, nor how they are selected, but paracrine factors within the ovary such as cytokines and epidermal growth factor may be involved.

In the early luteal phase of each menstrual cycle, a cohort of preantral follicles undergo further growth into antral follicles (*Box 6.46*). At this time, the follicles enlarge, the thecal cells become richly supplied with blood vessels and a fluid-filled cavity (the antrum) forms. The oocyte becomes surrounded by several layers of granulosa cells known as the cumulus oophorus. During the basal growth phase follicle diameter increases from about 0.2 mm to 2 mm. By the late luteal phase of the third cycle those follicles that have not degenerated have reached the selectable phase. In other words they may be recruited for further development. Over a period of about 5 days (termed the selection window) the follicles continue to grow but only one is selected to undergo final maturation. The mechanisms responsible for the selection of the dominant follicle are not well understood

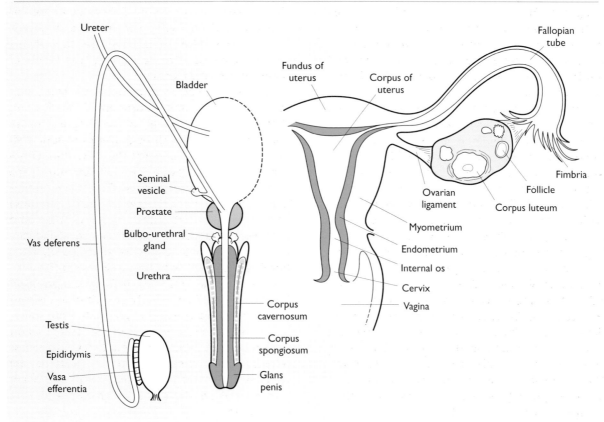

but may be determined by the number of FSH receptors or the concentrations of steroids or growth factors within the follicle. Over 15 days, the dominant follicle increases in diameter from 5 mm to around 20 mm, secretes increasing concentrations of estradiol and becomes a fully mature Graafian follicle (*Box 6.46*). Ovulation occurs in the third cycle.

The LH surge induces the ovum to complete its first meiotic division prior to ovulation producing two haploid daughter cells containing 23 chromosomes, one of which is the X chromosome. One cell, however, retains most of the cytoplasm and the smaller one (the first polar body) sits cramped in a small space, the vitelline space, between the secondary oocyte and the zona pellucida. Unlike the process of spermatogenesis, the secondary oocyte does not undergo its second meiotic division until after fertilization has occurred. Like the process of spermatogenesis, folliculogenesis occurs in waves and at any one time the ovary contains follicles at all stages of development, apart from the dominant follicle that is only present during the follicular phase of a cycle.

## Non-steroidal factors in the control of the hypothalamic-pituitary-gonadal axis

Whilst gonadotrophin-stimulated steroidogenesis is essential for the maintenance of gametogenesis, the ovary and testis elaborate a large variety of proteins

263

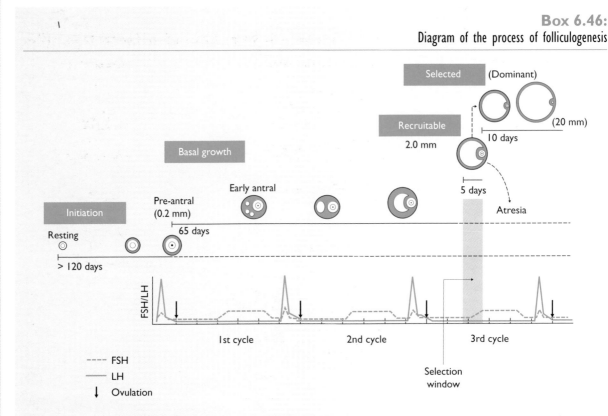

Box 6.46:
Diagram of the process of folliculogenesis

The development of a primordial follicle to a preovulatory follicle takes in excess of 120 days. After it has become a preantral follicle of about 0.2 mm diameter it takes about 65 days to develop into a preovulatory follicle. Cohorts of follicles continually develop but only one is 'selected' and becomes the dominant follicle. All others undergo atresia.

and peptides that can act as local paracrine agents within the gland or can exert central feedback effects.

One of the first non-steroidal factors to be isolated was inhibin and subsequently other glycosylated proteins were identified. Inhibin is a glycoprotein made up of a common α unit combined with one of two β units: $\beta_A$ (inhibin A) or $\beta_B$ (inhibin B). Various combinations of the two different β subunits gives rise to three forms of activins; activin, A, $\beta_A\beta_A$, activin B, $\beta_A\beta_B$ and activin C, $\beta_B\beta_B$ (Box 6.47). A third glycosylated protein, follistatin, is a high-affinity monomeric binding protein for inhibin and activin.

Inhibin synthesized in the Sertoli cells and granulosa cells exerts negative feedback effects on the secretion of FSH via actions on the pituitary gonadotroph. Within the gonads, and along with its other associated peptides, there is evidence for a role for inhibin in modulating steroidogenesis, cellular proliferation and differentiation. Other factors located in the testis and/or ovary include transforming growth factor α, basic fibroblast growth factor, transforming growth factor β, insulin-like growth factor-1 and its binding proteins and a number of cytokines. A variety of functions have been ascribed to these non-steroidal factors and it would appear they help to orchestrate the complex processes of spermatogenesis, oogenesis and folliculogenesis.

## Ovulation, menstruation and its problems

The average length of a menstrual cycle is approximately 28 days. Cycles do, however, vary consider-

Box 6.47:
Structures of the inhibins, activins and anti-Müllerian hormone (AMH)

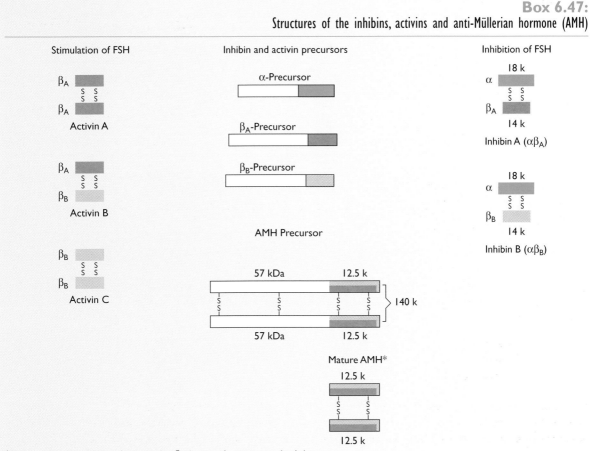

*Shows structural homology to the β chains of activins and inhibins.

ably in length although in 95% of women each cycle lasts between 25 and 34 days. Most of the variation is due to differences in the length of the first (follicular) phase of the cycle; the luteal phase is more likely to be about 14 days in length.

Menstruation occurs because of the effects of steroids on the endometrial lining of the uterus. During the follicular phase of the cycle, endometrial cells proliferate, glands enlarge and the endometrium becomes richly supplied with blood vessels (*Box 6.42*). Hence, it is termed the proliferative phase of the uterine cycle. After ovulation, progesterone secretion from the corpus luteum stimulates a further increase in endometrial thickness and secretion of a fluid to nourish a fertilized egg and encourage implantation of the conceptus.

This is the secretory phase of the endometrium. If fertilization occurs, the hCG secreted by the developing placenta maintains the corpus luteum and, hence, progesterone secretion. In the absence of fertilization, the steroid support of the endometrium is lost due to luteolysis. The spiral arteries that have grown up into the endometrium contract and cells, starved of their normal blood supply, break away and menstrual loss ensues.

There are several markers to indicate ovulation has occurred. Detection of the LH surge using commercial assays of the hormone in urine is both sensitive and robust. The increase in progesterone after ovulation results in a small rise in body temperature and whilst this small rise can be used to indicate when ovulation occurs, obtaining reliable temperature measurements is difficult. Some women feel mild pain in the abdomen, lasting from a few minutes to a couple of hours, around the time of ovulation. Known as *Mittelschmerz* (German for 'midpain') it is probably caused by irritation of the abdominal wall due to blood and fluid escaping from the ruptured follicle. Changes in the cervical mucus also occur around the time of ovulation.

The presence of cyclic menstruation does not necessarily indicate ovulation is occurring mid-cycle. In anovulatory cycles menstrual bleeding is due to estrogen withdrawal after the non-ovulatory follicles have degenerated. Measurement of circulating progesterone concentrations in the expected luteal phase of the cycle (usually day 21) is a reliable indicator of corpus luteum formation and, thus, previous ovulation. Total blood loss during each menstruation varies from cycle to cycle, and in different women at different stages of their reproductive life. However, the average blood loss is about 50–60 ml although this can vary from about 10 to 80 ml. Excessive loss of blood (menorrhagia) can lead to iron-deficiency anemia.

Disturbances in the menstrual cycle are not uncommon. Returning to *Clinical Case 6.2*, it can be seen that failure to start menstruating (primary amenorrhea) by the age of 16 years is rare and highly likely to have an organic cause (*Box 6.48*). Clearly, from the foregoing, it will occur as a result of any insult to the hypothalamo-pituitary-ovarian axis. It will also be seen if there is failure of Müllerian duct development or when there are more minor vaginal abnormalities (such as an imperforate hymen) preventing menstrual flow. A list of the causes of secondary amenorrhea will be very similar to that for primary amenorrhea except that the structural lesions of the Müllerian duct system will be excluded for the obvious reason that for menses to have occurred at all the system must be present. A number of syndromes of hypogonadism occur clinically; the commoner ones are detailed in *Box 6.49*.

Much more common than the cessation of menstruation is its irregularity. This is discussed in the context of *Clinical Case 6.8*.

# Polycystic ovary syndrome (PCOS)

## Clinical Case 6.8:

A 25-year-old Asian woman was seen in the Endocrine Clinic complaining of infrequent periods. Her menarche had been at the age of 13 years and her periods had always been infrequent and irregular with three or four each year. She had a family history of type 2 diabetes mellitus and was 1.65 m tall and weighed 62 kg. She had recently got married and was planning to have children in the near future. She had not noticed any excess hair growth and her serum testosterone was 1.9 nmol/l (NR < 2.5 nmol/l) and her serum progesterone on Day 21 of her menstrual cycle was 6 nmol/l (NR for ovulatory cycle >40 nmol/l). Ultrasound of her pelvis revealed polycystic ovaries, the definition of which is 10 or more cysts 2–8 mm diameter with a thickened stroma (*Box 6.50*).

---

**Box 6.48:**
Causes of primary amenorrhea[*]

**Gonadal** – these include:
- dysgenesis – e.g. Turner's syndrome
- damage – e.g. radiation
- failure of steroid synthesis – e.g. 17α-hydroxylase deficiency, or resistant ovary syndrome

**Genital tract** – these include:
- dysgenesis – failure of Müllerian duct development
- vaginal abnormalities

**Androgen insensitivity syndrome** (*Clinical Case 6.2*)
**Hypothalamo-pituitary disease** (*Box 7.9*)

[*]None are common.

---

PCOS is conventionally described as a combination of hyperandrogenism (often manifest as acne and hirsutism, anovulation (which may manifest, as in this case, with menstrual infrequency termed oligomenorrhea) and the appearances of polycystic

**Major clinical features of the more common genetic hypogonadal syndromes**

**Hereditary hemochromatosis** – HFE gene (1 in 10 European Caucasians heterozygous, 1 in 200 homozygous)

HFE gene mutations lead to increased iron absorption by unknown mechanisms

Clinical presentation in middle age, 10-fold more common in men (because women have menstrual iron loss). Other factors such as dietary iron intake may be important. Therapy involves regular venesection.

- Classical triad of skin pigmentation (~80%), diabetes mellitus (~90%, 'bronzed diabetes') and gonadal failure (~70%)
- Cardiac failure (~15%)
- Cirrhosis (~90%)
- Arthritis (~50%)

**Turner's syndrome** – 45XO*† (~1 in 2500 live births)

- Short stature (~100%)
- Delayed puberty (~100%) – dysmorphic 'streak' ovaries
- Dysmorphic features (~40%) – including broad chest, widely spaced nipples, short webbed neck
- Low set ears and micrognathia (~ 40%)
- Cardiovascular defects (~40%) – including coarctation of aorta, aortic stenosis
- Renal (30%) – abnormalities include horseshoe kidney
- Edema (~20%)
- Musculoskeletal (~90%) – including cubitus valgus, short 4th metacarpal, genu valgus
- Otolaryngological (~50%) – sensorineural deafness, recurrent otitis media
- Endocrine (~15%) – increased incidence of Graves' disease

*Patients require medical follow up due to the frequency of non-endocrine renal and cardiac features.

†Mosaicism occurs altering phenotype.

**Klinefelter's syndrome** – 47XXY† (karyotype surveys of neonates indicates ~1 in 600 live births but clinical presentation much less common).

- Male phenotype (~100%)
- Small testes (~100%)
- Normal/tall stature with eunuchoidal proportions (~100%)
- Reduced IQ (~80%)
- Reduced virilization at puberty + gynecomastia (~70%)
- Increased incidence of autoimmune thyroid disease and diabetes mellitus (~20%)

†Mosaicism occurs altering phenotype

**Prader–Willi syndrome** (1:20 000; 70% paternal 15q11-q13 deletion, 25% maternal uniparental disomy, 5% imprinting center defect)

- Obesity – associated with childhood hyperphagia (~100%)
- Short stature (~100%)
- Reduced IQ (~95%)
- Dysmorphic features – almond shaped eyes, triangular mouth (~90%)
- Delayed puberty and hypothalamic hypogonadism (~50%)
- Males – micropenis and cryptorchidism

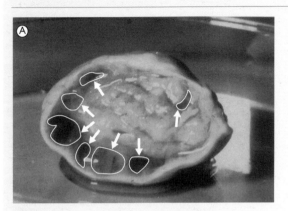

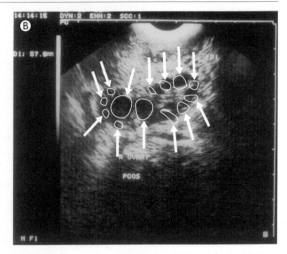

These images are available on the Website.

The cut section of an enlarged ovary Ⓐ demonstrates the multiple peripherally placed cysts (arrows). The capsule of the gland is thickened. The ultrasound scan Ⓑ facilitates the measurement of the size and also demonstrates non-invasively the multiple cysts and a central stroma that is denser than normal.

**Clinical features of PCOS***

- Hirsutism (~60%)
- Oligomenorrhea (~45%)
- Amenorrhea (~20%)
- Infertility (~20%)
- Obesity (~40%)
- Acne (~30%)

*The exact frequencies of the features vary according to the definition of PCOS, the ethnicity of the population and the clinical speciality collecting the data. For example, the frequencies of infertility and hirsutism will be different if the reported data comes from an infertility clinic or from a dermatology clinic.

ovaries on ultrasound scanning. It is very common, affecting some 20% of Caucasian women and being even more common in some ethnic groups e.g. Hispanic Americans or UK Asians. It is considered to arise during puberty and in 40% or so of cases it is associated with obesity. The high prevalence and variation in clinical features suggest that it is not a single disease entity and this may account for the variable endocrine findings in the condition.

Study of this condition is confounded because there is no animal model for PCOS, there is no male equivalent and ultrasound features are only present between the menarche and the menopause making multigenerational genetic studies very difficult. Additionally the ultrasound appearances of polycystic ovaries are found in any condition in which there is hyperandrogenism because androgen excess appears to prevent the final development of follicles (that subsequently form cysts). Thus, PCOS is seen universally in congenital adrenal hyperplasia (*Clinical Case 4.3*).

There are four main theories to explain the causation of PCOS – the adrenal, the ovarian, the pituitary and the metabolic. A role of the adrenal in the etiology of PCOS has been invoked because of the association of PCOS with increased DHEAS (a steroid secreted almost exclusively from the adrenal cortex). In a minority of patients, there is evidence for adrenal hyperandrogenism alone. More often, it is found in combination with excess androgens of ovarian origin. When patients with this syndrome are given tetracosactrin (a synthetic ACTH analog, see *Box 4.20*) or metyrapone (an inhibitor of 11β-hydroxylase which inhibits the final step in cortisol synthesis and hence causes a secondary increase in ACTH secretion, see *Box 4.19*) the increase in DHEAS and androstenedione secretion is higher than that in control subjects. In addition, there is evidence of increased activity of 11β-hydroxysteroid dehydrogenase (the enzyme that breaks down active cortisol into inactive cortisone). This would tend to reduce negative feedback effects, increase ACTH secretion and lead to increased production of adrenal androgens.

The ovarian and pituitary theories are difficult to disentangle because the two glands are functionally linked and because prospective studies of girls developing PCOS at puberty have not been done. It is not known which abnormality develops first. The ovarian hypothesis states that the prime etiology for PCOS is due to an increased capacity of the thecal cells to synthesize androgens. This is seen in ovaries of PCOS patients and thecal cells appear hyperplastic.

There are also clear abnormalities in gonadotrophin secretion. Serum LH concentration and the LH to FSH ratio are both elevated in PCOS patients and these are associated with an increase in the amplitude and frequency of LH pulses and loss of the nocturnal decrease in LH pulse frequency. This may be caused both by an increase in GnRH pulsatility from the hypothalamus and an increased sensitivity of the pituitary gonadotrophs to this neurohormone. Indeed, PCOS patients show an exaggerated LH response to a bolus injection of GnRH. Whilst reduction of endogenous gonadotrophin secretion by pituitary desensitization with a GnRH superagonist lowers circulating testosterone concentrations in patients with PCOS, it is not certain whether abnormalities in gonadotrophin secretion are the primary abnormality.

Many PCOS patients demonstrate insulin resistance that is exacerbated by obesity and the metabolic hypothesis suggests that the hyperandrogenism and the ovarian features of PCOS are the result of this insulin resistance. Indeed insulin resistance and hyperandrogenism are seen in a number of clinical situations, not just PCOS. The fasting serum insulin concentration is inversely related to SHBG concentrations and, thus, the higher the insulin concentration (as occurs in insulin resistance) the higher the free concentrations of circulating androgens. Additionally, in hyperandrogenic women, an acute increase in insulin leads to a rise in circulating testosterone concentrations.

Studies performed on cultured tissue have shown that insulin and the structurally similar insulin-like growth factor (IGF-1) act synergistically with LH to stimulate androgen production by theca-interstitial cells and with FSH to increase aromatase activity and induce LH receptors on granulosa cells. Thus, the pituitary and metabolic theories overlap in the ovary where the effects of insulin and gonadotrophins interact. Within the ovary, it is possible that a vicious cycle occurs in which atretic follicles produce more androgens (because they lack aromatase) and androgens favor further atresia. In the granulosa cells, insulin may sensitize the cells to LH leading to premature luteinization of small follicles and large follicles that are subject to down-regulation by LH.

*Clinical Case 6.9* did not have signs of hirsutism but she had oligomenorrhea and confirmed polycystic ovaries. She had a family history of type 2 diabetes and further investigations showed that she was markedly insulin resistant. Her serum progesterone concentrations in the luteal phase of her cycle showed that she was anovulatory. Over 70% women with PCOS are infertile and over 60% are hyperandrogenic and hirsute.

Hirsutism may be treated by suppressing androgen production or blocking androgen action (*Box 6.51*). Other treatments for PCOS are given in *Box 6.52*. Infertility is the other major problem facing women with PCOS and who, like *Clinical Case 6.9*, wish to conceive. Treatment is aimed at stimulating follicular development.

**Medical†**

| Drug | Use | Advantages | Disadvantages/side effects |
|---|---|---|---|
| Cyproterone‡ acetate | Antiandrogen (also decreases androgen production) | Improves hirsutism (~60%) | Requires contraception |
| Flutamide | Non-steroidal antiandrogen | Improves hirsutism (~50%) | Requires contraception. Occasional but serious hepatotoxicity (<0.5%), photosensitity (~<0.5%) |
| Finasteride | 5α-reductase competitor | Improves hirsutism (~45%) | Contraindicated in pregnancy |
| Ketoconazole§ | Inhibit androgen synthesis | Improves hirsutism (~40%) | Gastrointestinal symptoms, gynecomastia. Teratogenic, so requires contraception |
| Spironolactone | Antiandrogen (also decreases androgen production) | Improves hirsutism (~45%) | Weak antiandrogen. Frequently causes polymenorrhea |
| Eflornithine hydrochloride | Ornithine decarboxylase inhibitor | Topical cream improves hirsutism (~ 50%) by retarding hair growth | Caution in pregnancy |

**Other**

| Technique | Use | Advantages | Disadvantages/side effects |
|---|---|---|---|
| Electrolysis | Local dissolution of follicular epithelium | Effective for limited areas | Expensive, slow, painful, not permanent |
| Laser | Laser light absorbed by follicular eumelanin generates heat | Effective | Expensive, more effective on lighter skins |

*Not including local cosmetic measures (e.g. depilatory creams, plucking, waxing etc.) and also weight loss where this is a factor.
†Most of the clinical trials have not been technically rigorous and the assessments of hair growth neither objective nor blinded to the observer. As a result it is very difficult to compare efficacies of different agents.
‡Used with ethinylestradiol as a contraceptive.
§Regarded by many as too toxic for routine use.

## Contraception

The fertile couple is not a medical problem but, in global terms, contraception has important clinical and social implications not only regarding unwanted pregnancies but also in limiting the birth rate in overcrowded, socially deprived areas throughout the world. In this respect hormonal contraception, first marketed in the early 1960s, has had an important medical impact.

A large number of hormonal contraceptives containing synthetic estrogens and/or progestagens

**Medical[†]**

| Drug | Use | Advantages | Disadvantages/side effects |
|------|-----|------------|----------------------------|
| Antiandrogens e.g. cyproterone acetate | Treat hirsutism | Improves hirsutism | See Box 6.51 |
| Glucocortiocoid steroid e.g. dexamethasone | Decrease adrenal androgen synthesis | Used at night, orally active | Iatrogenic Cushing's possible |
| Estrogen e.g. oral contraceptive | Decrease ovarian androgen synthesis | Orally active | Side effects those of oral contraceptives |
| GnRH analog e.g. leuprolide | Decrease ovarian androgen synthesis | Effective in severely symptomatic | Requires low dose estrogen 'add-back' to avoid the effects of deficiency on bone etc. Expensive |
| Biguanide e.g. metformin | Insulin sensitizer | Improves insulin resistance (see Box 2.34) | Currently not licensed for use in PCOS |
| Thiazolidinedione e.g. rosiglitazone | Insulin sensitizer | Improves insulin resistance (see Box 2.34) | Currently not licensed for use in PCOS |
| Pancreatic lipase[‡] inhibitor e.g. orlistat | Weight loss | ~10 kg weight loss (see Box 2.35) | Currently not licensed for use in PCOS |
| Appetite suppressant[‡] e.g. sibutramine | Weight loss | ~10 kg weight loss (see Box 2.35) | Currently not licensed for use in PCOS |
| Ovulation induction, e.g. clomiphene | Fertility | Orally active | Ovulation induction and pregnancy rates less good in PCOS |

**Surgical**

| Procedure | Use | Advantages | Disadvantages/side effects |
|-----------|-----|------------|----------------------------|
| Laparoscopic ovarian surgery[§] | Clomiphene resistant infertility | Ovulation rates quoted ~80% and pregnancy rates ~50% | Few large-scale controlled trials by which to judge the veracity of claimed efficacy |

*With a prevalence of 20% in Caucasian women and up to 50% in UK Asian women it is clear that many women have the ultrasound appearances of PCO without symptoms requiring therapy.

[†]Treatments for hirsutism are given in Box 6.51

[‡]The clinical benefits of weight loss in obese patients with PCOS are indubitable and since it has many additional benefits it should be recommended as the first-line therapy in these patients.

[§]This includes a variety of techniques – electrocauterization, laser vaporization, multiple biopsies, resection.

are now available and some of the most widely used long-acting and orally active derivatives of estrogen and progesterone are shown in *Box 6.54*. Essentially there are two types of hormonal contraceptive preparations: combination pills in which estrogen and progesterone are either given sequentially, or as biphasic or triphasic combinations and progesterone only preparations which may be administered orally or as depot injections. Most popular today are the biphasic and triphasic oral contraceptives in which a combination of estrogens and progestagens are taken together for 21 days at differential doses which are most likely to resemble hormonal changes throughout the menstrual cycle. During the 7 steroid-free days a withdrawal bleed occurs.

The underlying principle of the combined estrogen/progesterone contraceptives is to suppress ovulation by negative feedback. Additionally, progesterone can exert direct anti-fertility effects on the female genital tract hence inhibiting implantation. Progesterone-only pills, which are taken continuously, or subcutaneous depot injections that release the steroid over a period of 8 weeks to 5 years, work principally by their effect on the cervical mucus and perhaps the endometrium preventing fertilization and implantation. Ovulation is also suppressed in about 20% women taking progesterone-only contraception. Compliance is important for women taking oral progesterone-only contraception because its effects on the cervical mucus only last for about 22–26 hours, after which time fertility returns.

Finally, there are the post-coital contraceptives (inappropriately named 'the morning after pill') in which high doses of estrogenic contraceptives in combination with a progestagen, are given within 72 hours of unprotected sex and in two doses 12 hours apart. Their action is to interfere with the transport and implantation of a possible conceptus.

## Infertility

Couples are considered to be infertile if they have not conceived after a year of unprotected sex. Infertility is related to age. About 4% of couples in their early 20s are infertile with the percentage rising to nearly 20% by their late 30s. In about 35% of these couples the problem is with the female, 35% the male, 20% both partners whilst about 10% have unexplained infertility.

Endocrine causes of infertility are frequently associated with menstrual irregularities. Thus, abnormalities in the basic pattern of menstrual bleeding in the post-pubertal adult is most likely to be due to hormonal disturbances and a consequent loss of ovulation. This can occur at all levels of the hypothalamo-pituitary-ovarian axis. Central disturbances can be induced by environmental changes, physical and emotional stress and extreme weight loss. For example, in anorexia nervosa LH pulsatility reverts to a prepubertal pattern and the LH response to an injection of GnRH is abnormally low. This is indicative of low levels of endogenous GnRH secretion.

High circulating prolactin concentrations e.g. from a pituitary adenoma or during lactation can also suppress ovarian activity as may all causes of hypopituitarism (see *Box 7.9*). There may be insufficient FSH secretion to produce adequate growth and maturation of follicles whilst continuous secretion of LH in the absence of maturing follicles may result in the over-production of androgens leading to amenorrhea and hirsutism. PCOS is the most common causes of anovulatory infertility.

## Ovulation induction and assisted conception

Treatments for infertility caused by endocrine abnormalities are based on simple application of the physiological principles inherent in the control of the hypothalamo-pituitary-gonadal axis. In anovulatory patients with functional ovaries, clomiphene citrate can be used to induce ovulation. The action of this partial estrogen agonist in reducing the negative feed-back of the more potent endogenous estradiol increases LH and FSH secretion. It is of no use in the treatment of primary ovarian failure or pituitary failure. An alternative therapy is with gonadotrophins but these are more complicated and expensive therapies compared

Orally active estrogens and progestagens (highlighted) used in many contraceptive agents

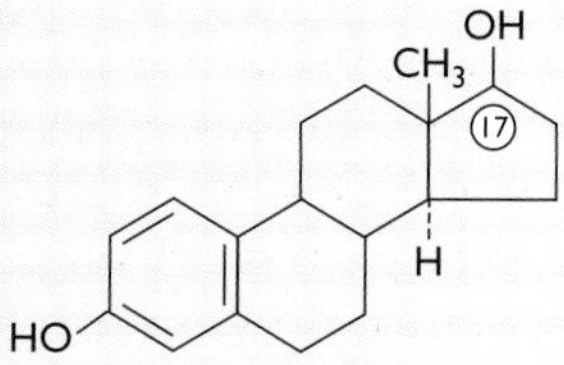

17β-Estradiol

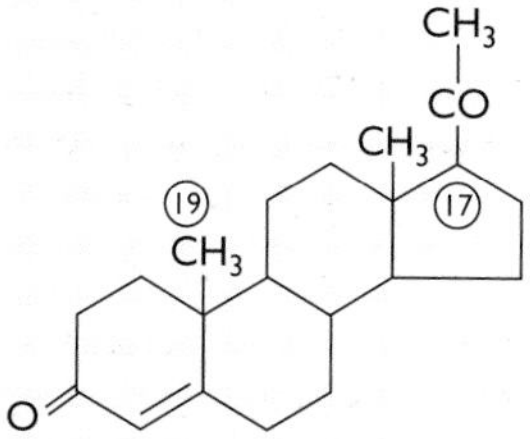

Progesterone

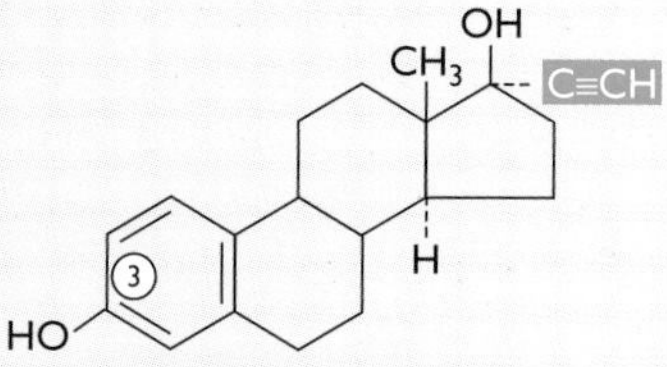

17α-ethinyl estradiol

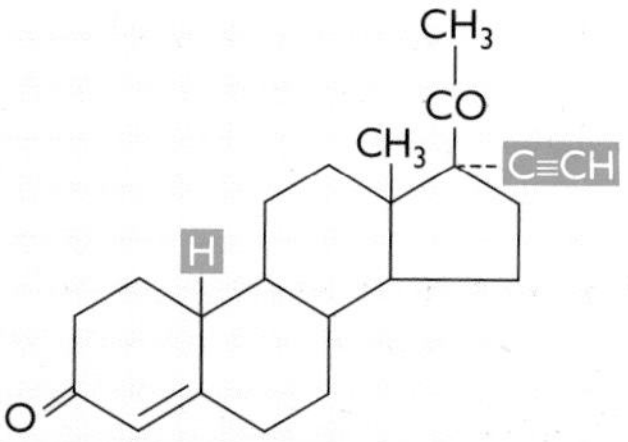

19 Norethinyl progesterone

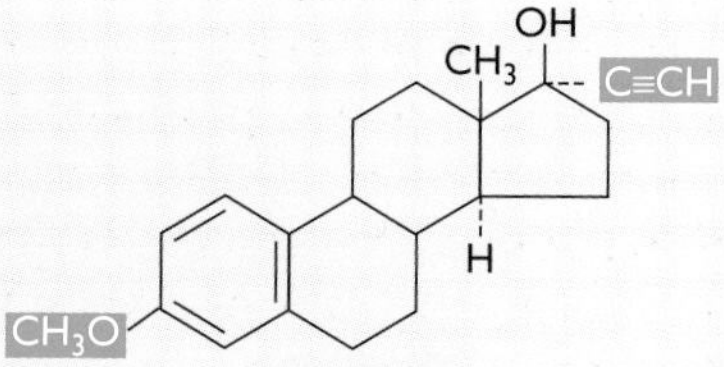

Mestranol

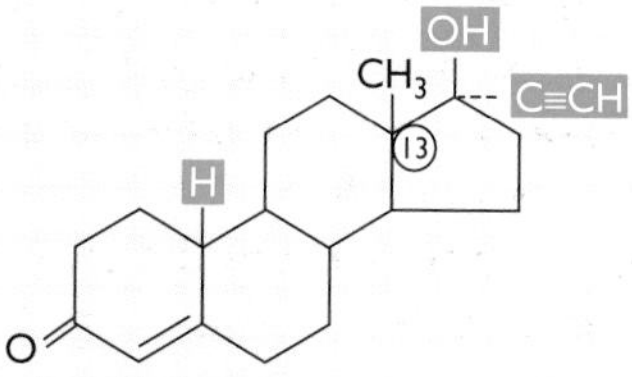

Norethidrone
(19 Nortestosterone)

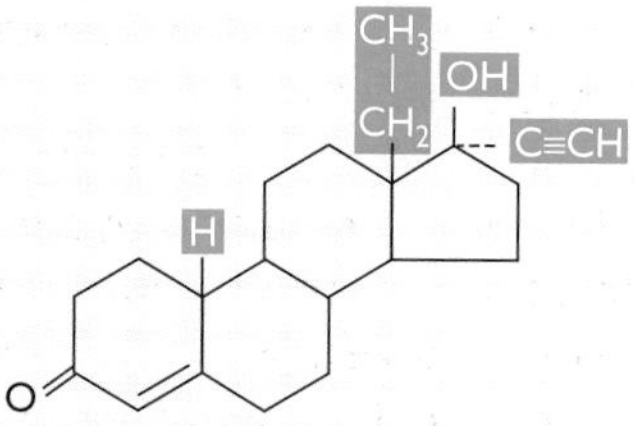

Norgestrel

The addition of an ethinyl group on $C_{17}$ makes estradiol orally active. Mestranol incudes an etherification on $C_3$. Removal of the $C_{19}$ methyl group[*] and addition of an ethinyl group on $C_{17}$ produces an orally active progestagen. Activity is increased by further modifications at $C_{17}$ and replacement of the methyl group with an ethyl group at $C_{13}$.

There are over 30 different combination pills that vary in the relative and absolute amounts of estrogen and progesterone. The estrogen is either ethinyl estradiol or mestranol and the progesterone can be one several types including ethynodiol diacetate, norethidrone, norgestrel, levonorgestrel, desogestrel or norgestimate. Norethindrone is the most widely used in different combined preparations and is also used in the mini-pill.

[*]This leads to a designation with a prefactory nor- in the name.

with clomiphene citrate and have an increased risk of multiple pregnancies.

Until the 1980s, gonadotrophins were exclusively extracted from the urine of menopausal women. First marketed in the 1960s, they contained both LH and FSH activity but subsequently the LH was removed and a 'pure', more effective, FSH product became available. However, demand for gonadotrophin therapy increased and by the 1980s literally hundreds of thousands of liters of urine a day were required to meet demand. Human recombinant FSH is now available for induction of follicular development and recombinant LH is in the final stages of clinical trials.

For the treatment of hypogonadotrophic hypogonadism resulting from hypothalamic dysfunction, pulsatile GnRH therapy using a programmable infusion pump is a more physiologic way of inducing ovulation. Though somewhat cumbersome, patients require less monitoring and ovarian hyperstimulation is less likely to occur than during gonadotrophin therapy.

The development of assisted conception techniques for infertile couples (where considered appropriate) required the developments in embryology of the 1970s. The first baby produced by *in vitro* fertilization was Louise Brown who was born on 25th July, 1978. Today there are a variety of techniques but these procedures are not always available and are not cheap for the patients. Endocrinologically, to obtain eggs for fertilization *in vitro* and subsequent placement into the womb for implantation, the follicular phase of the menstrual cycle must be controlled. The initial stage of treatment is to suppress endogenous gonadotrophin secretion by administering a long-acting GnRH agonist (see *Box 6.11*). As a result of receptor down-regulation, the pituitary gland becomes desensitized and endogenous production of LH and FSH minimal. Treatment with gonadotrophins (either a mixture of LH and FSH, or, more commonly, 'pure' FSH) induces multiple follicular development that is monitored by ultrasound scanning. When the follicles have reached an appropriate stage of maturation (judged by size), hCG is administered (to simulate a natural pre-ovulatory LH surge) and the eggs retrieved for fertilization by aspiration under ultrasound guidance.

# Ovarian failure, the menopause and andropause

## Clinical Case 6.9:

A 25-year-old nurse had attended the endocrine clinic for 4 years with autoimmune Addison's disease and hypothyroidism. She had usually attended annually but had brought forward her appointment, as she had not had a period for 6 months. Her menarche had been at 13 years of age and her periods had been regular with a cycle of 28 ± 4 days. She was not obese and she had taken her hydrocortisone, fludrocortisone and thyroxine replacement regularly. She had herself checked three negative pregnancy tests.

The loss of menstruation has usually signaled pregnancy or the loss of reproductive capability and has been welcomed or hated accordingly. *Clinical Case 6.9* was aware of the potential diagnoses and had sought confirmation. The circulating concentration of estradiol was very low (<37 pmol/l, NR 130–500 pmol/l) and the FSH and LH concentrations were high 67 IU/l (NR 2–9 IU/l) and 58 IU/l (NR 2–9 IU/l) respectively. These results indicated hypergonadotrophic hypogonadism due to ovarian failure and blood was taken for autoantibody studies in view of her pre-existing diagnoses of autoimmune Addison's and Hashimoto's diseases. This confirmed that she had autoantibodies to ovarian tissue (see Website). The diagnosis in this patient was autoimmune ovarian failure and a premature menopause. She was treated with sex steroid replacement. Unlike the situation for *Clinical Case 6.6* (cyclophosphamide induced permanent azoospermia), the implications for fertility for *Clinical Case 6.9* are not so final because of the potential availability of assisted conception and oocyte donation.

The menopause is defined as the cessation of menstruation at the end of a woman's reproductive life. Since menstrual periods may become very irregular perimenopausally, the menopause is operationally defined as the absence of menstruation for a year. A variety of terms is associated with that of the menopause. It has been recommended that the term climacteric be avoided and the term peri-menopause be used for the time both prior to and just after the menopause. The term menopausal transition is used to refer to the period of menstrual cycle irregularity prior to the menopause.

Currently, the mean age of the menopause in the UK is about 53 years and average female life expectancy is 81 years. A woman may thus spend nearly 40% of her life in an estrogen-deficient state. Occasionally, women may undergo a premature menopause (defined as <40 years) as seen in *Clinical Case 6.9*. It occurs because there are no ovarian follicles to develop and secrete estrogen under the influence of gonadotrophins. As a result, there is also no formation of a corpus luteum to secrete progesterone. The lack of female sex steroid hormones normally produced by the ovaries results in a loss of negative feedback and high circulating concentrations of gonadotrophins. The only source of female sex hormones after the menopause comes from the adrenal androgens converted peripherally to estrogens.

The loss of estrogen has several profound effects, not only physically but also psychologically. Some of these symptoms are limited to the peri-menopausal period when a woman is adjusting to the loss of her hormones. Others may become manifest at the menopause but can have serious consequences in the long term. Common symptoms associated with the peri-menopausal period are hot flushes and night sweats, vaginal dryness and depressive episodes. Hot flushes and night sweats affect about 70% of all menopausal women with about 25% seeking medical help due to the severity of symptoms. There is now increasing evidence that estrogens affect blood flow and dilatation of arterioles and thus symptoms linked with altered control of blood flow during estrogen withdrawal are not surprising. Loss of estrogen also leads to the thinning of the vaginal walls and loss of vaginal secretions. This causes vaginal dryness and sexual intercourse may become painful.

Psychological symptoms are often linked with the menopausal years, particular in those women who have a history of depression. To what extent these are due to social changes (e.g. children leaving home, marriage becoming dull) and negative cultural influences (aging and loss of reproductive status and sexuality) are difficult to determine. Nevertheless women do suffer from tiredness, lack of concentration, anxiety, tearfulness and loss of interest in sex.

Bone is severely affected in post-menopausal women so that during 2–5 years after the menopause there is an increased loss of bone mass (see *Box 5.35*). In both men and women, peak bone mass is usually achieved between the ages of 20 and 30 years. Thereafter there is a gradual age-related loss in both sexes. After the withdrawal of estrogens at the menopause, this bone loss is accelerated for several years, thereafter continuing at a similar rate to men. The result of this accelerated bone loss means women are more likely than men to suffer from fractures related to osteoporosis. Common fractures are those of the wrist, hip and spine (vertebrae). Compression fractures of vertebrae can occur without trauma and may cause the loss of several inches in height of an individual. Sex steroid replacement therapy can not only stop this accelerated bone loss but lead to an increase in bone density. When therapy is withdrawn, however, bone loss occurs again at an accelerated rate.

The other major long-term adverse affect of the menopause is on the cardiovascular system. This has been attributed to the metabolic effect of the loss of sex steroids increasing the atherogenic potential of circulating lipids leading to coronary artery disease and stroke. Epidemiologically, before the menopause women appear to be protected against cardiovascular disease by their sex hormones. Observational studies indicate the same is true for women taking HRT. The results of large-scale prospective studies of HRT in the primary prevention of coronary disease are awaited. A recent large prospective study on the effect of combined estrogen and progesterone in secondary prevention of cardiac events in older women with established coronary disease failed to show benefit. After the menopause or after withdrawal of HRT, their risk of developing cardiovascular disease becomes the same as that of men.

Hormone therapy at the menopause has also been suggested in epidemiological studies to reduce cognitive decline, Alzheimer's disease, cataract formation and colon cancer.

Whilst loss of female sex hormones, notably estrogens, do have profound physiological effects, there are clearly cultural influences on the way in which women experience and cope with menopausal symptoms. In Western cultures, social influences on the menopause are largely negative and women are left with the choice of being 'saved' by HRT or becoming old, sexless and a useless member of society. In contrast, in cultures where menopausal women achieve status and social advantages, the reported incidence of menopausal symptoms are often negligible or even absent. For example amongst the Rajput of Northern India, women who are past their menopause are no longer in purdah and are able to move freely within their community. Similarly, the New Zealand Maoris view their post-menopausal years as a relief from child-bearing and thus the menopause is an attribute. Japanese women report a lower frequency of menopausal symptoms compared with American and Canadian women and the same is true for the Navaho Indians. Thus, whilst the menopause can be considered as the beginning of an estrogen-deficient state and will become an increasing health problem as longevity increases, cultural influences can affect the way women experience their menopause.

There is a question as to whether there is an equivalent 'andropause' in men. Testicular function and sperm production continues throughout life although loss of libido, impotence and failure to achieve orgasm do occur with higher frequency at increasing age. Whilst there is some evidence for a decrease in circulating concentrations of free testosterone, there is no evidence of a consequent rise in LH (or FSH) to suggest that this is sensed as abnormal by the hypothalamo–pituitary feedback loop. As a result, although the use of adjunctive androgen replacement therapy has been recommended by some, the 'andropause' cannot be seen in any way as analogous to the cataclysmic fall in female sex steroids that occurs with ovarian failure in all women.

# Hormonal replacement therapy (HRT) and selective estrogen receptor modulators (SERMS)

Hormone replacement therapy may either be taken over a relatively short period of time to alleviate menopausal symptoms, such as hot flushes, or be taken prophylactically for several years or more to offset changes in bone density and cardiovascular risk. It must be noted, however, that when HRT is stopped the same physiological changes that accompany the untreated menopause still occur, but later in life. The time at which HRT should be started to prevent osteoporotic fractures is not known.

The usual estrogenic preparations are conjugated estrogens (glucuronides and sulfates), that are extracted from pregnant mares' urine or synthetic estrogens such as estradiol or estradiol valerate. For women who have not undergone a hysterectomy, these estrogens need to be taken in combination with a progestagen because unopposed estrogen action causes excessive proliferation of the uterine lining and so increase the risk of developing endometrial cancer. The C-21 progesterone derivatives (e.g. medroxyprogesterone) or the C-19 derivatives of nortestosterone (i.e. norethisterone) may be used though they differ slightly in metabolic and androgenic effects. In cyclic HRT preparations, estrogen is given for about 25 days with a progestagen added for the last 10–14 days. A withdrawal bleed occurs.

For those women who object to the cyclic bleeding, continuous estrogens plus a progestagen (e.g. medroxyprogesterone) or a progestagen-impregnated intrauterine coil (Mirena coil containing levonorgestrel) can be used as an alternative. Others may use preparations such as tibolone, a synthetic steroid that has weak estrogenic, androgenic and progestagenic effects. It relieves menopausal symptoms, maintains skeletal integrity and does not cause endometrial hyperplasia.

Estrogens may also be given transdermally (as patches) to avoid the metabolic effects on the liver as they are absorbed from the gut or topically as intravaginal pessary, ring or cream. Progestagens are generally not given if a woman has had a hysterectomy.

Over the last few years there has been debate about HRT safety particularly with regard to the risk of developing breast cancer. In this regard, it has to be borne in mind that, although breast cancer is an emotive subject, the life time risk for the average Caucasian woman is 12% whilst the life time risk of coronary death is 35% and the risk for any osteoporotic fracture is 40%. Statistically, the increased risk is small and it has to be balanced against the adverse cardiovascular and skeletal effects of estrogen deficiency. Absolute contraindications to HRT include undiagnosed vaginal bleeding, active thromboembolic disease and *active* breast or endometrial cancer. Its use in cured breast cancer patients with marked menopausal symptoms remains under discussion. Estrogen use increases thromboembolic disease some 3-fold.

Drugs active at the estrogen receptor such as tamoxifen have been used for some time in the treatment of breast cancer. Around the menopause, this partial estrogen agonist/antagonist stabilizes bone loss and produces estrogen-like changes in plasma lipid profiles but has little, if any, action on breast tissue or the endometrium. It may, however, make vasomotor effects worse in the perimenopausal period. The large trials that established tamoxifen benefit in breast cancer failed to show any cardiovascular benefits. Whilst it has been in use for many years, its mode of action has only recently been understood. It binds the estrogen receptor but prevents the activity of one of the transcription domains on the receptor (*Box 6.54*). Thus, it has partial agonist/antagonist properties and these depend on the target tissue.

There is now intense investigation to develop SERMS, like tamoxifen, that exert selective estrogenic effects (e.g. on bone and plasma lipids) and anti-estrogenic or no effect on tissues where estrogen stimulation may be undesirable (e.g. breast and endometrium). One important current contender is raloxifene that has been shown to reduce fracture risk. The results of large-scale trials in the primary prevention of coronary disease are ongoing.

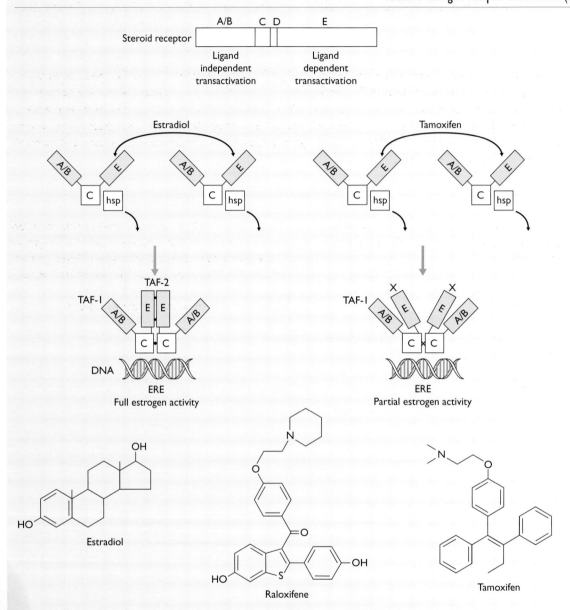

Estradiol

Tamoxifen

Full estrogen activity

Partial estrogen activity

Estradiol

Raloxifene

Tamoxifen

The estrogen receptor has two regions that have a transcriptional activating function (TAF). One in the A/B domain is independent of ligand binding and the other in the E domain is dependent on ligand binding. Estradiol binding induces dimerization of receptors, DNA binding and activation of both TAF-1 and TAF-2 functions. Tamoxifen, which has both agonistic and antagonistic estrogen actions also induces receptor dimerization and DNA binding (pure estrogen antagonists do not) but only TAF-1 is active. Thus, the agonistic/antagonistic potency of tamoxifen depends on the ability of TAF-1 to synergize with other transcription factors that can bind to a promoter. The actions of tamoxifen and raloxifene are both gene and tissue specific.

Abbreviations: ERE, estrogen response element; hsp, heat shock proteins.

# CLINICAL CASE QUESTIONS

The following are examples of applied pathophysiology and these clinically based questions can be answered with the information provided in this chapter. Answers and additional material are available on the website.

---

### Clinical Case Study Q6.1:

A 6-year-old boy of non-consanguinous Pakistani medical parents was brought to the clinic because of pubic hair increasing over the previous 6 months. The only past medical history was of asthma for which he took no regular medication. On examination, he was lean with a blood pressure of 90/50 mmHg. He was Tanner stage 3 for genitalia and pubic hair and stage 1 for axillary hair. He had 3 ml testes bilaterally. It was noted that he was 'needle-phobic' because his brother had had to undergo previous medical treatment (for a different medical condition) requiring multiple infusions.

---

**Question 1:** What are the possible diagnoses? Given his 'needle-phobia', which investigations would you perform initially?

**Question 2:** Which investigations would you perform next?

**Question 3:** What is the likely diagnosis and how would you treat him?

**Question 4:** The growth curve is shown in *Box Q6.1* (see Website). How do you interpret his growth between the ages of 7 and 10.5 years? Which investigations would you perform at the age of 10.5 years?

**Question 5:** How should he be treated?

Clinical Case Study Q6.2:

An otherwise healthy neonate has the external genitalia shown (*Box Q6.3*).

Genitalia of neonate in *Clinical Case Study Q6.2*

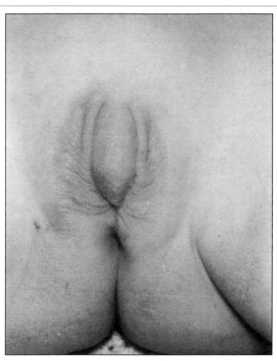

Question 1: What are the possible causes of these appearances and how would you investigate the child?

Question 2: No masses are palpable in the groins. What is the most likely diagnosis and what investigations would you perform?

**Clinical Case Q6.3:**

A 40-year-old man was seen in a psychiatric sexual dysfunction clinic with erectile dysfunction of 2 years duration. He was married and had two children. He drank $1/2$ bottle of wine per week and jogged 2 miles per day. He was noted to have 'small testes', a serum testosterone of 4.8 nmol/l (NR 9–25 nmol/l) and he was treated with intramuscular testosterone esters with symptomatic benefit. After 2 years, he was referred to the Endocrine Clinic because he had developed a rash (erythema multiforme) and a link with his testosterone treatment was suspected.

**Question 1:** He was seen having had no androgen replacement for 3 months. What are the possible endocrine diagnoses and which investigations would you perform?

**Question 2:** Given these results what is the diagnosis and which further investigations would you perform?

**Question 3:** What conclusions would you draw from these results and which further investigations would you perform?

**Question 4:** How should he be treated?

## CHAPTER 7

# The pituitary gland

## Chapter objectives

*Knowledge of*

1. Anatomical and functional connections of the hypothalamo-pituitary axis
2. Causes of hypopituitarism, their investigation and treatment
3. Control of post-natal growth and its abnormalities
4. Pathophysiology of pituitary adenomas and their treatment
5. Regulation of circadian rhythms
6. Pathophysiology of obesity
7. Physiological regulation of water balance

> *"'Do you know who made you?'*
> *'Nobody as I knows on,' said the child, with a short*
> *laugh … 'I 'spect I grow'd'."*
> *Uncle Tom's Cabin, Harriet Beecher Stowe.*

The pituitary gland sits below the brain in a midline pocket or fossa of the sphenoid bone known as the sella turcica, imaginatively named by anatomists because of its likeness to a Turkish horse saddle. Embryologically, anatomically and functionally the human gland is divided into two lobes. The anterior lobe constitutes two thirds of the volume of the gland and the posterior lobe one third. As with all other endocrine glands, symptoms arise as the result of either hypo- or hypersecretion of hormones.

## Clinical Case 7.1:

The Neurosurgeons referred a 31-year-old man to the Endocrine team. Until some 3 years previously, he had been an international level canoeist but his abilities began to deteriorate gradually, despite the attentions of his coach. He fell from the national rankings. He only came to medical attention because as a computer programmer he had noted deteriorating visual acuity.

An optician reported a bitemporal field defect and recommended neurosurgical referral. MR scan showed a large suprasellar tumor (*Box 7.1*) that was removed by transsphenoidal surgery. Histologically, it was reported to be a craniopharyngioma. On post-operative examination, he was found to be grossly hypothyroid and hypogonadal and these were confirmed using biochemical tests. His serum free T$_4$ was 4 pmol/l (NR 10–24 pmol/l), TSH 0.9 mU/l (NR 0.5–4.0 mU/l) and testosterone <0.5 nmol/l (NR 9–25 nmol/l).

The clinical features of secondary hypothyroidism and hypogonadism are discussed in detail elsewhere, but to understand the clinical presentation of this particular case requires knowledge of both the anatomy and the embryology of the pituitary gland.

## Anatomical and functional connections of the hypothalamo-pituitary axis

The posterior part of the pituitary gland (the neural lobe or neurohypophysis) is embryologically and

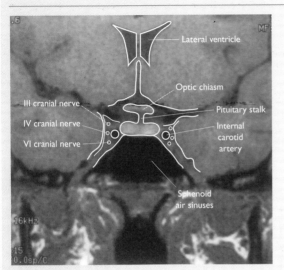

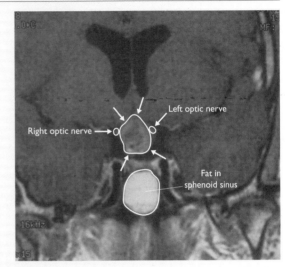

Coronal scans

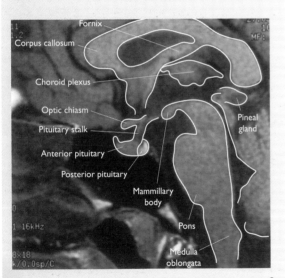

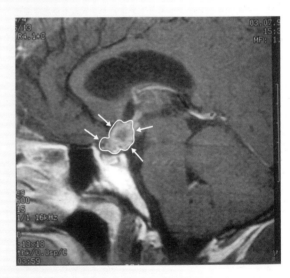

Sagittal scans

Coronal and sagittal scans of *Clinical Case 7.1* are shown with normal scans for comparison. For clarity, anatomical features have been marked on the normal scans.

The large craniopharyngioma causing a bitemporal hemianopia and hypopituitarism is clearly shown (arrowed).

Note that on the coronal scan of the patient in *Clinical Case 7.1* the fat within the sphenoid sinus shows up as a bright ('high signal intensity') area that draws the eye but is a normal finding.

These images are available on the Website.

anatomically continuous with the hypothalamus, an area of gray matter in the basal part of the forebrain surrounding the third ventricle (*Box 7.2*). Neurons in the hypothalamus project directly to the posterior pituitary gland and approximately 100 000 axons form the hypophyseal nerve tract (*Box 7.3*). The posterior pituitary gland is thus formed from axons and nerve terminals of hypothalamic neurons; hormones stored in the terminals are released into the general circulation in response to electrical excitation. Surrounding the nerve terminals are modified astrocytes known as pituicytes and these cells appear to have an important role in the local control of hormone release.

The anterior lobe (or adenohypophysis) is anatomically distinct from the hypothalamus (*Box 7.2*) and consists of a collection of endocrine cells. Originally three different cell-types were identified according to their ability to take up general histological stains; these were chromophobes, acidophils and basophils (*Box 7.4*). Newer immunohistochemical techniques allow classification of cells by their specific secretory products. About 50% of adenohypophyseal secretory cells are somatotrophs (synthesizing somatotrophin or GH), 10–25% lactotrophs (making prolactin), 15–20% corticotrophs (ACTH), 10–15% gonadotrophs (LH and FSH), and 3–5% thyrotrophs (TSH). Some cells, usually chromophobes, do not stain with any of the antibodies to the various anterior pituitary hormones although electron microscopy reveals that these cells contain secretory granules.

Whilst the anterior pituitary gland is not anatomically connected with the hypothalamus, it is functionally connected with this part of the brain (*Box 7.3*). Nerve cells in the hypothalamus secrete neurohormones that, via a system of hypophyseal portal vessels in the median eminence, act on the endocrine cells of the anterior lobe to stimulate or inhibit their synthesis and secretion.

Within the hypothalamus, there are discrete groups of nerve cells, termed nuclei, arranged bilaterally around the third ventricle (*Box 7.5*). Those concerned with hormone secretions from the pituitary gland tend to be distributed more medially whilst those concerned with autonomic functions, such as temperature regulation, food intake and satiety and sympathetic stimulation of adrenomedullary secretions, tend to be located more laterally.

The pituitary gland maintains its anatomical and functional connections with the brain yet sits outside the blood–brain barrier (*Box 7.5*). The anterior part of the sella turcica is the tuberculum sellae which is flanked by wing-like projections of the sphenoid bone known as the anterior clinoid processes. The posterior part, known as the dorsum sellae, is flanked by the posterior clinoid processes. These clinoid processes are the points of attachment of the diaphragma sellae, a reflection of the dura mater surrounding the brain. In this way, the entire pituitary gland is surrounded by dura such that the arachnoid membrane, and thus the cerebrospinal fluid, cannot enter the sella turcica.

As a whole, the hypothalamus is bound rostrally (towards the nose) by the optic chiasm, caudally by the mammillary bodies, laterally by the optic tracts and dorsolaterally by the thalamus. Clinically, (and demonstrated by *Clinical Case 7.1*), it is noteworthy that the optic chiasm lies about 5 mm above the diaphragm sellae and anterior to the pituitary stalk, though there is some anatomical variability. Thus, it is clear that any mass lesion of sufficient size in the area of the pituitary gland will cause visual field defects. The tumor in *Clinical Case 7.1* was a craniopharyngioma and an understanding of the origin of this tumor requires more detailed knowledge of the embryology of the pituitary gland.

## Embryology of the pituitary gland

The anterior lobe of the gland develops from an evagination of ectodermal cells of the oropharynx in the primitive gut and its anlage is recognizable at 4–5 weeks gestation. The evagination is known as Rathke's pouch (*Boxes 3.21 and 7.2*) and it is eventually pinched off from the oral cavity and becomes separated by the sphenoid bone of the skull. The lumen of the pouch is reduced to a small cleft whilst the upper portion of the pouch surrounds the neural stalk and forms the pars tuberalis. This, together with the anterior lobe, is called

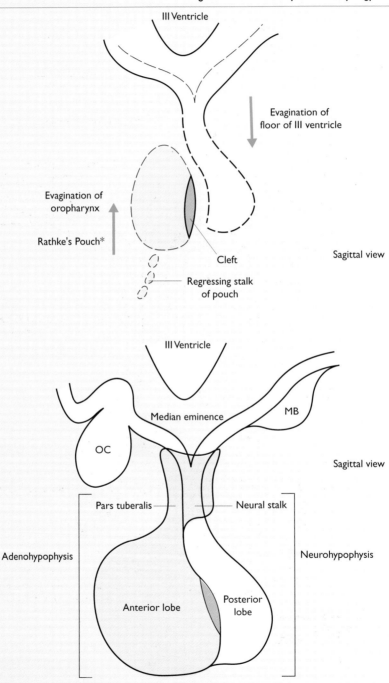

III Ventricle

Evagination of
floor of III ventricle

Evagination of
oropharynx

Rathke's Pouch*

Cleft

Sagittal view

Regressing stalk
of pouch

III Ventricle

Median eminence

MB

OC

Sagittal view

Pars tuberalis — Neural stalk

Adenohypophysis

Neurohypophysis

Anterior lobe

Posterior
lobe

Abbreviations: MB, mammillary body; OC, optic chiasm
*Originating from pharyngeal endoderm (see Box 3.21)

Anatomy of the functional connections between the hypothalamus and pituitary gland

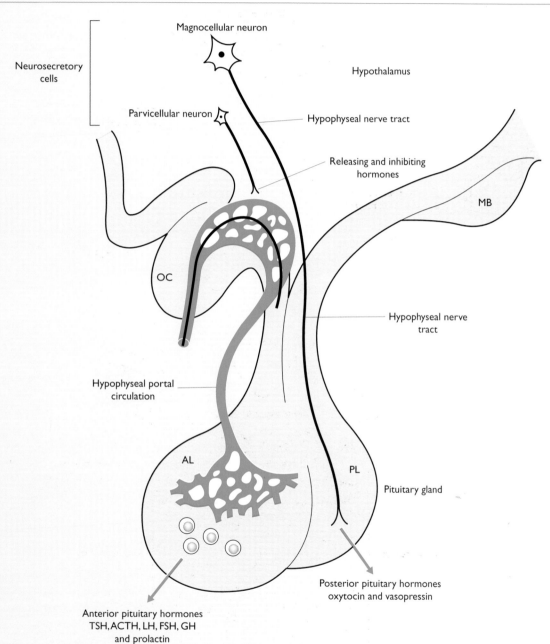

Neurosecretory cells

Magnocellular neuron

Hypothalamus

Parvicellular neuron

Hypophyseal nerve tract

Releasing and inhibiting hormones

MB

OC

Hypophyseal nerve tract

Hypophyseal portal circulation

AL

PL

Pituitary gland

Posterior pituitary hormones oxytocin and vasopressin

Anterior pituitary hormones TSH, ACTH, LH, FSH, GH and prolactin

Abbreviations: AL, anterior lobe; PL, posterior lobe; OC, optic chiasm; MB, mammillary body

Box 7.4:

Hormone secretions of the anterior lobe of the pituitary gland and their control

| Cell type | Hormone | % Pituitary cell population | Hypothalamic hormone | Predominant hypothalamic nucleus of synthesis |
|---|---|---|---|---|
| Thyrotroph[†] | TSH | 3–5% | TRH (+) Somatostatin (–) | Paraventricular, anterior periventricular |
| Corticotroph[†] | ACTH | 15–20% | CRH (+) Vasopressin (augments CRH) | Paraventricular, supraoptic |
| Gonadotroph[†] | LH FSH | 10–15% | GnRH (+) | Arcuate |
| Somatotroph[*] | GH | 40–50% | GHRH (+) Somatostatin (–) | Arcuate, anterior periventricular |
| Lactotroph[*] | Prolactin | 10–25% | Dopamine (–) TRH (+) PRF's (+) | Arcuate, paraventricular, unknown |

[†]Basophils – stain with basic dyes
[*]Acidophils – stain with acidic dyes
(+), stimulatory; (–), inhibitory

the adenohypophysis. When some cells from Rathke's pouch are left behind, forming tumors, these are craniopharyngiomas.

The posterior lobe develops from neural crest cells as a downward evagination of the floor of the third ventricle of the brain (*Box 7.2*). The lumen of this pouch closes as the sides fuse to form the neural stalk while the upper portion of the pouch forms a recess in the floor of the third ventricle known as the median eminence. The neural stalk together with the median eminence form the infundibular stem and this, together with the posterior lobe, is collectively termed the neurohypophysis.

The cleft-like remnant of Rathke's pouch demarcates the boundary between the anterior and posterior lobes of the pituitary gland. In some animals, but not in humans, cells in this area form an anatomically distinct intermediate lobe and secrete a hormone (melanocyte-stimulating hormone, MSH) that stimulates melanocytes in the skin and,

thus, alters skin color (see *Box 4.30*). In humans, these cells become interspersed with cells of the anterior pituitary gland and secrete hormones derived from pro-opiomelanocortin, notably ACTH. The hypothalamo-pituitary axis is established by 20 weeks gestation and in the adult the gland weighs 500–900 mg and measures about $15 \times 10 \times 16$ mm.

Pituitary morphogenesis and the development of different cell types involves a number of genes that code for transcription factors and their sequential expression is now known to be crucial. They involve the sequential expression of at least five homeobox genes and also the actions of a number of inductive signals from the diencephalon (*Box 7.6*).

## Craniopharyngioma

The size of the craniopharyngioma of *Clinical Case 7.1* produced damage to the anterior pituitary

Diagram of the anatomy of the hypothalamo-pituitary axis showing the major hypothalamic nuclei and the pituitary gland, enclosed in dura mater, sitting within the sella turcica and outside the blood—brain barrier

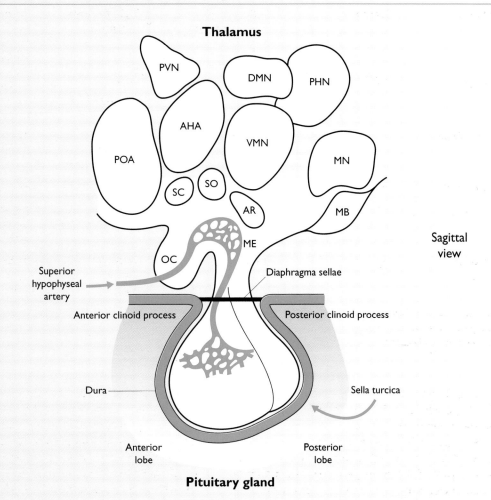

Abbreviations: AHA, anterior hypothalamic area; AR, arcuate nucleus; DMN, dorsomedial nucleus; MB, mammillary body; ME, median eminence; MN, medial nucleus; OC, optic chiasm; PHN, posterior hypothalamic nucleus; POA, preoptic area; PVN, paraventricular nucleus; SCN, suprachiasmatic nucleus; SO, supraoptic nucleus; VMN, ventromedial nucleus.

gland and the optic chiasm. Such tumors are rare with only a few hundred cases in the UK presenting each year, and usually in patients under the age of 20 years. They are nearly always cystic (sometimes lobulated) and filled with oily green fluid that has a characteristic appearance on MR scan. They may also calcify and appear as suprasellar calcification on a plain skull X-ray. There is some normal anatomical variability in the position of the optic chiasm (*Box 7.7*) and it is clear that the clinical presentation of such tumors depends on local anatomy and the structures damaged. For example,

Box 7.6:
Transcription factors involved in pituitary gland development[*]

**Pit-1** – termed POU1F1 in newer terminology.
- Expression begins about the 14th day of fetal development (in the mouse) and continues throughout life.
- Activates transcription by forming dimers with a number of other transcription factors including Zn-15, HESX-1, P-Lim and also the thyroid hormone, estrogen and retinoic acid receptor.
- Activates transcription from the GH, prolactin and β-TSH and Pit-1 promoters.
- Loss of function mutations affecting Pit-1 in humans and mice (Snell and Jackson dwarf mice) causes loss of somatotrophs, lactotrophs and thyrotrophs

**PROP-1** – name derived from 'prophet of Pit-1' indicating that the gene product is required for Pit-1 expression.
- Expression begins at embryonic day 10.5 in the mouse and is reduced by day 14.
- PROP-1 binds as a dimer to affect transcription.
- Loss of function mutations in the mouse (Ames dwarf) results in lack of GH, prolactin and TSH. Those in the human result in additional deficiencies of LH and FSH.

**HESX-1** – named to denote a 'homeobox gene expressed in embryonic stem cells' but also called Rpx for 'Rathke's pouch homeobox' gene
- Expression begins before that of PROP-1 and is more widespread. Expressed in cells that become Rathke's pouch and in the precursors of all pituitary cell types.
- Important in the development of the optic nerves.
- Mice with HESX-1 knock-out have microphthalmia (small eyes), abnormalities of the corpus callosum and septum pellucidum and small pituitary glands. Patients with loss of function mutations have clinical features of septo-optic dysplasia.

**TTF-1** – homeodomain thyroid transcription factor-1.
- Normally expressed in the brain and posterior pituitary gland.
- Targeted disruption in mice leads to pituitary gland aplasia; a role in inducing Rathke's pouch has been suggested

**LHX3 and LHX4** – Lim class homeodomain transcription factors
- LHX3 is involved in the early development of Rathke's pouch which forms but fails to thicken in the absence of LHX3.
- Lack of LHX4 in mice leads to mild hypopituitarism with a marked reduction in the numbers of lactotrophs and somatotroph cells.

[*]Pit-1 and PROP-1 mutations account for a large proportion of the familial cases of multiple pituitary hormone deficiencies.

occasionally tumors extend into the cavernous sinuses and damage eye movements due to palsy of the left 3rd (occulomotor), 4th (trochlear) or 6th (abducens) cranial nerves (see *Clinical Case 7.4*).

The usual treatment for craniopharyngiomas is surgical with post-operative radiotherapy recommended for any residual tumor. Medical treatment involves the replacement of missing hormones. The role of the adenohypophysis in regulating the

functions of the various endocrine organs is discussed in Chapters 3, 4 and 6.

In most circumstances, it is not the trophic anterior pituitary gland hormones that are replaced but those of the target tissues. Thus, thyroxine (not TSH), hydrocortisone (not ACTH), testosterone (not LH) were given to *Clinical Case 7.1* with improvement in his symptoms. However, when seen in the out-patient department at follow-up it was noted

Diagram to illustrate the normal variation in the position of the optic chiasm (OC) relative to that of the pituitary gland

Optic nerve

Prefixed        Normal        Postfixed

that since initiating endocrine replacement he had started to pass large volumes of urine and to complain of intense thirst. In addition, he was always lacking energy and, although he could keep up with a full-time sedentary job, he went to bed early at about 9 p.m. and had virtually no social life. The pathophysiological explanation for the appearance of these new symptoms is explored in more detail on page 327.

## Blood supply of the hypothalamo-pituitary axis

The importance of the blood supply of the axis is demonstrated by the next clinical case of Sheehan's syndrome.

### Clinical Case 7.2

A 26-year-old Afro-Caribbean woman had given birth to a 3.8 kg baby boy at 39 weeks gestation. Though the antenatal progress had been unremarkable, the delivery had been difficult, necessitating the use of obstetric forceps and complicated by a very large post-partum hemorrhage. As a Jehovah's Witness she had refused blood transfusion and, since bleeding

continued and despite all other measures, she had required an emergency hysterectomy. Several times during the operation her systolic blood pressure had been measured at 50 mm Hg. The post-operative period had been complicated by a transient period of renal failure but after a further 2 weeks she was discharged. She bottle fed her son because she had failed to lactate. Her 6 week postnatal assessment had been unnoteworthy but 3 months later she was referred to the Endocrine team as she had developed hot flushes.

The blood supply to the hypothalamo-pituitary axis is complex but defines the functional relationship between the hypothalamus and adenohypophysis. Any interruption of blood flow impairs the hypothalamic control of adenohypophyseal secretions. The hypothalamus receives its blood supply from the circle of Willis whilst the neurohypophysis and adenohypophysis receive blood from the inferior and superior hypophyseal arteries respectively (Box 7.8). The capillary plexus of the inferior hypophyseal artery drains into the dural sinus although some of these capillaries in the neural stalk form 'short' portal veins that drain into the anterior pituitary gland.

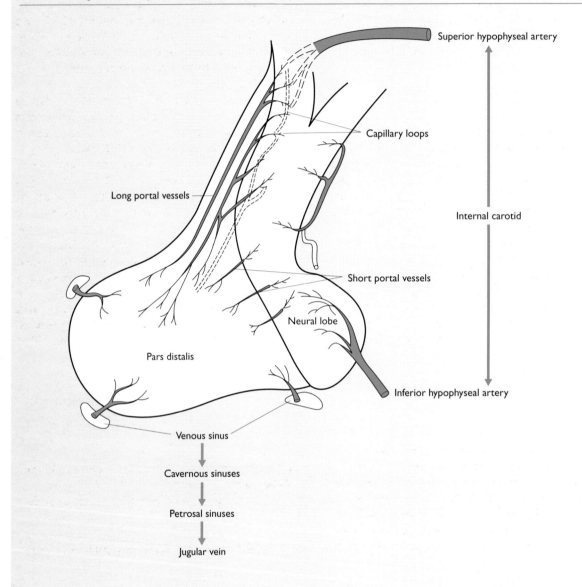

Diagrammatic representation of the blood supply and venous drainage of the median eminence and pituitary gland

Superior hypophyseal artery

Capillary loops

Long portal vessels

Internal carotid

Short portal vessels

Neural lobe

Pars distalis

Inferior hypophyseal artery

Venous sinus

Cavernous sinuses

Petrosal sinuses

Jugular vein

This constitutes only a small fraction of the circulation of the anterior lobe, which is one of the best vascularized mammalian tissues. The major portion of the circulation arises from the 'long' portal veins. These are formed from the capillary network of the superior hypophyseal arteries that invest the nerve endings of the neurosecretory cells in the median eminence. Thus, the hypothalamic releasing and inhibiting hormones are released into these hypophyseal portal veins, through which they are transported to the endocrine cells of the anterior pituitary lobe. Here, the portal veins form a secondary capillary network into which the hormones of the anterior pituitary are secreted. The capillaries in the hypophyseal portal system are fenestrated improving the delivery of hormones to the adenohypophyseal cells. The venous channels from the anterior pituitary gland drain into the cavernous sinuses and, thence, into the superior and inferior petrosal sinuses and into the jugular vein (*Box 7.8*).

# Sheehan's syndrome

During pregnancy, there is an approximately 50% increase in the volume of the pituitary gland. This is primarily due to hyperplasia of the lactotrophs that secrete prolactin to prepare the breasts for lactation. Thus, whilst the volume of the pituitary increases, the fossa in which the pituitary gland sits does not increase to accommodate this growth. A sudden fall in blood pressure after an event such as a post-partum hemorrhage causes ischemia of the gland, cellular damage and edema. In turn, the edema results in swelling of the pituitary gland (which is already enlarged by the lactotroph hyperplasia) further restricting the normal blood flow to the gland. The result is an infarct in the gland that causes loss of its secretions. This is initially manifest by failure of lactation (lack of prolactin) and amenorrhea (loss of gonadotrophins) but may also variably demonstrate hypothyroidism (TSH) and hypoadrenalism (ACTH). This has been termed Sheehan's syndrome and, it is to be emphasized, improvements in routine obstetric care have rendered it very rare.

Three important clinical observations may be made. The first is that destructive lesions of the pituitary gland, whether they be due to a tumor, infarct, radiotherapy or, indeed, basal meningitis (*Box 7.9*) all have similar effects. They reduce secretions from the anterior pituitary gland leading to hypopituitarism (the severity of which depends on the lesion). The second is that the sequence of the loss of trophic hormones due to progressive lesions tends to be the same. Thus, somatotrophin-secreting cells are lost first, then gonadotrophs, whilst thyrotrophs seem to survive till last. The third is that such lesions rarely cause a deficiency of the posterior pituitary hormone secretions, oxytocin and arginine vasopressin (AVP). Indeed, it is to be emphasized that the polyuria and intense thirst

---

**Box 7.9:**
Causes of pituitary failure*

**Developmental abnormalitites** – These include:
- Holoprosencephaly – abnormal development of the embryonic forebrain resulting in hypothalamic abnormalities and facial dysmorphism e.g. cleft palate, hypertelorism (widely spaced eyes), absent nasal septum.
- Septo-optic dysplasia – hypoplasia or absence of the optic chiasm, optic nerves or both, agenesis or hypoplasia of the septum pelluciudum, corpus callosum or both.
- Transcription factor mutations – e.g. Pit-1 (see *Box 7.6*).
- 'Idiopathic' hypopituitarism – often associated with abnormalities on MR scan including ectopic or hypoplastic pituitary glands.

**Other**
- Trauma (see *Clinical Case 4.6*)
- Inflammation – bacterial, viral or fungal infections of the base of the brain.
- Infiltrative disease – e.g. sarcoidosis (see *Clinical Case 7.7*), Langerhans cell histiocytosis.
- Tumors of the brain or hypothalamus – e.g. meningiomas, germinomas, gliomas (see *Clinical Case 7.6*).
- Radiation of the brain and hypothalamus – effects depend on the age at irradiation, the dose and the degree to which it is fractionated (and to some extent the sex of the patient).
- Tumors of the pituitary gland (see *Clinical Case 7.5*)

*It may be difficult to distinguish damage to the hypothalamus from that to the pituitary gland. All are rare.

seen in *Clinical Case 7.1* resulting from a deficiency of AVP (causing diabetes insipidus, see below) was related to damage to the neural stalk or the hypothalamus and *not* to the posterior pituitary gland.

Clinical Cases *7.1* and *7.2* illustrate how lesions of the pituitary gland cause loss of several hormone secretions. There are also diseases in which there is a deficiency of a single anterior pituitary hormone. One of the most common is a relative lack (or insufficiency) or complete deficiency of somatotrophin or growth hormone (GH), affecting approximately 1 in 4000 live births. This may be caused either by a failure in the hypothalamic control mechanisms or by a defect in the pituitary gland.

# Growth and somatotrophin deficiency

## Clinical Case 7.3:

A 2-year-old boy was referred to the general Pediatric clinic because of 'failure to thrive'. He had been born weighing 2.79 kg after a normal pregnancy and delivery. Developmental milestones (such as the age of speaking and walking) were normal. Both parents were about the 25th centile for height. In the clinic, he was noted to be short (well below the 3rd centile, but also dysmorphic with a short body (sitting height SDS −5, subischeal leg length SDS −2). (*Box 7.10*). He weighed 10.03 kg (3rd centile). He was noted to be kyphotic with a short neck. X-rays revealed shortening of the cervical spine but MR imaging of the spine was normal. An endocrine cause of his short stature was thought unlikely. Review of his clinical appearance and the radiological findings by clinical geneticists failed to suggest an underlying diagnosis. One year later, he was referred to the Pediatric Endocrine clinic for the very practical reason that he was too short to use the toilets at his nursery school. He was indeed very short (*Box 7.12*) and the skeletal disproportion still present.

The young boy in this case was initially referred with 'failure to thrive', a term generally used for

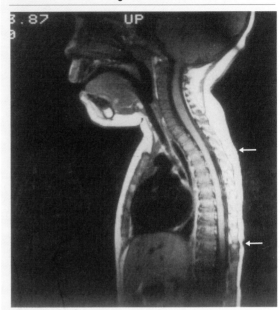

Note the short thorax (arrowed), a major factor in his short spine.

children under the age of 2 years who are failing to put on weight (i.e. lean for their height). To interpret this case it is necessary to understand the use of growth charts (*Boxes 7.11* and *7.12*). As can be seen from the charts, at initial presentation he was nearer the 3rd centile for weight than he was the 3rd centile for height. Thus, he was not failing to thrive, he was failing to grow. With parents on the 25th centile, he would have been expected, all other things being equal, also to grow along that line.

The fastest relative growth rates occur in embryonic and fetal life when a single fertilized ovum progresses, as in this case, to 2.79 kg of live baby after 40 weeks. This represents an increase in fetal mass of about $44 \times 10^7$ fold whilst length increases 3850-fold. Post-natal growth never matches this with only a 20-fold increase in mass and 3–4-fold increase in length. In early childhood, there is a period of rapid growth followed by a period of steady growth with a mid-childhood acceleration, a pubertal growth spurt and a phase of deceleration to final height. In the involutionary years, there is

- The growth of a child is multifactorial and complex but, fortunately, predictable. Postnatal growth is rapid in infancy (~15 cm/year rapidly decelerating at age 3 years), a childhood rate of about 6 cm/year (with an adolescent deceleration), followed by a pubertal growth spurt.

- Evaluation of a child's growth is made using cross-sectional and longitudinal standards derived from the normal population. Carefully documented and accurate auxological data obtained using an appropriate calibrated stadiometer are invaluable. The most frequently used charts are for height and weight though additional charts for height velocity are available. Charts for patients with clinical conditions associated with deficient growth such as achondroplasia or Turner's syndrome (gonadal agenesis) are also available.

- Some disorders give rise to disproportionate growth (as was seen in *Clinical Case 7.3*). This can be assessed using charts for sitting height and lower body segment length.

- Since genetic factors are very important in determining final height, parental heights should also be plotted. Generally, a child can be expected to reach mid-parental height ± 6.5 cm. Deviation from the growth patterns of parents or sibs is a reason for investigation of an underlying cause.

- Adult final height may be empirically (and approximately) calculated by consideration of chronological age, parental heights and the degree of skeletal maturity. The latter is referred to as the 'bone age' and is best determined by an experienced user of the method of Tanner & Whitehouse from an X-ray of the left hand and wrist.

a period of shrinkage, reflecting the changes of spinal shortening.

Intrauterine growth is regulated by endocrine, maternal and genetic factors, though the determinants of prenatal growth are poorly understood. Fetal plasma GH concentrations are very high and yet infants with GH hormone deficiency, and even those with anencephaly, may have normal body length at birth. Loss of human chorionic somatotrophin (hCS) secreted by the placenta (see below) does not appear to affect intrauterine growth. Mothers lacking the hCS gene have given birth to infants of normal birth weight. In contrast, excessive serum insulin may be associated with increased length in infants of diabetic mothers (see *Clinical Case 2.3*). The related insulin-like growth factors (IGFs) are also important in fetal growth (see *Box 7.19*) and, though their precise role is not established, when IGF-1 is lacking (e.g. Laron dwarfs) the reports of birth length show a wide variability, including normality, suggesting that IGF-1 is not a major factor.

Maternal (intrauterine) influences have been difficult to define but poor maternal nutrition is the most important factor leading to low birth weight and length world-wide (*Box 7.13*). Maternal alcohol ingestion and smoking are other adverse factors on fetal growth, and maternal infections such as rubella, toxoplasmosis and cytomegalovirus lead to many abnormalities, as well as short stature. Congenital HIV infection also retards fetal growth. Intrauterine growth retardation (IUGR) is usually defined as a birth weight of less that the 10th percentile for gestational age but of these about 10% are not truly abnormal.

## Growth hormone – secretory patterns and control

Growth hormone or somatotrophin is a single chain polypeptide containing 191 amino acids, two disulfide bridges and four helical structures (*Box 7.14*). The position of the helices and the three-dimensional structure of this hormone are important for binding to its receptor. It shares structural homologies with prolactin and hCS, the latter being a GH variant synthesized exclusively in the placenta. There is a cluster of five genes from which these polypeptide hormones may be synthesized although normally there is a tissue-specific expression of only one gene. The binding of the tissue-specific transcription factor Pit-1 (*Box 7.6*) to the promoter region of the GH gene results in only one form of GH being secreted by the anterior pituitary gland.

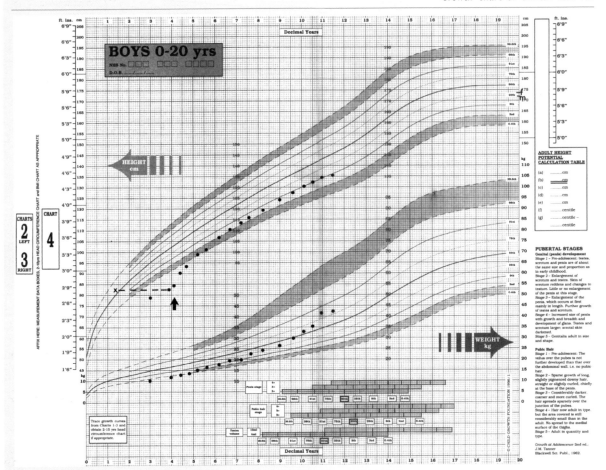

- Age is plotted on the horizontal (X) axis.
- Two sets of normal data are plotted. Height (the upper set of curves) is plotted on the left-hand vertical (Y) axis and weight (the lower set of curves) on the right-hand Y-axis. The curves are centiles of the normal population (thus, the 50th centile is average since 50% of the population lie above it and 50% below it).
- The bottom bar-plots allow the Tanner stages of puberty to be plotted.
- Parental heights are plotted on the right-hand axis (f = father's actual height and m = mother's height 'corrected' for the mean difference between the sexes).
- Measurements of height and weight are plotted as dots (enlarged in his case for visibility) against chronological age (which is decimalized).
- Bone age calculated from Tanner-Whitehouse data for X-rays of the left hand and wrist is plotted as an X with an interrupted line connecting to the chronological age to which it refers.
- There are three observations before the arrow that marks the onset of growth hormone therapy. Note the marked discrepancy between chronological age (~3.9 years) and bone age (~1.4 years, termed bone age 'delay'). This is characteristic of GH deficiency as is the tendency for weight to be relatively more normal than height.
- Growth rate is visible as the slope of the lines plotted. It is clear that GH therapy led to a marked increase in growth velocity, termed 'catch-up' growth. In *Clinical Case 7.3*, this is somewhat unusual in being manifest as 'crossing centiles' some 6 years after starting treatment.

**Common (~90%)**
- Genetic short stature – includes normal children born to normal short parents.
- Intrauterine growth retardation – approximately 2% of infants are small for gestational age. This results from a number of possible factors including those affecting the fetus (e.g. congenital abnormalities), the placenta (e.g. vascular insufficiency) or the mother (e.g. hypertension).
- Malnutrition – a common cause in developing countries.
- Constitutional delay – a term used to describe short but otherwise normal children with a delay in growth and pubertal development. By definition, examination and investigations are normal. Males fail to achieve Tanner stage G2 by 14 years and girls B2 by 13 years (see *Box 6.19*). Bone age is also delayed.

**Uncommon (~10%)**
- Chromosomal abnormalities – includes Trisomy 21 (Down's syndrome, 1 in 600 births), 45X0 (Turner's syndrome see *Box 6.49*),
- Chronic disease – malabsorption (e.g. celiac disease), renal failure, liver disease, congenital heart disease, chronic anemia (e.g. sickle cell disease), pulmonary disease (e.g. cystic fibrosis), infection (e.g. HIV).
- Endocrine – includes hypothyroidism (see *Clinical Case 3.3*).

**Rare (<1%)**
- Osteochondrodysplasia – a group of more than 100 individually rare inherited conditions giving rise to abnormalities in the size and shape of bones.
- Endocrine – Cushing's syndrome, pseudohypoparathyroidism, rickets (see *Clinical Case 5.5*), GH deficiency, GH insensitivity

*These are often divided into those that are primary i.e. due to a defect in the growth plates themselves and those that are secondary to a chronic disease.

Classically, the synthesis and secretion of GH has been thought to be controlled by two hypothalamic neurohormones; growth hormone-releasing hormone (GHRH) that is stimulatory and somatostatin that is inhibitory of GH secretion (*Box 7.15*). However, the view that only two hormones are involved in the control of GH secretion has been challenged by the finding of another hormone, ghrelin, that also causes GH release (*Box 7.16*). In the human hypothalamus, both the 40 and 44 amino acid forms of GHRH are synthesized and secreted by neurosecretory neurons whose cell bodies predominantly reside in the arcuate nucleus of the hypothalamus (*Box 7.5*). Released from nerve terminals in the median eminence and transported to the anterior pituitary gland via the hypophyseal portal capillaries, GHRH acts on the somatotrophs

of the anterior pituitary gland via a G-protein linked receptor to stimulate cAMP synthesis and eventually activates Pit-1 promoter. Thus, mutations in the gene coding for Pit-1 result in hypoplasia of the pituitary gland and deficient secretion of GH as well as that of prolactin and TSH (*Box 7.6*).

Somatostatin is a 14 amino acid peptide (the somatostatin variant released by δ cells in the pancreatic islets is a 28 amino acid peptide) synthesized in hypothalamic neurons mainly located in the anterior periventricular nuclei. Somatostatin acts on the somatotrophs to inhibit cAMP generation.

Both GH and prolactin are partly regulated by a 'short' feedback loop i.e. each can feedback directly on the hypothalamus to inhibit its own release (*Box 7.15*). The GH-stimulated release of IGFs from

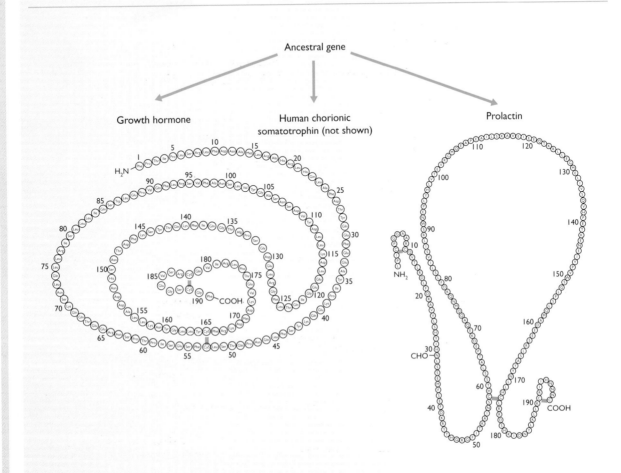

GH and prolactin contain disulfide bonds bridging two cysteine residues and they both contain between 190–200 amino acids and have regions of identical amino acid sequences. Along with human chorionic somatotrophin, this family of homologous hormones is thought to have evolved from a common ancestral gene.

the liver also has important feedback effects on the control of GH.

Pulsatile GH secretion represents the sum activity of GHRH and somatostatin-secreting neurons. These are regulated by an integrated system of neural, metabolic and hormonal signals (*Box 7.17*) and the metabolic factors include all fuel substrates. The overall metabolic effect of this hormone is to raise blood glucose concentrations. Hypoglycemia stimulates its release, whilst hyperglycemia sup-presses it. Oral glucose administration (a glucose tolerance test, see *Box 7.24*) lowers GH secretion in healthy subjects and this provides a useful test in differentiating a state of GH excess (acromegaly) from normality (see below).

In the adult human, approximately five pulses of GH are secreted during a 24 h period with a larger peak occurring at the onset of sleep at night (*Box 7.18*). Between these pulses circulating GH concentrations are too low to be detected even by

Summary of the actions of GH and prolactin and the feedback mechanisms controlling their secretions

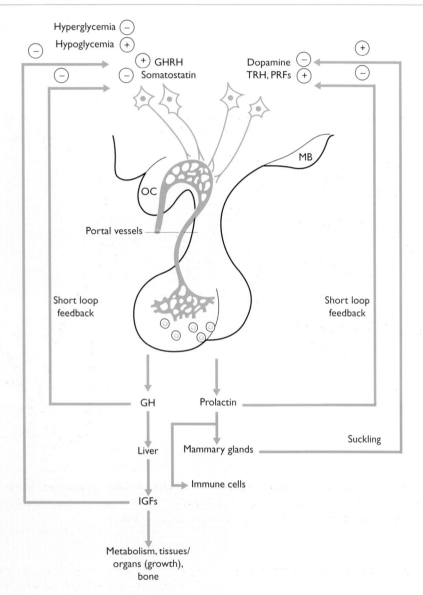

The synthesis and secretion of GH and prolactin are controlled by two opposing hypothalamic neurosecretory hormones, although the predominant hypothalamic control of GH is stimulatory (by GHRH) while that of prolactin is inhibitory (by dopamine).

Abbreviations: GHRH, growth hormone releasing hormone; TRH, thyrotrophin releasing hormone; PRFs, prolactin releasing factors, as yet unidentified.

## Box 7.16:
### Ghrelin — birth of a hormone

- The small synthetic hexapeptide hexarelin (GH releasing peptide-6, GHRP-6) was shown in the 1980s to cause the release of GH from somatotroph cells of a number of species.
- Its mechanism of action was shown to be different from that of GHRH.
- The production of analogs led to the cloning of the receptor mediating the actions on somatotroph cells, a highly conserved 366 amino acid protein.
- The search for the endogenous ligand for the receptor proved difficult and was only solved by cloning the receptor into chinese hamster ovary (CHO) cells and testing extracts of a number of tissues for activity. The highest concentration of the putative ligand was found in stomach not hypothalamic extracts.
- Ghrelin is a 28 aminoacid peptide with a lipid n-octanoic acid on serine 3.
- Studies are now required to establish its possible role in the control of GH secretion and its role in other tissues.
- Interestingly, the ghrelin gene knock-out mouse grows normally.

## Box 7.17:
### Major factors controlling GH secretion

| Stimulation | Inhibition |
|---|---|
| GHRH | Somatostatin |
| Hypoglycemia | Hyperglycemia |
| Decreased free fatty acids | Increased free fatty acids |
| Increased amino acids | |
| Starvation | |
| | |
| Sleep | IGFs |
| Exercise | Senescence |
| Stress | |
| | |
| Puberty | Growth hormone |
| Estrogens | Progesterone |
| Androgens | Glucocorticoids |
| | |
| α-adrenergic agonists | β-adrenergic agonists |
| Serotonin | Serotonin antagonists |
| Dopamine agonists | Dopamine antagonists |

sensitive two-site immunoradiometric assays (IRMA, *Box 3.25*), though more sensitive assays are under development. The mean concentration of circulating GH varies throughout life (*Box 7.18*). It rises after birth reaching concentrations higher than that of adults. A peak period is observed during puberty and there is a marked decline in old age. The reduction in old age has been termed the 'somatopause', by analogy with the menopause, and this concept will be discussed further in the context of GH replacement in adults (see Website).

## Actions of growth hormone and insulin-like growth factors

*Clinical Case 7.3* illustrates the importance of GH in post-natal growth and development but, apart from growth, this hormone has other important metabolic functions. It is an anabolic hormone with widespread actions, many of which are mediated via the production of insulin-like growth factors, IGF-1 and 2, that are synthesized by the liver and in target tissues (*Box 7.19*).

Its most profound effect is on linear growth by stimulating proliferation of the cartilage in the epiphyseal plates of long bones before they fuse. In addition to stimulating linear growth, GH also increases total bone mass and mineral content by increasing the activity and probably the number of bone modeling units (see *Clinical Case 5.6*). GH increases lean body mass, reduces adiposity by its lipolytic effects, and increases organ size and function, the latter effect being mediated by IGFs as in bone (*Box 7.20*). Normal

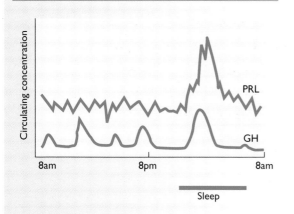

Diagrammatic representation of the daily pattern of growth hormone (GH) and prolactin (PRL) secretion in adult humans. There is a sleep-related increase in both GH and prolactin secretion.

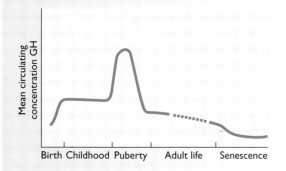

Life-time pattern of growth hormone secretion, in which the mean daily secretions are higher in childhood, reaching a peak at puberty and falling to lower concentrations in adulthood.

- The IGF family consists of 3 members (insulin, IGF-1 and IGF-2) sharing common structural similarities. There are variant forms of the IGFs (see website).
- IGF-1 and IGF-2 also have metabolic functions but also play important roles in cellular proliferation and the functions of differentiated tissues (mediated by the IGF-1 receptor).
- Each agonist binds its cognate receptor with high affinity but IGF-2 binds the insulin receptor with higher affinity than does IGF-1. The IGF-2 (or mannose 6-phosphate) receptor does not mediate cellular functions but plays a role in clearing IGFs.
- The circulating concentrations and the biological effects of the IGFs (but not insulin) are modulated by the IGF-BPs.
- Hepatic production of IGF-1 plays a major feedback role in regulating the secretion of GH by the pituitary gland. GH receptors and both IGFs are expressed in virtually every tissue. Mice in which genes have been rendered non-functional generally, or only in specific tissues (targeted disruption), have allowed elucidation of the relative roles of the production of IGFs by the liver and also locally.
- IGF-2 is a major fetal growth factor. IGF-1 is more important for post-natal growth and indeed is more important than GH. Specific loss of hepatic IGF-1 production does not impair post-natal growth indicating the importance of local IGF production.
- Insulin is generally regarded as having metabolic functions (mediated by the insulin receptor) but also plays a role in fetal growth.

concentrations of GH are also required to sustain normal pancreatic islet function. Thus, in GH deficiency insulin secretion declines whilst an excess of GH reduces insulin-dependent glucose uptake causing a rise in insulin secretion to compensate for the GH-induced resistance. On balance, GH is a diabetogenic hormone (see *Box 7.20*).

The $t_{1/2}$ of GH in the circulation is about 20 minutes. It circulates in several forms that vary according to size (molecular weights of 20 000 and 22 000), isoelectric point (acidic forms), oligomers (up to pentamers) and fragments (molecular weights of 12 000 and 16 000). In addition, approximately 50% is bound to the extracellular domain

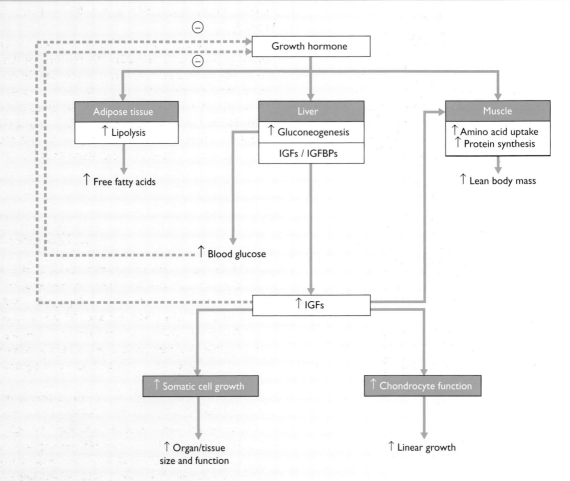

GH has direct actions on the liver, adipose tissue and muscle although many of its actions are mediated by increasing the synthesis and release of insulin-like growth factors (IGFs). These stimulate DNA, RNA and protein synthesis in many organs and tissues increasing both their size and function. Growth hormone also stimulates the synthesis and release of insulin-like growth factor binding proteins (IGFBPs) which bind circulating IGFs. This binding provides a reservoir of circulating IGFs. Dashed lines represent some of the feedback factors resulting from the action of GH on peripheral tissues.

of its receptor (also termed the GH-binding protein GHBP). There are two molecules of the GH receptor, full-length and truncated forms. The full-length form belongs to the Class I cytokine receptor family. These are all proteins with single transmembrane domain in which the intracellular domain is associated with a protein tyrosine kinase

known as JAK that, in turn, phosphorylates STAT kinase initiating a cascade of protein phosphorylations (*Box 7.21*). The GH receptor is cleaved by a metalloproteinase enzyme and the amount of GHBP circulating has been used as a measure of GH receptor in cases where GH insensitivity is suspected. The truncated form of the GH receptor (GHRtr)

## Box 7.21:
### Growth hormone and prolactin receptors

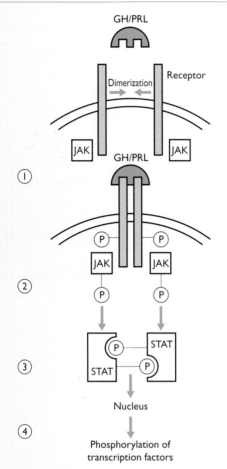

The receptors for growth hormone and prolactin, as for most of the cytokines, activate the JAK/ STAT pathway of signal transduction. Such hormone/cytokine receptors have no inherent tyrosine kinase activity, as seen in the receptors for many growth factors. Instead binding of the hormones to their receptors causes receptor dimerization and the consequent binding of one or more associated JAK tyrosine kinases ①. This induces self-phosphorylation ℗ of the JAK kinases as well as the receptor ②. The phosphorylated JAKs subsequently phosphorylate the STAT kinases ③ which, as dimers, translocate to the nucleus and activate transcription factors ④.

Abbreviations: JAK, just another kinase; STAT, signal transducers and activators of transcription.

also produces circulating GHBP and has a dominant negative effect on the activity of the full-length form. Thus, patients with predominantly GHRtr are GH insensitive but have circulating GHBP.

IGFs are also bound in the circulation to IGF-binding proteins (*Box 7.22*). The binding of IGF-1 to IGFBP$_3$, in particular, forms a very stable complex and this provides a circulating reservoir of these growth factors. Thus, unlike the rapid fluctuations seen in the concentration of circulating GH, IGF-1 concentrations are relatively stable and their circulating $t_{1/2}$ is much longer. Receptors for IGFs,

## Box 7.22:
### IGF-binding proteins

- The six IGF BPs share structural homologies of gene structure and have three domains, the conserved amino and carboxyl terminals being cysteine rich. All but IGF BP6 bind IGF-1 and IGF-2 with equal affinities; BP6 binds IGF-2 with much greater affinity.
- The IGF BPs bind to cells and also intercellular matrix and this alters their affinities for the growth factors.
- IGF actions on mitogenesis, substrate uptake and metabolic activity, modulation of cellular function are, by and large, mediated through the IGF-1 receptor. The effect of the BPs binding IGFs is generally to inhibit these effects. Since the circulating concentration of the IGFs is ~100 nmol/l and the IGF-1 receptor is saturated at ~5 nmol/l, the BPs play a major role in regulating IGF bioavailability.
- IGF BPs are subject to the action of cellular endoproteases that produce fragments that bind the IGFs with much lower affinity, thus reducing their effects on IGF action.
- IGF BP1, IGF BP3 and IGF BP5 may have paradoxical effects potentiating the actions of IGF. The mechanism is uncertain.
- The IGF BPs also exert actions that are independent of the IGF-1 receptor.
- GH regulates the concentration of IGF BP3 that binds ligands other than the IGFs e.g. acid labile subunit (ALS) and plasminogen.

like those of GH, are single transmembrane proteins but, in this case, their receptors have inherent tyrosine kinase activity (*Box 1.18*). When phosphorylated by IGF binding, the receptor initiates a series of further kinase phosphorylations and subsequent cytoplasmic or nuclear effects.

From the foregoing, it is obvious that GH deficiency and resistance to GH, caused by a genetic defect in the GH receptor, leads to a deficiency in IGF-1 (*Box 7.23*). Somatotrophin resistance, known as the clinical syndrome of Laron dwarfism, is char-

acterized by high plasma GH and low IGF-1 concentrations and absence of GHBP in most patients. The clinical picture is associated with dysmorphism particularly affecting the central face (prominent forehead and depressed nasal bridge) and marked short stature, the degree being to some extent related to the severity of the functional defect in the receptor. Other features include obesity and delayed puberty. It is rare and treatment with recombinant human IGF-1 markedly improves growth.

## GH replacement therapy

Isolated somatotrophin deficiency affects approximately 1:4000 children and the exact lesion giving rise to the GH deficiency is not usually discovered. Lesser degrees of GH lack are termed insufficiency and these are due to a number of possible causes (*Box 7.23*). The patient in *Clinical Case 7.3* underwent testing of anterior pituitary gland function and was shown to have a very poor somatotrophin response to provocative tests (*Box 7.24*). The rest of pituitary function was normal as was an MR scan of the brain. It was, therefore, concluded that he had isolated GH deficiency and he was started on replacement GH (*Box 7.25*). The clinical result was very significant 'catch-up' growth (*Box 7.12*).

It is clearly imperative that GH deficient children receive replacement therapy if they are to have any chance of reaching a normal final height. The question as to whether treatment should be continued in lower doses once final height has been attained or whether adults, with an acquired GH deficiency, should also be treated has only recently been raised. Adult GH deficiency certainly can cause marked symptoms and clinical features (*Box 7.26*) and the beneficial effects of somatotrophin in some deficient adults have been noted for nearly 40 years.

---

**Box 7.23:**
Causes of IGF-I deficiency[*]

**GH deficiency**

- Any cause of hypothalamo-pituitary dysfunction (see *Box 7.9*).
- GHRH deficiency – to date no mutations have been reported in the GHRH gene itself.
- GHRH resistance – loss of function mutation in the receptor (reported in the Pakistan province of Sindh and in the *little* mouse).
- Isolated GH deficiency – e.g. loss of function mutations in the GH-I gene. These patients develop antibodies to GH when treated with the recombinant protein.
- Neurosecretory dysfunction – this is said to be present in short patients growing poorly but otherwise normal who have low serum IGF-I concentrations, normal GH concentrations to pharmacological tests but low GH concentrations on nocturnal profiles.

**GH resistance**

- Loss of function mutations of the GH receptor e.g. Laron syndrome. The question has been raised as to whether heterozygosity for these mutations has a dominant negative effect given the need for the biologically active GH receptor to dimerize.
- Acquired GH resistance occurs in malnutrition and liver disease.
- Mutations leading to truncation of the IGF-I molecule and loss of function.

[*]All are rare.

---

*'Replacement therapy with thyroid, adrenocortical hormone and estrogen in females or androgens in males is usually satisfactory treatment for adult hypopituitarism. One patient, a thirty-five year old teacher, treated in this way for eight years, was treated in addition with human growth hormone, 3 mg three times a week. After two months of GH she noted*

- GH is secreted in a pulsatile fashion and has a diurnal variation. Its secretion is stimulated by exercise and affected by food (being stimulated by amino acids and inhibited by hyperglycemia). Randomly taken GH measurements should be avoided.
- Physiological tests of GH secretion include those requiring frequent blood samples overnight to determine the magnitude and frequency of GH pulses.
- IGF-I is synthesized by the liver in response to GH but the correlation between the serum concentrations of the two may be poor. The serum concentration of IGF-I is dependent on age and puberty status.

**When GH deficiency is suspected**, provocative pharmacological tests to stimulate GH secretion include:

Insulin induced hypoglycemia (generally regarded as the 'gold standard' and also cheap)

Glucagon

GHRH

Intravenous arginine infusion

Insulin-induced hypoglycemia is contraindicated in patients with seizures or ischemic heart disease and should only be performed by appropriately trained staff. Glucagon can be unpleasant, causing nausea. Recently, a combination of GHRH and arginine or GHRH and hexarelin has been advocated. GH secretion depends on pubertal stage so when investigating children it is recommended that the tests be 'primed' with estrogen treatment.

- Peak serum GH of >25 mU/l is regarded as a normal response to a pharmacological stimulus in children whilst a peak of <9 mU/l is diagnostic of GH deficiency in adults.
- Interpretation of the provocative tests requires the following considerations:

All pharmacological tests have false positive and false negative rates

The separation of normality from GH insufficiency or deficiency is somewhat arbitrary since they lie on a biological continuum

Growth is more important than the results of biochemical tests (that are notoriously difficult to reproduce)

**When GH excess is suspected**, suppression of GH secretion with glucose is regarded as the gold-standard test.

- Normal subjects usually respond to a glucose load with a serum GH less than 2 mU/l.
- Failure to suppress to this level may be seen in diabetes mellitus, anorexia nervosa, renal and hepatic disease and in normal adolescence. Additional tests with TRH or GnRH have been recommended but their place in assessment remains uncertain.
- Measurement of serum IGF-I and IGF BP3 concentrations has been used as a surrogate measure of GH secretion.

*increased vigor, ambition and sense of well-being. Observations in more cases will be needed to indicate whether the favorable effect was more than coincidental.'*

[Raben MS. Growth hormone 2: clinical use of human growth hormone. New England Journal of Medicine 1962, 266: 82–6.]

The lack of adequate supplies of the hormone until 1985 (the onset of industrial supplies of recombinant protein) precluded such therapy.

*Clinical Case 7.1* had a craniopharyngioma and developed pan-hypopituitarism as a result. Despite his adrenal, thyroid, and gonadal hormone replacement therapy he suffered from fatigue and weight gain (*Box 7.26*). Although he was just able to hold down a job, he got no social or sporting enjoyment out of life. When he was started on low-dose GH replacement, he noted a spectacular improvement. He lost 15 kg of fat and was able to get back to vigorous training so that he is now competing and coaching again. As will be seen *Clinical Case 7.4* was not so fortunate.

**Medical**

| Drug | Use | Advantages | Disadvantages/side effects |
|------|-----|------------|----------------------------|
| Growth hormone | Growth hormone deficiency | Human recombinant GH available from several manufacturers | Single daily subcutaneous injection usually at night. Regarded as expensive |
| | For children | Dose calculated according to body surface area or body weight. Auxological monitoring | Thyrotrophin deficiency may be 'unmasked'. ~10% may develop GH antibodies |
| | For adults | Dose titrated against assays of serum IGF-1 and/or IGF BP3. Mean dose ~0.5 mg/d | Rarely fluid retention. Benign intracranial hypertension. Higher doses needed in women. *Potential* risk of increase in malignancy rates |
| GHRH e.g. somatorelin | Improve endogenous GH secretion | Advantages over GH to be established | Daily subcutaneous injections Expensive |
| IGF-1 | Treatment of GH insensitivity | Recombinant IGF-1 as 'orphan drug' Daily subcutaneous injection. Improves growth and other aspects of the condition | Not commercially viable. Hypoglycemia, edema, Hyperandrogenism. Does not normalize growth (indicating the importance of GH acting directly) |
| Oxandrolone | Constitutional delay | Orally active. Effective without reducing final height | Few side effects in low dose used |

**Surgical**

| Procedure | Use | Advantages | Disadvantages/side effects |
|-----------|-----|------------|----------------------------|
| Leg lengthening+ | Increase final height | ~5 cm increase in final height | Painful, slow, expensive and prone to complications |

*The treatment of other medical conditions leading to poor growth (*Box 7.13*) requires other treatments not given here.
+Requires the patient to be at final height and extremely motivated.

# GH excess – gigantism and acromegaly

Excessive secretion of somatotrophin before the epiphyses have fused results in excess linear bone growth and gigantism. The tall record holders documented in the Guinness Book of Records are in all likelihood (for the most part undiagnosed) pituitary giants. Such excess is usually the result of somatotrophin-secreting pituitary tumors that are, fortunately, rare. Excessive secretion after epiphyseal fusion results in acromegaly.

## Adult GH deficiency and the 'somatopause'

**Adult GH deficiency**
**Symptoms***
- Decreased energy levels
- Social isolation
- Lack of positive well being
- Depressed mood
- Increased anxiety

**Clinical features***
- Increased body fat, particularly central adiposity
- Decreased muscle mass and exercise tolerance
- Decreased bone density, associated with an increased risk of fracture
- Increased LDL cholesterol and apolipoprotein B. Decreased HDL cholesterol
- Decreased cardiac muscle mass (especially in childhood-onset somatotrophin deficiency) with impaired cardiac function
- Decreased total and extracellular fluid volume
- Decreased insulin sensitivity and increased prevalence of impaired glucose tolerance
- Increased concentration of plasma fibrinogen and plasminogen activator inhibitor type I
- Accelerated atherogenesis

*Note that in clinical trials these are improved or normalized.

**Somatopause**
- There is a natural decline in GH secretion with increasing age
- This has been termed by some the 'somatopause' in comparison with the menopause
- This has led to the use of GH in the elderly in a number of studies
- As a result, GH has appeared for sale as a rejuvenating hormone

## Clinical Case 7.4:

A 58-year-old carpenter attended an orthopedic surgeon because he had difficulty in holding the tools of his trade. For the previous 12 years, he had seen his primary care physician repeatedly complaining of 'pins and needles' and numbness in both hands. The orthopedic surgeon confirmed the clinical diagnosis of bilateral carpal tunnel syndrome and performed bilateral decompression of the median nerve at the wrist. Clinical examination showed the hands to be broad and spatulate (Box 7.27) and the surgeon referred him to the Endocrine outpatient clinic.

Acromegaly affects approximately 50 people in a million with an annual incidence of about 3 per million. It affects males and females equally and is an insidious disease being present for a number of years before clinical suspicions are aroused. It tends to present in the fifth decade of life. The patient in Clinical Case 7.4 typifies this delay in diagnosis.

Excess somatotrophin results in raised circulating concentrations of IGF. Thus, the growth promoting effects of IGF-1 leads to the characteristic proliferation of bone, cartilage and soft tissues and an increase in the size of other organs to produce the classic signs and symptoms of acromegaly (Box 7.27). Carpal tunnel syndrome, due to pressure on the median nerve in the wrist, is commonly associated with acromegaly and, indeed, this led to the diagnosis in Clinical Case 7.4. The other endocrine condition giving rise to carpal tunnel syndrome is hypothyroidism, though peripheral nerves in patients with diabetes mellitus are more susceptible to compression syndromes.

Glucose intolerance and hyperinsulinemia are common metabolic complications of acromegaly affecting 50–70% patients. Hypogonadism is also frequently associated with excess growth hormone secretion. This may be the result of a GH-secreting tumor impairing gonadotrophin secretion or the excess GH interacting with the prolactin receptor owing to its structural homology with prolactin. Excess prolactin secreted by some tumors impairs pituitary and gonadal function, and also cause galactorrhea (and gynecomastia in men). Another possibility is that excess IGFs stimulated by GH have a negative effect on the gonads where they normally exert paracrine control of gonadal function.

The vast majority of cases of acromegaly (>99%) are due to pituitary tumors although occasional

*Clinical Case 7.4* and the clinical features of acromegaly*

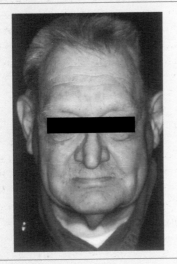

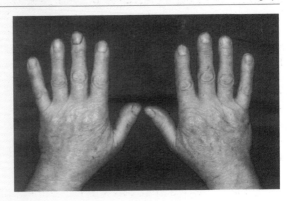

Clinical photographs of the hands and face of *Clinical Case 7.4*

These images are available in color on the website.

## Clinical features of acromegaly

| Symptoms | | Signs |
|---|---|---|
| | **Skeletal** | |
| Carpal tunnel syndrome (~50%) | | Enlarged hands, feet (~100%) |
| | | Jaw protrusion (~90%) |
| | | Dental malocclusion (~80%) |
| Arthralgia/arthritis (~85%) | | Osteoarthritis (~30%) |
| | **Skin** | |
| Excessive sweating (~85%) | | Greasy skin, skin tags (~60%) |
| | **Cardiovascular**[†] | |
| Angina | | Hypertension (~50%) |
| | | Cardiomyopathy (~5%) |
| | **Respiratory** | |
| Diurnal drowsiness (~30%) | | Obstructive sleep apnea (~30%) |
| | **Metabolic**[‡] | |
| Polydipsia, polyuria, recurrent infections | | Retinopathy, neuropathy |
| | **Renal** | |
| Renal colic (~20%) | | Renal stones (~20%) |
| | **Other endocrine** | |
| Menstrual irregularity (~50%) | | Hypogonadism (~40%) |
| Impotence (~40%) | | |

*These are the effects of excess somatotrophin. The effects of a mass lesion are the same whatever the tumor secretes. There is also an increased risk of colonic polyps and neoplasia (~2 fold).

[†]The effects of GH excess alone are difficult to disentagle from the effects of secondary diabetes mellitus and hypertension.

[‡]The clinical features and complications of diabetes mellitus (~35%).

cases due to hypothalamic or ectopic production of GHRH (or, even more rarely, ectopic soma-totrophin) have been described. It is noteworthy that most of these rare cases were not diagnosed prospectively. The pituitary tumors are benign (adenomas) and tend to be macroadenomas (i.e. above 10 mm diameter). A number of histological types has been described that may correlate with growth rate and tendency to recur postoperatively. Some tumors are made up of two cell types e.g. one secreting somatotrophin and the other prolactin whilst others contain cells that co-secrete both hormones. It has been suggested that such tumors arise from a presumed precursor cell type.

The diagnosis of acromegaly was confirmed in *Clinical Case 7.4* when his serum GH concentrations remained more than 90 mU/l after an oral glucose load (*Box 7.24*). A pituitary tumor was revealed on a MR scan and the patient underwent treatment (*Box 7.28*). Transsphenoidal surgery to remove the tumor resulted in a considerable reduction in the somatotrophin response to glucose but the serum concentrations remained elevated. He, therefore, underwent cranial irradiation and 8 years later his somatotrophin responses to insulin-induced hypoglycemia were all less than 2 mU/l (*Box 7.24*). He subsequently developed hot flushes and was found to be hypogonadal (serum testosterone 2.3 nmol/l, NR 9–25 nmol/l). He also complained of increasing fatigue and weight gain, as was seen in *Clinical Case 7.1*. By this time, he had no measurable somatotrophin response to insulin-induced hypoglycemia. His hypogonadism was treated with androgens, but, unlike *Clinical Case 7.1*, somatotrophin replacement was not sanctioned by his Health Authority. The fact he was treated for growth hormone excess and is now clinically affected by its deficiency and yet his Health Authority refused to pay for the treatment, raises number of ethical and political issues (see Website).

## Pituitary adenomas – incidence and treatment

In post-mortem series about 25% of the population has pathological evidence for a pituitary tumor and about 40% of these stain for prolactin.

However, clinical presentations of pituitary tumors are much less common. It is evident from the foregoing cases that pituitary tumors cause clinical problems by any of three mechanisms: unregulated production of a hormone, interference with the normal production of hormones or damage to local structures. It is self-evident that these effects are governed to a large extent by the size of the tumor. As a result, pituitary adenomas are classified by the hormones they produce and by size. Microadenomas are less than 10 mm in diameter and macroadenomas larger than this. Pituitary microadenomas tend to present with symptoms of hormonal excess and usually such tumors can be successfully treated surgically (*Box 7.28*). More problematic are the large macroadenomas that cause general sellar enlargement, suprasellar damage, visual loss and hypopituitarism (of variable degree) and may extend laterally into the cavernous sinuses. These are much less likely to be curable by surgery alone.

Pituitary tumors may be treated medically, surgically, radiotherapeutically or with any of these in combination (*Box 7.28*). The use of each of these modalities of therapy varies with the type of tumor and the availability of expertise. Generally speaking microadenomas are treated with transsphenoidal microsurgery with success rates reaching about 90%.

Macroadenomas are treated with surgery and, if appropriate, radiation therapy after incomplete removal of the adenoma. Medical treatment can include dopamine agonists such as cabergoline or bromocriptine for GH and prolactin-secreting tumors or the somatostatin analog octreotide for GH secreting adenomas.

Prolactinomas account for about 30% of primary pituitary tumors whilst GH hypersecretion accounts for approximately 15% and ACTH excess 10%. Those producing no biologically active hormone (null-cell) account for about 30% with gonadotrophinomas about 10% and thyrotrophinomas <1%. *Clinical Case 7.5* is a patient with a prolactinoma illustrating some of the problems and treatment associated with pituitary adenomas and serves to introduce the subject of prolactin and its control.

## Medical

| Drug | Use | Advantages | Disadvantages/side effects |
|---|---|---|---|
| Dopamine agonist e.g. cabergoline | Prolactinoma Acromegaly | Orally active. First line therapy for prolactinomas. Normalizes serum prolactin (~95%) and shrinks tumors (~95%) | Nausea, postural hypotension Less effective (and higher doses needed) in acromegaly. Reduces serum GH (~80%) but rarely normalizes IGF-1, shrinks some tumors (~20%) |
| Somatostatin analog e.g. octreotide | Acromegaly | Reduces GH concentrations (~ 80%) Shrinks tumors (~30%) | Given by subcutaneous injection. Expensive. Gastrointestinal upset. Gallstones (~30%). Reduced insulin secretion |
| GH receptor antagonist e.g. pegvisomant | Acromegaly | Mutated human GH that prevents GH receptor activation. Adjunctive to other therapies Pegylation improves duration of action. Normalizes IGF-1 in ~80% | Currently experimental. Requires injection. Likely to be expensive when marketed |

## Surgical

| Procedure | Use | Advantages | Disadvantages/side effects |
|---|---|---|---|
| Transsphenoidal† | Removal of pituitary mass lesions | Reduces excess hormone secretion. Improves mass effects e.g. visual fields (~80%). 'Curative' in microadenomas (~60%) | Expensive. Death (<1%), visual loss (0.5%), CSF leak (~0.5%), diabetes insipidus (~5%), meningitis (0.5%), hypopituitarism (~30%). Recurrences in ~10% of microadenomas and ~90% of macroadenomas |

## Radiotherapy

| Conventional, supervoltage (45 Gy) | All forms of tumor in the pituitary region | Relatively well tolerated. No anesthetic or surgical risks. Effective | Slow effect in reducing tumor secretion of hormones and tumor shrinkage (many months or years). Optic atrophy, vasculitis, cognitive effects. Risk of second tumor in radiation field (~1%) Hypopituitarism (~90% at 20 years). |
|---|---|---|---|

*Treatment of Cushing's is given in *Box 4.24*. The outcomes of treatment depend on a multitude of factors including the size of tumor, its inherent tendency to grow, biological variation and technical expertise, previous therapy especially surgery.
†Transfrontal procedures are used if there are technical difficulties in the transsphenoidal approach, the tumor is very large or there is doubt as to the nature of a mass lesion. They are associated with higher rates of operative mortality and morbidity.

# Prolactinomas

## Clinical Case 7.5:

A 47-year-old bank clerk woke one morning with severe chest pain radiating to both arms. He was taken to his local hospital and, although his electrocardiogram was normal, he was considered to have suffered an acute myocardial infarction. He was treated intravenously with an infusion of streptokinase and subsequently heparin and oral aspirin. Two hours after finishing the streptokinase, he complained of a sudden severe headache, diplopia (double vision) and blurred vision. On examination, he was fully conscious but with right 3rd and 6th cranial nerve palsies and a left temporal visual field defect. On transfer to Neurosurgery, a CT scan revealed a large pituitary mass with suprasellar extension and evidence of a recent hemorrhage within the mass Box 7.29. This hemorrhage into his existing pituitary tumor was caused by his treatment for a suspected myocardial infarction. As a result there was a sudden swelling of the tumor into the cavernous sinus that caused compression of the 3rd and 6th cranial nerves. His sudden onset of headache caused by the hemorrhage is termed pituitary apoplexy.

Measurement of his serum prolactin (213 000 mU/l, NR <400 mU/l) indicated he had a prolactin-secreting tumor, a prolactinoma. Concerns that he may have suffered a recent myocardial infarction, coupled with the recent therapy with fibrinolytic drugs resulted in medical treatment being preferred to surgical decompression of the optic chiasm and 3rd and 6th cranial nerves. He was treated with the dopamine agonist, cabergoline, to inhibit prolactin secretion. Within hours, clinical improvement was seen and after 3 days the headache disappeared; the cranial nerve palsies recovered after one month. Six months later his serum prolactin concentration was 84 mU/l, fluid within the tumor was no longer visible and the tumor was much reduced in size.

Prolactinomas are benign, clonally expanded tumors and clinical presentation is different in

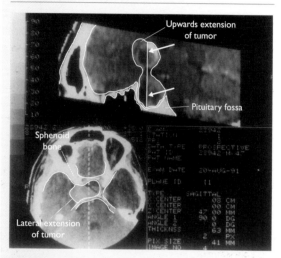

The lower axial scan demonstrates the expansion of the mass into the right cavernous sinus leading to the cranial nerve lesions.

The upper, reformatted image demonstrates the extension of the mass above the pituitary fossa. It also shows a vertical line (arrowed) roughly bisecting the contents of the pituitary fossa. As the CT scan was performed with the patient lying on his back this line was caused by the horizontal fluid level of blood within the tumor.

These images are available on the website.

males and females; females tend to have smaller tumors that come to light earlier because of their predilection for causing amenorrhea due to the inhibitory effects of excess prolactin on the pituitary gland and ovaries. Males tend to have larger tumors that come to light late, perhaps because males are reluctant to discuss gradually deteriorating gonadal and sexual function.

In the UK, the use of dopamine-agonist drugs (including cabergoline or bromocriptine) is recommended as first line treatment for prolactinomas, even in the presence of visual field defects. This is because they lower serum concentrations of prolactin and shrink the tumors. However, in those who cannot tolerate these drugs, or those in whom the drugs fail to shrink the tumors sufficiently, surgery and/or radiotherapy have been used with results similar to those of other tumor types (*Box 7.28*). In countries in which other forms of health care funding are used, surgery (that may be curative) may be recommended to minimize ongoing medical costs. In pituitary apoplexy associated with mass effects such as visual loss, surgical intervention may be recommended to decompress the optic chiasm.

## Prolactin and its control

Prolactin is a single chain protein made up of 199 amino acids with three disulfide bridges and, as noted above, it shares strong structural homologies with GH. Their cell-surface receptors are also similar, although the intracellular domain of the prolactin receptor is different and shorter than that for GH. The intracellular signal transduction pathway is similar to that of GH involving the JAK-STAT kinase pathway (see *Box 7.21*) and like the GH receptor, truncated forms of the prolactin receptor are found in a number of tissues.

The main function of prolactin is stimulating breast development and milk production. However, more than 300 functions have been attributed to prolactin (more than for all the other pituitary hormones combined), including salt and water balance, cell growth and proliferation (*Box 7.30*). Recently prolactin has emerged as a stimulatory modulator of immune function but the clinical relevance of this function has yet to be established.

It also has effects on the hypothalamo-pituitary-gonadal axis and can inhibit pulsatile GnRH secretion from the hypothalamus and alter the activity of certain steroidogenic enzymes. In women, its actions depend on the phase of the menstrual cycle. Excess prolactin secretion is associated with infertility and menstrual irregularity or even complete amenorrhea. In men, it causes decreased testosterone and sperm production. In addition, excess prolactin can cause galactorrhea (inappropriate milk production) in women and gynecomastia (breast development) in men.

Like GH, prolactin secretion is regulated by a dual hypothalamic inhibitory and stimulatory system and can regulate its own secretion through a short-loop feedback (*Box 7.15*). In contrast, its

---

### Box 7.30:
### Actions of prolactin

**In the human the established actions are:**
- Preparing the female breast for lactation.
- Other roles poorly understood though widespread tissue expression of prolactin receptors.
- Males have the same circulating concentrations of prolactin as non-lactating females.
- No clinical condition associated with loss of the prolactin gene or its receptor has been described raising the possibility that it is an absolute requirement for life. The mouse prolactin gene knock-out is viable.

**In animal species, prolactin has very diverse actions including:**
- Water and electrolyte balance – reduces $Na^+$ and water loss in kidney and gut.
- Growth and development – many actions on body growth, cellular proliferation and development (e.g. metamorphosis in amphibians).
- Endocrinology and metabolism – widespread actions affecting lipid, carbohydrate and steroid metabolism.
- Brain and behavior – altering brain biochemistry and modifying behavior in a wide variety of species.
- Reproduction – lactation as well as altering the biochemistry of the ovary, testis, uterus, prostate of a number of mammalian species.
- Immunoregulation – widespread effects on the thymus and spleen and specific leukocytes including macrophages and lymphocytes.

---

hypothalamic control is unique in that the predominant hypothalamic influence is inhibitory whereas for all other hormones the predominant influence is stimulatory. Thus, damage to the hypothalamic control causes increased prolactin secretion rather than decreased secretion, as seen with all other anterior pituitary hormones.

Dopamine, released into the hypophyseal portal veins from the nerve terminals of the intrahypothalamic tuberoinfundibular tract, is the main neurohormone inhibiting prolactin secretion although somatostatin also has an inhibitory effect. Whilst thyrotrophin releasing hormone has a potent stimulatory action on prolactin release, it is clear that other, but as yet undefined, factors are also involved. For example, suckling is a potent stimulus for prolactin secretion but this does not coincide with a rise in TSH secretion. Inhibition of dopamine release or antagonism at the dopamine D2 receptor also increases prolactin secretion. A list of the main factors that stimulate or inhibit prolactin secretion is given in *Box 7.31* as well as the causes of hyperprolacinemia. Note that dopamine antagonist drugs and hypothyroidism are the most common causes of hyperprolactinemia.

---

**Box 7.31:**

Major factors controlling prolactin secretion and causes of hyperprolactinemia

---

**Factors controlling prolactin secretion**
Inhibitory – Dopamine.
Stimulatory – TRH, other releasing factors, pregnancy, lactation (suckling), estrogen, opioids, dopamine D2 receptor antagonists, sleep, stress.

**Causes of hyperprolactinemia**
Common (~90%)
- Drugs – e.g. dopamine D2 receptor antagonists used as antiemetics (metoclopramide) or neuroleptic agents (phenothiazines).
- Primary hypothyroidism – as a result of increased hypothalamic-hypophyseal portal concentrations of TRH.

Uncommon (~10%)
- Macroprolactinemia – a result of the binding of an immunoglobulin to the prolactin.
- 'Stalk syndrome' – interference in the supply of dopamine to the normal lactotrophs usually associated with moderately elevated circulating concentrations of prolactin (<3000 mU/l)
- Pituitary tumor – micro or macroprolactinoma usually associated with markedly elevated circulating concentrations of prolactin (>5000 mU/l).

Rare (<1%)
- Renal failure – a result of impaired clearance of prolactin.

Whilst the secretory patterns of GH and prolactin differ (*Box 7.18*), both hormones show a sleep-related increase in their secretions. This diurnal rhythm does not occur in the absence of sleep and contrasts with the endogenous circadian rhythm of ACTH/cortisol secretion that normally occurs irrespective of social cues and habits.

# Circadian rhythms and the suprachiasmatic nucleus

Many physiological functions such as core temperature, bronchodilation, blood pressure and hormone secretions show daily rhythms. Some of these variables, like ACTH and melatonin secretion (see below), are directly driven by the body's internal 'clock'. This is thought to reside within the suprachiasmatic nuclei (SCN) of the hypothalamus (*Box 7.5*) and studies on isolated brain slices from this region have shown that neurons of the SCN show inherent cyclical activity (metabolic and electrical), independent of any input. In animals, lesions of the SCN abolish all circadian rhythms, including those of ACTH/cortisol and melatonin.

In humans, this clock has a natural, free-running periodicity of about 24.5 hours but normally it is entrained to the light–dark cycle (a 'zeitgeber') so that its cycle is complete in 24 hours; the body clock is, thus, in time with the environment. The next case illustrates what happens when the endogenous body clock is not entrained.

---

## Clinical Case 7.6:

A 7-year-old boy was seen in the long-term follow up clinic. He had initially presented at the age of 5 years with poor vision and on MR scan found to have a large tumor of the optic nerve (an optic nerve glioma, *Box 7.32*). Following treatment, he had been left blind with no perception of light. His parents were finding day to day life very difficult. In particular, it was evident that his sleep pattern was disrupted and he disturbed the whole family by getting up repeatedly in the middle of the night to play.

---

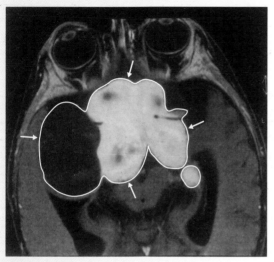

The axial MR scan shows a large tumor mass and the diagram shows the normal structures that it has replaced.

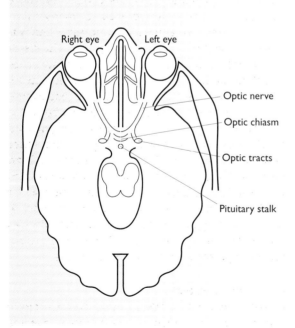

Right eye    Left eye

Optic nerve

Optic chiasm

Optic tracts

Pituitary stalk

Brain tumors, together with leukemia, are the most common tumors of childhood and approximately 1 in 2000 20-year-olds are survivors of child-hood cancer. The sequelae of these treatments are very important and in this case it was not only the loss of vision (a considerable handicap in itself) but also loss of normal sleep patterns. The disruptions to sleep, meals and school work were major for the family of *Clinical Case 7.6* and were caused by the boy's 'free-running' clock having lost the synchronizing effects of light. Hormone rhythms such as cortisol also become desynchronized with the environment and whilst societal factors and physical activity can exert some resynchronizing effects the main influence is undoubtedly the light–dark cycle.

This occurs because the SCN receives a direct input from the retina (the retino-hypothalamic tract); it is the only part of the brain, apart from the visual cortex, to receive a direct input from the eye. Neurons from the SCN project to wide areas of the brain including the hypothalamic nuclei, the mid-brain raphe nucleus and the ventral lateral geniculate nucleus. It also projects indirectly to the pineal gland that, nestling between the rostral part of the cerebral hemispheres, secretes melatonin (*Box 7.33*).

## The pineal gland and melatonin

In submammalian species, the pineal gland is sensitive to light and has direct neural connections with the brain. In man, these features have been lost. Instead, the SCN projects to the pineal via hypothalamic connections to the brain stem and spinal cord. From thence, the innervation is sympathetic to the superior cervical ganglion and pineal itself. The human pineal weighs approximately 150 mg and, apart from melatonin, contains a large number of chemical agents (including biogenic amines such as norepinephrine and serotonin, peptides such as GnRH and TRH and the neurotransmitter gamma amino butyric acid, GABA). The endothelial cells in the vasculature of the pineal are fenestrated so the organ is outwith the blood–brain barrier.

Pinealocytes are specialized secretory cells controlled by the norepinephrine output from the sympathetic system. In animals, the pineal controls a number of functions primarily to do with the timing of puberty and reproduction and removal of the pineal causes precocious puberty and disrupts the annual breeding patterns of seasonal breeders. Melatonin seems to be the main agent involved in this and it is thought that the duration of the melatonin signal (it is synthesized and secreted primarily during the dark phase of the cycle) is important in such control. The SCN and the pars tuberalis are rich in melatonin receptors.

Melatonin is synthesized from tryptophan (*Box 7.33*) and is greatest at night in the absence of light. Exposure to natural or bright artificial light rapidly reduces the activity of the enzyme *N*-acetyltransferase. Melatonin treatment in humans reduces LH and GH secretion, causes sleepiness and alters the electroencephalogram. Tumors of the pineal region in man are rarely (~20%) composed of pinealocytes (forming pinealcytoma or pinealblastoma according to differentiation) and such tumors are very rarely associated with precocious puberty.

Recent studies have shown that melatonin can be used beneficially to improve sleep patterns in patients such as *Clinical Case 7.6*. Many studies have used very large doses, such as 50 mg, but those using physiological doses of 0.1–1 mg have demonstrated effects on sleep latency and duration and also lower body temperature. Melatonin is now widely available throughout the world as a food additive, though not the UK, where it is treated as a drug (see Website). It is used to treat the sleep disturbance that occurs as a result of modern travel across time-zones – giving rise to the phenomenon of 'jet-lag' – and it has also been used to help shift-workers adapt their sleeping patterns. Studies in animals and *in vitro* have suggested that melatonin also has antioxidant effects and that it can influence immune responses and have an effect on malignant cells. Such effects at physiological concentrations or in humans remain unproven.

## Autonomic functions of the hypothalamus

The hypothalamus is important in regulating pituitary functions, but it also has a number of other functions generally attributed to autonomic control. These include temperature regulation, food intake, emotion and memory.

An important aspect of hypothalamic autonomic control with regard to the endocrine system is the control of food intake. The effects of obesity on endocrine function can be widespread and endocrine abnormalities can cause obesity. A number of hormones play central roles in the control of food intake.

## Obesity

Obesity is defined as an 'excess of body fat' and is one of the least specific definitions in medicine. It can be determined scientifically using a variety of techniques (*Box 7.34*) with greater or lesser degrees of accuracy. For clinical practice the less sophisticated determination of body mass index (BMI) and waist–hip circumference ratios are undemanding and (given their simplicity) remarkably useful. Using these simple measures obesity may be graded in severity and its epidemiology determined (*Box 7.35*).

In general obesity increases with age, and is higher in women and (in Western countries) those from lower socio-economic strata. In many countries, it has reached epidemic proportions and it is more prevalent in certain ethnic groups. The distribution of fat is sexually dimorphic with more subcutaneous fat in women in general and an increase in intra-abdominal fat in men. There is good experimental evidence that these two types of adipose tissue behave metabolically differently. The gynecoid distribution leads to low waist–hip circumference ratios whilst android distribution leads to a high ratio. Android obesity is particularly associated with insulin resistance and increased cardiovascular morbidity and mortality (i.e. risk of heart attacks). It is the etiological association with other diseases that makes obesity important (*Box 7.36*), shortening life-expectancy and reducing its quality.

### Etiology of obesity

Obesity occurs when caloric intake exceeds caloric expenditure. In a sedentary adult with an average daily intake of 2300 kcals (9700 kilojoules) basal metabolism will account for 60–70% energy expenditure, dietary and obligatory thermogenesis for 5–15% and spontaneous activity for 20–30%.

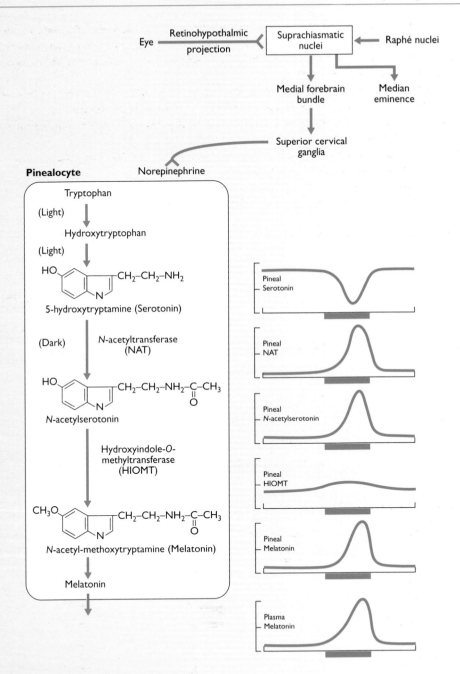

The synthesis of hydroxytryptamine from tryptophan is stimulated by light whilst the activity of NAT is stimulated by darkness. Dark bars indicate the dark phase of the light–dark cycle.

Box 7.34:
Measures of obesity

- Three main experimental measures of fat mass in man have been used for many years. They require the determination of body density, water or potassium content and the assumption that the body composition can be divided into fat and fat-free or lean body mass with certain characteristics. These techniques are relatively costly, time-consuming and do not give information on the distribution of the fat.
- Techniques such as bioelectrical impedance rely on the fact that fat is not as good an electrical conductor as lean body mass. It is cheap but also does not allow an assessment of the distribution of the fat mass.
- Imaging techniques such as CT or MR allow the determination of fat from a number of tomographic 'slices' of the body. The distribution of the fat mass can be calculated.
- Simple anthropomorphic measurements such as height and weight allow the calculation of body mass index (BMI), whilst calipers can be used to measure subcutaneous fat.

BMI = body weight (in kg)/height$^2$ (in m)

Waist/hip circumference$^*$ = ratio of waist circumference to that of the hips

$^*$Note this can be difficult to do accurately in the very obese. Waist is said to be at the umbilicus while hips are 4 cm below iliac crest.

Box 7.35:
Grades of obesity and its epidemiology

**Grades**

| BMI (kg/m$^2$) | WHO class | General term |
|---|---|---|
| <18.5 | Underweight | Thin |
| 18.5–24.9 | – | 'Normal' |
| 25.0–29.9 | Grade 1 overweight | Overweight |
| 30.0–39.9 | Grade 2 overweight | Obese |
| >40 | Grade 3 overweight | Morbid obesity |

**Epidemiology (Prevalence of BMI >30 kg/m$^2$)**

| Country | Year | Ages (years) | Men (%) | Women (%) |
|---|---|---|---|---|
| England | 1980 | 16–64 | 6 | 8 |
| | 1987 | | 7 | 12 |
| | 1991 | | 13 | 15 |
| | 1997 | | 17 | 20 |
| USA | 1960 | 20–74 | 10 | 15 |
| | 1973 | | 11 | 16 |
| | 1978 | | 12 | 15 |
| | 1991 | | 20 | 25 |
| Netherlands | 1987 | 20–59 | 6 | 8 |
| | 1990 | | 7 | 9 |
| | 1995 | | 8 | 8 |

## Box 7.36:
### Effects of obesity

**Effects on life expectancy**[*]

| BMI (kg/m²) | % increase in mortality rate |
|---|---|
| 25 | 0 |
| 30 | 25 |
| 35 | 50 |
| 40 | 150 |
| 45 | 200 |
| 50 | 300 |

[*]These have been difficult to determine because of the counfounding issues of smoking and the decreased life expectancy of very thin people.

**Diseases caused by obesity**
- Diabetes mellitus
- Coronary disease
- Hypertension
- Obstructive sleep apnea
- Cancers (e.g. endometrial)
- Arthritis
- Gallstones

Additional energy may be used for physical work and exercise. Thus:

Total energy expenditure = basal (resting) metabolic rate + thermogenesis + physical activity

For any person to gain weight, food intake (energy) must exceed energy expenditure.

The factors that control food intake are complex and not only involve physiological control mechanisms but also social, cultural and cognitive aspects to eating as well as physical activity. A very powerful billion pound food industry (supported by food technology) has generated highly palatable food and made it ubiquitous and cheap (at least in Western industrialized nations). It is, by and large, rich in fat as this is one of the mechanisms generating palatability (whilst also reducing satiety). Fat is also energy dense at 9 kcal/g compared with carbohydrate or protein at 4 kcal/g. High-fat foods are readily available from fridges, food dispensers or fast-food outlets in a society that is losing the concept of fixed meal-times (resulting in 'snacking' and 'grazing').

There is no evidence that the obese have a low resting metabolic rate. Indeed, as the total body mass increases, resting metabolic rate increases (*Box 7.37*). Thus, an obese person has a higher rate than a lean person of the same height. Furthermore, most studies show that the obese do about the same physical activity as lean individuals. Weight gain in some populations (e.g. the Pima Indians of Arizona) is predicted by a lower physical activity but in most instances it seems unlikely that reduced physical activity accounts for more than 40% of the weight gain. However, in a society that becomes progressively more sedentary, it should not be ignored.

It is noteworthy that, for most people, body weight remains remarkably constant over many years despite the intake of prodigious numbers of calories. This together with experimental work in both animals and humans has indicated that body fat mass is very tightly regulated around a 'set-point'. For example, the weight of the cafeteria-fed rat returns to that of its standard-feed litter-mate as soon as the food is returned to normal lab chow and in studies in which American prisoners were deliberately overfed, the weight gain that occurred was lost when they returned to 'normal' prison life.

## Control of appetite, food intake and satiety

*Clinical Case 7.7* is an example of a patient in whom the appetite/feeding 'set-point' has been disturbed by neurological damage to his hypothalamus; it will introduce the neural and endocrine control of food intake.

### Clinical Case 7.7:

A 22-year-old man was referred to the obesity clinic. With a height of 1.79 m he had weighed 73 kg until 2 years previously. Over the succeeding 2 years his

---

The formulae of Schofield may be used to calculate resting metabolic rate (kcal/d) in adults.

| Age (years) | Men | Women |
| --- | --- | --- |
| 18–30 | RMR = 15.1BW + 693 | RMR = 14.8BW + 488 |
| 31–60 | RMR = 11.5BW + 872 | RMR = 8.13BW + 846 |
| >60 | RMR = 11.7BW + 588 | RMR = 9.08BW + 680 |

*These are useful in preventing fruitless discussion. Thus, a 35-year-old female patient who weighs 123 kg and claims that 'she gains weight even on 800 kcal/d, is significantly underestimating intake since her RMR = 8.13 x 123 + 846 = 1846 kcal/d.

Abbreviations: BW, body weight; RMR, resting metabolic rate.

---

weight had progressively increased to 170 kg and over the same period he had become more withdrawn and had lost his job as a handyman. He had been treated by his primary care physician for depression with little success. There was no family history of obesity. On examination, he looked withdrawn and initiated little spontaneous conversation. In the light of his neurological symptoms, an MR scan of the brain was performed that revealed a large hypothalamic mass with an additional lesion in the brain stem (Box 7.38). The list of possible diagnoses for such multiple lesions includes the granulomatous disease sarcoidosis that affects many organs. Chest X-ray was normal and serum biochemistry showed normal calcium concentration but abnormal tests of liver function. A liver biopsy was, therefore, performed and the typical appearances of sarcoid (non-caseating granulomata) were seen on light microscopy. Psychometric testing showed a major problem with short-term memory. He was treated with oral glucocorticoid steroids with considerable improvement in his mental state and memory. His appetite remained unchanged however, and he lost very little weight despite documented shrinkage of the hypothalamic sarcoid tissue (Box 7.38). Additional endocrine replacement treatment for panhypopituitarism was also required.

Regulation of food intake and satiety is a complex process involving the co-ordination of sensory stimuli, circulating hormones (e.g. cortisol, insulin, gut hormones and leptin secreted by adipocytes), and vagal afferents from the gut relayed via the nucleus tractus solitarus (NTS). The hypothalamus co-ordinates this information through a complex network of orexigenic and anorexigenic peptides that have been summarized in Box 7.39.

## Genetics of obesity

Obesity runs in families. Studies on identical and non-identical twins and also on adults who were adopted have shown a strong genetic component to the development of obesity (accounting for about 80% of the effect). Experimental rodent models of obesity have been extremely useful and recently the human equivalents have been described. These include (with the human equivalent in brackets): the *ob/ob* mouse (loss of function mutation in leptin gene); the *db/db* mouse (loss of function mutation in leptin receptor); MC4 receptor knock-out mouse (melanocortin 4 receptor defects); POMC knock-out mouse (POMC cleavage defect leading to loss of MSH). Such patients are rare but they throw considerable light on the biochemical mechanisms underlying appetite, illustrating a general applicability between species. There are a number of other rare disorders associated with obesity such as Prader–Willi or

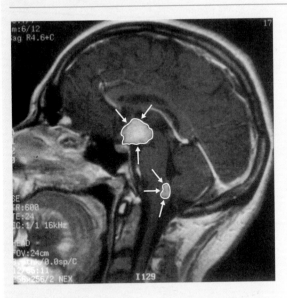

At presentation the sagittal section shows the large hypothalamic mass (upper arrows) together with a smaller brain stem mass (lower arrows).

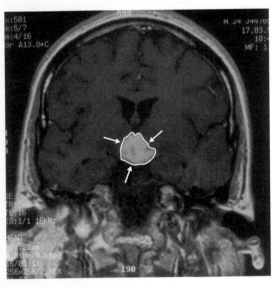

The first coronal section shows the extent of the involvement of the hypothalamus at presentation.

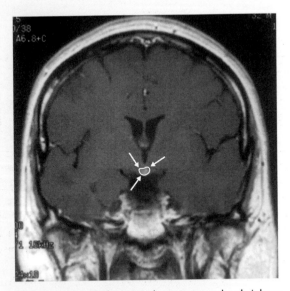

The second coronal section demonstrates the shrinkage of the sarcoid tissue with high doses of oral prednisolone, a synthetic glucocorticoid steroid.

These images are also available on the website

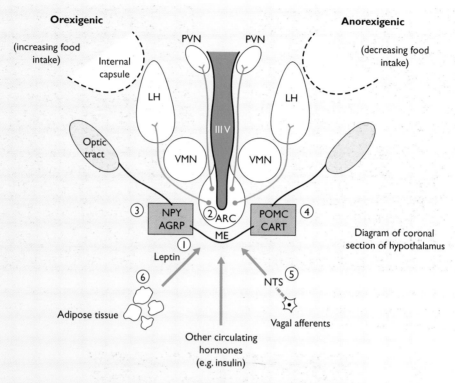

Diagram of coronal section of hypothalamus

① Leptin secreted by adipocytes is transported across the blood-brain barrier. Fasting or loss of body fat mass lowers serum and CSF leptin concentrations.

② The arcuate nucleus (ARC) is rich in leptin (and insulin) receptors.

③ Leptin inhibits neuropeptide Y (NPY) and agouti-related protein (ARGP) neurones in the ARC, whose axons project to the lateral hypothalamus (LH) and the paraventricular neuclus (PVN). Both NPY and ARGP are potent orexigenic agents.

④ Leptin activates pro-opiomelanocortin (POMC) neurones that produce α melanocyte stimulating hormone (αMSH). αMSH acts at the melanocortin-4 (MC4) receptors and is co-expressed with the cocaine and amphetamine-regulated transcript (CART). POMC/CART neurones also project to the LH and PVN and there is a reciprocal innervation from these nuclei to the ARC. Both αMSH and CART are potent anorexigenic agents

⑤ The nucleus of the tractus solitarius (NTS) is involved in the termination of food intake, termed satiation. Afferent inputs related to satiety include neurological signals from the vagus and sympathetic systems together with chemical signals such as the endocrine factor from the gut cholecystokinin. There are reciprocal connections between hypothalamic nuclei including the PVN and the NTS.

⑥ Obesity is associated with high circulating leptin concentrations. This has given rise to the idea that obesity is a condition marked by leptin (and insulin) resistance.

*A large number of orexigenic and anorexigenic molecules has been described. To simplify the diagram only NPY/AGRP and POMC/CART are shown.

Abbreviations: ME, median eminence; VMN, ventromedial nucleus; III V, 3rd ventricle.

Bardet–Biedl syndromes. For the most part, the exact genes involved in 'common or garden' obesity remain to be elucidated. It is clear that a large number of genes is likely to be implicated and current likely contenders in the human include POMC and CART (*Box 7.39*). It is to be noted that genome-wide linkage studies for polygenic obesity in mouse strains has implicated at least 70 loci, indicating the magnitude of the likely problem in the human.

Not all congenital causes of obesity are genetic. It has been suggested that obesity, together with hypertension and coronary disease result from the intrauterine environment. The 'thrifty phenotype' hypothesis is discussed in *Box 2.22*.

For *Clinical Case 7.7*, there is no evidence of a genetic cause of obesity and all the clinical information implicates the hypothalamic deposition of sarcoid. It has been recognized for many years that destructive lesions of the midline ventromedial hypothalamus cause this problem whilst more lateral hypothalamic lesions cause anorexia and weight loss. Some of the hypothalamic pathways involved in the regulation of appetite and satiety are shown in *Box 7.39*. *Clinical Case 7.7* showed evidence of the loss of appetite control together with evidence of the loss of satiety. When admitted to the hospital ward, he stole food from other patients at every meal.

**Treatment of obesity**

Obesity is a disease. It has major effects on morbidity and mortality that are directly related to the severity of the obesity. In general, in the present state of knowledge it is not worth investigating severely obese patients for a cause of their obesity. Exclusion of hypothyroidism or Cushing's often appears in textbooks of endocrinology but they are not causes of severe (also termed morbid) obesity.

The indications for the investigation of hypothalamic disease in *Clinical Case 7.7* were the rapid weight gain in adult life, lack of family history and the associated neurological features. The more typical case is of long-standing obesity with a history of repeated partially successful 'diets', virtually always ending in a return to the same degree of obesity or worse. Clearly, cases in which there are associated features (e.g. polydactyly and retinitis pigmentosa in Bardet–Biedl syndrome and small hands and feet in Prader–Willi syndrome) suggest an underlying syndrome and, thus, a Mendelian genetic causation will be diagnosed on the associated features. The vast majority of the cases of adult onset obesity will not warrant investigation. Indeed, to do so would be to suggest that treatment lies in any other direction than caloric restriction. The treatment of morbid obesity is extremely difficult and at present the only long-term successful forms of treatment are surgical (*Box 7.40*).

## The neural lobe of the pituitary gland – AVP and oxytocin

Arginine vasopressin (AVP) and oxytocin are small peptides with strong structural homologies. They consist of nine amino acids arranged in a ring structure with a short 'tail' (*Box 7.41*). It is likely that both evolved from a common ancestral gene and the uses ascribed to the gene products have been related to the emergence of land-living amphibia (water retention by AVP) and suckling of young in mammalian species (oxytocin). AVP is mainly synthesized in the supraoptic nuclei and to a lesser extent the paraventricular nuclei while the reverse is true for oxytocin. The hormones synthesized in the large (or magnocellular) neurosecretory cells of these nuclei are transferred to the posterior pituitary gland whilst those in the smaller cells (or parvicellular neurons) control the hormone secretions of the anterior pituitary gland.

Like all other peptide and protein hormones, they are synthesized as a large prohormone and after packaging into secretory granules, the prohormones pass by axonal flow to the nerve terminals (Herring bodies) in the neurohypophysis. During this passage, the prohormones are cleaved into the biologically active AVP or oxytocin and a larger polypeptide fragment. Neurophysin II is the product cleaved from the vasopressin pro-hormone and neurophysin I from the oxytocin pro-hormone. Both neurophysins are co-secreted with the active hormones upon electrical activation of the neurosecretory cells.

Treatment of obesity

## Medical

| Drug | Use | Advantages | Disadvantages/side effects |
|---|---|---|---|
| Pancreatic lipase inhibitor e.g. orlistat | Decreases dietary fat absorption | Orally active. Not absorbed. Effective in studies lasting >2 years 10% weight loss | Effects depend on patient compliance. Marked gastrointestinal effects if low fat diet not adhered to. May reduce fat-soluble vitamin concentrations |
| Serotonin reuptake inhibitor e.g. sibutramine | Decreases food intake. ± increase thermogenesis | Orally active. Effective in studies lasting >2 years, ~5% weight loss | Sympathomimetic side effects include dry mouth-insomnia, fatigability, increase in heart rate and blood pressure |
| Ephedrine and caffeine | Decrease appetite and increase thermogenesis | Effective in clinical trials. ~40% of the effect is due to increased thermogenesis and ~60% due to decreased appetite | Loss of lean body mass as well as fat. Increased heart rate giving palpitations |
| Experimental agents e.g. leptin | Decrease appetite | A large number of agents have been tried in experimental studies. These include leptin | Not commercially available |

## Surgical

| Procedure | Use | Advantages | Disadvantages/side effects |
|---|---|---|---|
| Jaw wiring | Decrease food intake | No anesthetic risk. Effective in motivated patient | All weight regained when wiring removed, so no longer recommended |
| Gastric* restriction | Decrease food intake | Laparoscopic adjustable banding has lower risks than vertical banded gastroplasty and is probably the treatment of choice | Morbidity and mortality rates depend on procedure and operator |
| Jejuno-ileal* bypass | Decreases food intake | Loss of 30–50% body weight | Multiple metabolic sequelae |

*See Website for details of the operations.

## AVP – actions and control

AVP derives its name from the first action ascribed to it nearly 100 years ago, an increase in systemic blood pressure (i.e. a pressor agent). Its actions on water balance in the kidney (where it is effective in very low concentrations) gave rise to the alternative name antidiuretic hormone (ADH) and the terms tend to be used interchangeably. AVP has three known receptors and, whilst this chapter will consider exclusively the actions of AVP on these

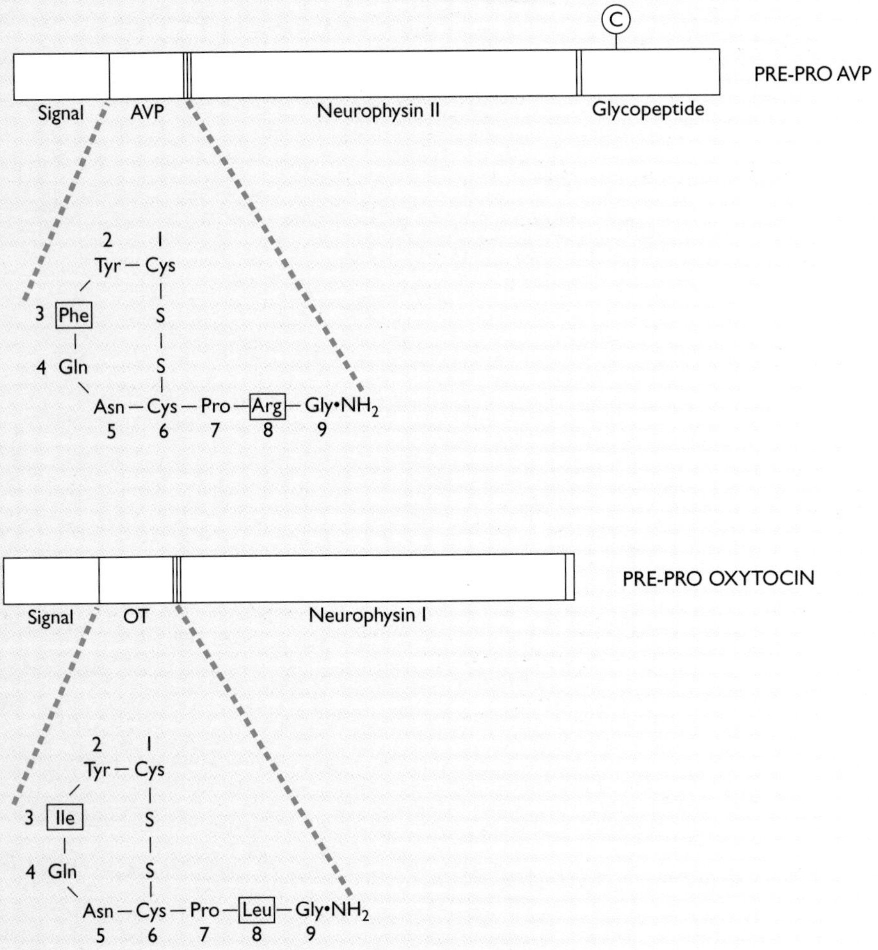

AVP and OT are co-secreted with their associated neurophysins.

receptors, this hormone acts in concert with aldosterone and atrial natriuretic peptide to control blood volume and pressure (*Box 7.42*).

In the kidney, it acts on the G-protein linked $V_2$ receptors on the capillary (basal) side of the distal convoluted and collecting ducts and stimulates the synthesis of cAMP. The cAMP activates a kinase on the luminal (apical) side of the ducts that initiates a series of events culminating in the insertion of water channels, known as aquaporins, into the luminal membrane (*Box 7.43*). Water passes into the collecting duct cells and, by osmosis, across the basal membrane, into the interstitial fluid and, hence, back into the circulation. There is also an osmotic gradient (set up by the counter-current activity of the loop of Henle) from the cortex to the medulla of the kidney. Thus, as the collecting ducts pass through the cortex to the medulla increasing

Integrated action of arginine vasopressin (AVP) with other hormones regulating blood volume and pressure

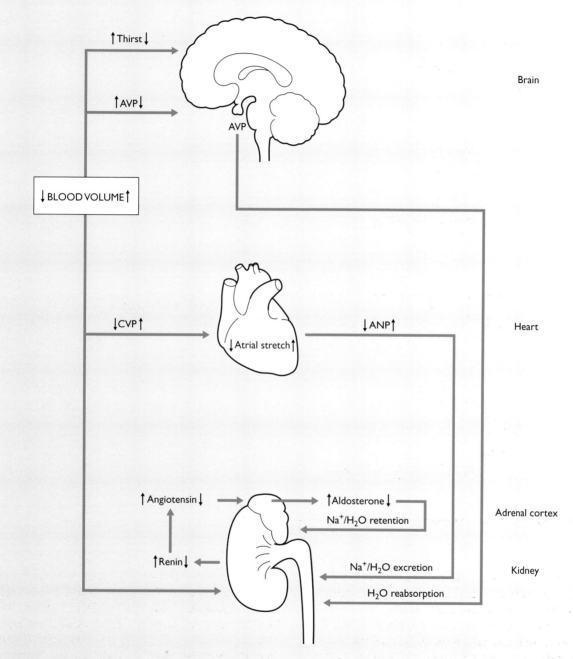

Arrows to the left indicate changes in hormone secretion in response to a reduction in blood volume, those on the right the changes in response to an increase in blood volume.
Abbreviations: ANP, atrial natriuretic peptide; CVP, central venous pressure.

The actions of arginine vasopressin (AVP) secretion and mechanisms of control

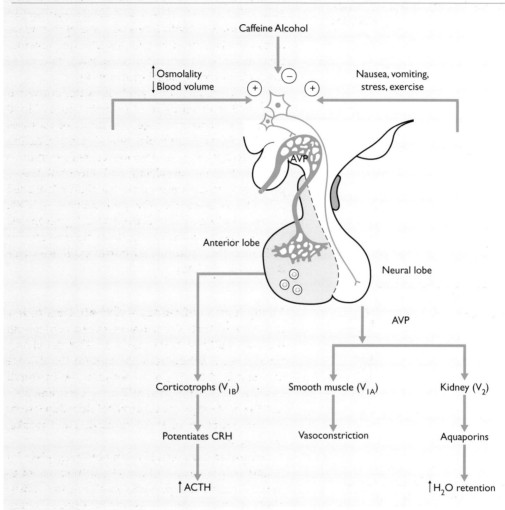

amounts of solute-free water (also termed 'free water') can be reabsorbed by the osmotic gradient. This is governed by the aquaporins and, hence, AVP.

Increased osmolality of the extracellular fluids stimulates AVP release. Changes in osmolality are detected by osmoreceptors. Osmotically sensitive cells were first described in the hypothalamus but it is now known that there are additional osmoreceptors in the circumventricular organs and in systemic viscera. These are not only important in

regulating AVP secretion but also in stimulating thirst. As a result, AVP induces increased water retention and a reduction in serum osmolality, the relationship of which is shown in *Box 7.44*.

Another potent stimulus to AVP secretion is a reduction in effective blood volume and AVP secretion is stimulated by a volume reduction of just 5–10% (*Box 7.44*). This is controlled by so-called stretch receptors that detect changes in blood volume/pressure. These include the baroreceptors and other receptors in the cardiovascular system. Thus,

The relationship between serum arginine vasopressin concentration and blood volume depletion or plasma osmolality

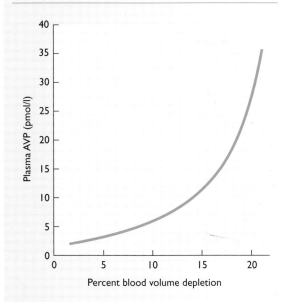

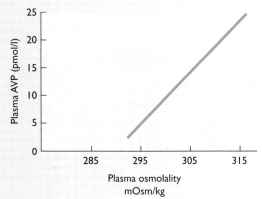

may be important in situations such as the post-operative state, affecting water balance. In contrast, alcohol is a potent inhibitor of AVP release (as little as 30–90 ml of whiskey is sufficient) resulting in inappropriate dehydration and some of the symptoms associated with a 'hang-over'. The preventative measure is to drink a restorative volume of water after excess ethanol consumption.

Apart from its primary role in water conservation, AVP is also important in maintaining blood pressure after hemorrhage as a result of its vasopressive effects on arteriolar smooth muscle. Acting on $V_{1A}$ receptors on smooth muscle cells it induces vasoconstriction via calcium and phospholipase-C generated second messengers. The final established role of vasopressin is the potentiation of CRH action on pituitary corticotrophs via $V_{1B}$ receptors. AVP is released from parvicellular neurosecretory cells into the hypophyseal portal capillaries (see *Boxes 4.14* and *7.43*).

### Vasopressin deficiency – diabetes insipidus

It is evident that AVP is important in controlling the osmolality of body fluids. In AVP deficiency there is loss of solute-free water and (in the absence of a matched intake) a consequent rise in serum osmolality. Patients with AVP deficiency, and subject to constant polyuria are absolutely dependent on the sensation of thirst to guide fluid intake, resulting in polydipsia.

Returning to a consideration of *Clinical Case 7.1* (a patient presenting with a visual field defect as the result of a craniopharyngioma), it is now possible to interpret the events and additional symptoms that occurred after the initiation of replacement hormones. This patient noted polyuria and polydipsia soon after starting hydrocortisone and thyroxine replacement therapy. Both thyroxine and cortisol (i.e. hydrocortisone) are required by the kidney to ensure the ability to excrete free water normally. In the absence of these, the patient was protected from the effects of AVP deficiency. Once these were replaced, the increase in free water clearance could not be matched by AVP secretion (because of hypothalamic damage) and as a result the patient developed diabetes insipidus (DI).

for example, after a hemorrhage AVP secretion is stimulated and water is retained, increasing blood volume. The reverse occurs in response to an increase in blood volume/pressure.

Other stimulants to AVP secretion include emotional stress, pain and a variety of drugs. Nausea and vomiting are also extremely potent stimulators of its release (*Box 7.43*). The effects of these stimuli

Patients such as that of *Clinical Case 7.1* are said to have 'central' DI due to a lack of AVP that can occur as a result of any of the causes of hypothalamo-pituitary damage (see *Box 7.9*). However, DI can also occur when the kidneys are insensitive to the action of AVP, termed nephrogenic DI. This may be acquired or congenital and mild or severe (*Box 7.45*). Cranial DI is usually diagnosed using a water-deprivation test (that includes the response to a long-acting AVP analog) or hypertonic saline infusion. The latter is more expensive but may aid the diagnosis of milder forms of AVP deficiency (*Box 7.46*). *Clinical Case 7.1* underwent a water deprivation test to confirm cranial DI and was treated with desmopressin, a long-acting analog of vasopressin that can be given intranasally, subcutaneously or orally.

Nephrogenic DI does not, by definition, respond to vasopressin or its analog. It has been treated primarily by maintaining fluid intake. Nonsteroidal anti-inflammatory drugs have also been used as have mild thiazide diuretics.

## Vasopressin excess – syndrome of inappropriate antidiuresis (SIAD)

A variety of disorders are associated with serum AVP concentrations that are inappropriately high for the serum osmolality. This is discussed in relation to *Clinical Case 4.5*.

## Oxytocin – actions and control

The major action of oxytocin is in lactation when, through a neuroendocrine reflex, it initiates the 'let down' of milk by inducing contractions of the myoepithelial cells surrounding the alveoli of the mammary gland (*Box 7.47*). In animals, there is evidence that it plays a major role in parturition but in the human, there is much less evidence to support this role. It does, however, play a contributing role in that it induces powerful contractions of the uterine muscle. Thus, synthetic oxytocin is widely used therapeutically in obstetrics not only to induce labor and maintain progression but also to reduce post-partum bleeding.

Oxytocin can have stimulatory effects at the AVP $V_2$ receptor in the kidney. There is no naturally occurring disease associated with excess oxytocin secretion but in obstetric situations, when given in high doses as an intravenous infusion in 5% dextrose, it can cause water retention and iatrogenic hyponatremia.

---

**Box 7.45:**
*Causes of diabetes insipidus*[*]

**Lack of AVP (central DI)**
- Any cause of hypothalamo-pituitary damage (see *Box 7.9*) – Note that these have to cause damage to the pituitary stalk or hypothalamus.
- Mutation of the AVP-neurophysin gene – none to date affects the coding region for AVP

**Resistance to AVP action in the kidney (nephrogenic DI)**
- Familial[†] – X-linked or autosomal recessive, this arises as the result of loss of function mutations in either the $V_2$ receptor or in the aquaporin 2 gene.
- Acquired – this includes a large number of possible causes:
   Renal disease – e.g. polycystic kidney, sickle cell hemoglobin
   Electrolyte disorder – e.g. hypercalcemia (see *Clinical Case 4.1*)
   Drugs – e.g lithium carbonate, demeclocycline
   Pregnancy – due to increased expression of a vasopressinase

[*]All are rare.
[†]This presents in infancy with or without a family history, with persistent thirst unresponsive to exogenous AVP analog.

**Box 7.46:**

Tests to diagnose causes of polyuria and polydipsia: central diabetes indipidus (CDI) versus nephrogenic diabetes insipidus (NDI)

## ① Water deprivation test

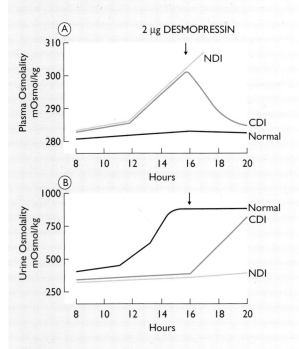

## Interpretation of results:

- In a normal person urine osmolality after 8 hours water deprivation and after desmopressin is >750 mosmol/kg.
- In patients with diabetes insipidus urine osmolality is typically <300 mOsmol/kg after 8 hours water deprivation despite raised plasma osmolality
- In patients with CDI, urine osmolality increases and plasma osmolality decreases after desmopressin but there is no response in patients with NDI.
- Patients with partial CDI, NDI or primary polydipsia often have urine osmolality between 300 and 750 mosmol/kg and thus this test does not distinguish between these different causes of polyuria.

## ② Osmotic stimulation test

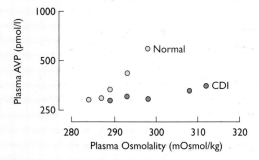

**Data**:

Schematic diagram showing typical changes in plasma Ⓐ and urine Ⓑ osmolality in subjects during 8 hours water deprivation and after an intramuscular injection of desmopressin.

**Procedure**:

- Patients must not drink tea, coffee or alcohol or smoke 12 hours prior to the test, though fluid intake encouraged the night prior to testing.
- No fluids, only dry snacks are allowed for 8 hours during which patient is supervised at all times.
- Urine is sampled hourly for measurment of osmolality and volume and the patient is weighed regularly. Venous blood is sampled every 2 hours for measurement of plasma osmolality.
- After 8 hours 2μg desmopressin (long-acting analog of AVP) is administered and urine and blood samples are taken every hour for a further 2 hours. For safety reasons the test is terminated if the patient loses ≥ %5 body weight

**Data**:

Graph shows the vasopressin response of 2 subjects to an osmotic stimulus induced by a constant infusion of hypertonic saline.

**Procedure**:

Patients are infused with 3–5% sodium chloride for 120–150 minutes at a constant rate during which time venous blood samples are taken every 30 minutes for measurement of plasma osmolality and the concentration of circulating vasopressin (measured by radioioimmunoassay).

**Interpretation of results**:

Patients with CDI may have a higher plasma osmolality compared with controls and there is no AVP response to an osmotic simulus.

The test is useful in distinguishing mild forms of CDI

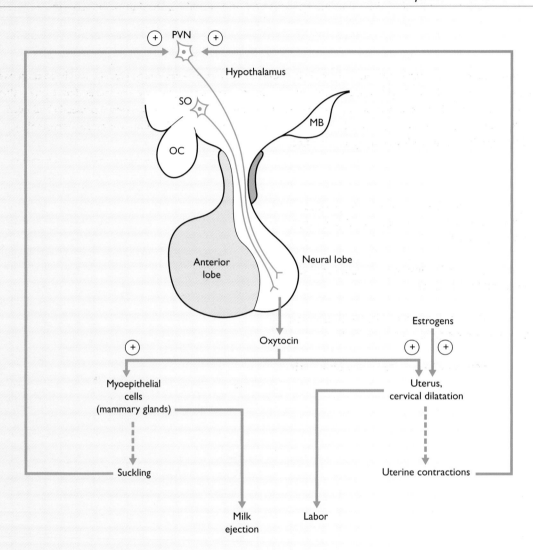

Abbreviations: MB, mammillary body; OC, optic chiasm; PVN, paraventricular nucleus; SO, supraoptic nucleus

# CLINICAL CASE QUESTIONS

The following are examples of applied pathophysiology and these clinically based questions can be answered with the information provided in this chapter. Answers and additional material are available on the website.

---

## Clinical Case Study Q7.1

A 35-year-old patient was seen in the outpatient clinic with amenorrhea of 4 years standing. She had been diagnosed as having paranoid schizophrena 8 years previously and had since received regular intramuscular depot phenothiazine treatment since. Some 2 years previously, she had been seen in the Ob-Gyn clinic and a serum prolactin had been 2457 mU/l (NR <400 mU/l). The serum LH had been 1.2 IU/l and the FSH 1.3 IU/l. The Ob-Gyn made a diagnosis of drug-induced hyperprolactinemia with secondary amenorrhea.

---

Question 1: Were Ob-Gyn correct? In particular, does the hyperprolactinemia account for the hypogonadotrophic hypogonadism?

Question 2: What other investigations might have been considered by Ob-Gyn?

Question 3: How may these results be interpreted and what further investigations are required?

Question 4: How may these results be interpreted?

---

### Clinical Case Study Q7.2

A 71-year-old woman was referred to the lipid clinic with a serum cholesterol of 8.2 mmol/l (recommended <5.2 mmol/l) and triglycerides of 3.3 mmol/l (NR <2 mmol/l). She had a past medical history of bilateral carpal tunnel decompressions performed some 15 years previously and was being treated for systemic hypertension by her primary care physician. She was 1.65 m tall and weighed 99 kg. Noting her facial features, the physician elicited the fact that her wedding ring had been enlarged twice and that her shoe size had increased 2 sizes. It was noted that her son had diabetes mellitus type 2 at the age of 40 years. She was requested to supply a series of old photographs from the family album (*Box Q7.2a*, see website).

**Question 1:** What initial tests would you perform?

**Question 2:** What interpretation do you make of these results?

**Question 3:** What further tests would you perform?

**Question 4:** In the light of these results, what is the differential diagnosis and how would you treat her?

## Clinical Case Study 7.3

A 28-year-old female secretary developed hyperthyroidism and was treated at another hospital. At initial presentation, the serum sodium concentration was 130 mmol/l (NR 135–145 mmol/l). Hyperthyroidism recurred 2 years later when therapy with carbimazole was discontinued and she was admitted to another hospital for a sub-total thyroidectomy. The preoperative serum sodium concentration was 128 mmol/l (NR 135–145 mmol/l). Two days post-operatively, the serum sodium concentration had fallen to 108 mmol/l (NR 135–145 mmol/l) and she became confused. She was not edematous and there was no evidence of heart failure. Serum biochemical tests of liver and renal function were otherwise normal. Her lying and standing blood pressures were normal with no postural drop.

**Question 1:** What are the most likely diagnoses and what investigations would you perform?

**Question 2:** What treatment would you institute and what further investigations should be performed?

## CHAPTER 8

# Cardiovascular and renal endocrinology

## Chapter objectives

*Knowledge of*

1. Hormones secreted by and acting on the cardiovascular system and kidney
2. Paracrine and autocrine control of vascular homeostasis
3. Endocrine basis of heart failure and its treatment
4. Endocrine changes in response to sepsis
5. Hormonal control of erythrocyte cell mass and its abnormalities
6. Clinical features of carcinoid syndrome, its investigation and treatment

---

*'I pant, I sink, I tremble, I expire'*
*Epipsychidion, Percy Bysshe Shelley.*

The cardiovascular system and the kidneys play an indispensable role in maintaining the biochemical constancy of the extracellular fluid. Not only are they responsive to many hormones (most of which are concerned with maintaining blood flow to tissues and organs), they are also major endocrine organs in their own right. The hormones secreted by or acting on the cardiovascular and renal systems are summarized in *Box 8.1*. These diverse hormones effect the regulation of blood pressure and serum electrolyte concentrations through complex interactions. *Clinical Case 8.1* serves to focus on those hormones, some of which have already been discussed in Chapters 5 and 7.

## Endocrinology of heart failure

---

### Clinical Case 8.1:

A 45-year-old woman presented to the Emergency Room with acute shortness of breath such that she was barely able to give a history. She was a life-long non-smoker and had a past history of moderately severe asthma requiring on average two courses of oral glucocorticoid steroids per year. In addition, over the previous year she had noted deterioration in her exercise tolerance that was unrelated to her asthma. Non-invasive cardiac investigations (an echocardiogram) 6 months previously had demonstrated impaired left ventricular function. Over the day prior to admission, use of her $\beta_2$-adrenergic agonist inhalers had not proved beneficial. When seen, she had a blood pressure of 130/75 mmHg, a tachycardia of 130/min, a respiratory rate of 30/min and widespread wheeze in her chest. No cardiac murmurs were heard. The peak expiratory flow rate was 120 l/min (normal for her age and height 450 l/min). Chest X-ray showed borderline cardiomegaly (*Box 8.2*).

The dilemma for the medical team in this case was to distinguish the cause of her dyspnea when she clearly had two possible causes; asthma or pulmonary edema due to poor left ventricular (LV) function. In this case, knowledge of the endocrinology of heart failure facilitated the differential diagnosis.

Hormones produced by and acting on the cardiovascular system and kidney

| Produced by: | | | | |
|---|---|---|---|---|
| **Cardiovascular system** | | | **Kidney** | |
| **Hormone** | **Function** | **Hormone** | **Function** | |
| Atrial natriuretic peptide (ANP) | ↑ Filtration rate / ↓Na$^+$ reabsorption | Renin (enzyme) | ↑ Angiotensin-aldosterone system | |
| Endothelins (ET-1, ET-2, ET-3) | Vasoconstriction / ↑NO | Prostaglandins | ↓ Na$^+$ reabsorption | |
| Nitric oxide (NO) | Vasodilatation | Erythropoietin | ↑ Erythrocyte production | |
| | | 1,25 (OH)$_2$ vitamin D | Calcium homeostasis | |
| | | Prekallikreins | ↑ Kinin production | |

| Acting on: | | | | |
|---|---|---|---|---|
| **Cardiovascular system** | | | **Kidney** | |
| **Hormone** | **Function** | **Hormone** | **Function** | |
| Angiotensin II | Vasocontriction | Aldosterone | ↑Na$^+$ reabsorption | |
| Arginine Vasopressin | Vasoconstriction | Arginine Vasopressin | Water retention | |
| Catecholamines | Vasocontriction/dilatation in skeletal muscle | Catecholamines | Varied | |
| Bradykinin/nitric oxide | Vasodilatation | 1,25(OH)$_2$ vitamin D | ↑Ca$^{2+}$ reabsorption | |
| Thromboxanes | Vasoconstriction | | | |

Impaired LV function causes a primary decrease in cardiac output and, as a result, arterial blood pressure falls. Venous pressure rises because of the inability of the heart to match input to output. This can cause edema due to increased pre-load on the venous side of the circulation and this is usually manifest as pulmonary edema. The arterial underfilling, due to failure of the LV, activates the baroreceptor reflex via stretch receptors in the aortic arch and carotid sinuses as well as several neurohumoral reflexes. Increased sympathetic tone in the CVS results in increased myocardial contractility, tachycardia and arterial vasoconstriction thus increasing cardiac afterload.

Increased sympathetic stimulation of the juxtaglomerulosa apparatus of the kidney, as well as decreased perfusion pressure, induces release of renin that activates the angiotensin-aldosterone system (see *Box 4.34*). This, together with increased sympathetic vasoconstrictor tone, leads to increased renal sodium (and, hence, water) retention. Thus, in heart failure the renin-angiotensin-aldosterone system is activated and the peripheral blood concentration of renin can be used as an indicator of its severity. Furthermore, the effectiveness of aldosterone on salt and water retention in the kidney in such patients is maintained (i.e. there is no mineralocorticoid 'escape').

Apart from stimulating aldosterone secretion, angiotensin II has direct vasoconstrictor effects on both afferent and efferent renal arterioles and a constrictor effect on mesangial cells reducing glomerular filtration surface. It also has direct mitogenic effects on cardiac myocytes and may also play a role in increasing thirst in heart failure via a central CNS effect. There is considerable evidence for local tissue renin-angiotensin systems and increasing experimental work indicates that angiotensin II plays an intracrine role in the heart to affect cell proliferation and apoptosis.

Non-osmotic release of AVP also occurs in heart failure as a result of activation of carotid baroreceptors. This (combined with an increase in thirst) leads to a decrease in free water excretion and potentially hyponatremia (see *Box 7.42*). Hyponatremia in heart failure is an ominous prognostic sign.

LV dysfunction results in increased left atrial pressure and atrial natriuretic peptide (ANP) is secreted from the atria in response to increased distension (*Box 8.3*). This 28 amino acid peptide increases glomerular filtration, decreases collecting duct sodium reabsorption and inhibits the renal renin-angiotensin-aldosterone system. Brain natriuretic peptide (BNP), belonging to the same family of peptides, is a 32 amino acid hormone (*Box 8.3*). It is not only synthesized in the brain but also in the ventricles and is released into the circulation in response to ventricular failure. It has the same effects as ANP and can act on the same receptors. Circulating concentrations of BNP are sensitive measures of heart failure and were used in *Clinical Case 8.1* to clarify the cause of dyspnea. The serum BNP was markedly elevated (21 pmol/l, NR 0.5–6.1 pmol/l) strongly supporting a diagnosis of pulmonary edema. In clinical studies, measures of BNP have the ability to detect heart failure with a sensitivity of nearly 100% and a specificity of about 85%.

Apart from activation of the renal renin-angiotensin-aldosterone system and the counter-regulatory ANP/BNP peptides, the reduced cardiac output seen in heart failure also activates local hormones involved in the control of vasoconstriction. These include the endothelins (see below) that are very potent hormones working, primarily via paracrine actions, to increase vasoconstrictor tone. High circulating concentrations may be seen in heart failure and again are indicative of a poor prognosis.

The treatment for heart failure is to reduce peripheral resistance (antagonize vasoconstriction) and to reduce total plasma volume so as to decrease preload on the heart. Whilst diuretics remain a therapeutic mainstay, the involvement of the endocrine system means that the vast majority of treatments for heart failure are in fact related to its endocrine control (*Box 8.4*). *Clinical Case 8.1* was treated with inhaled $\beta_2$-adrenergic agonist and parenteral glucocorticoid steroid for her asthma; an intravenous diuretic (furosemide) and an oral angiotensin converting enzyme inhibitor was given for her heart failure.

## Paracrine and autocrine regulation of blood pressure: the endocrinology of sepsis

The vascular endothelium that provides the barrier between the blood and the vascular wall is the site of production of several hormones in the control of blood pressure. These include the endothelins,

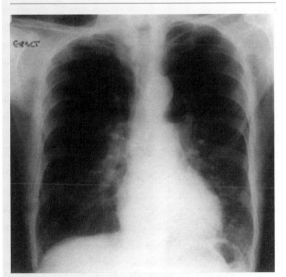

**Box 8.2:**
Chest X-ray of *Clinical Case 8.1*

This postero-anterior film shows overexpanded lung fields compatible with asthma and borderline cardiomegaly (the ratio of the radiological width of the cardiac shadow to that of the thorax is 0.5) and with upper lobe blood diversion (that reproduces poorly). This image is available on the Website.

Structures and sites of synthesis of the natriuretic family of peptides and their receptors

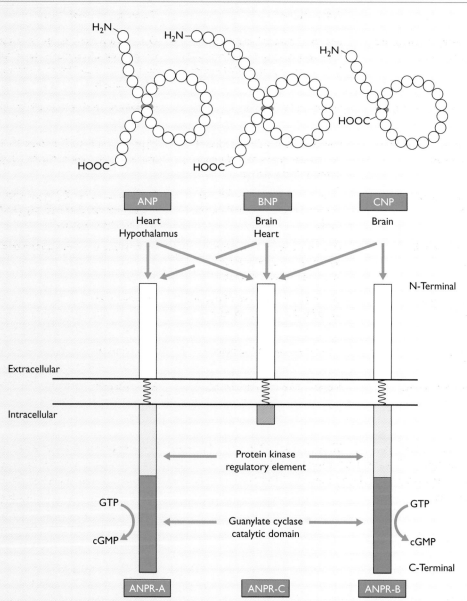

There are three natriuretic peptides: atrial (ANP), brain (BNP) and C-type (CNP). All three hormones have a 17 member amino acid ring formed by a disulfide bridge between cysteine residues though they are products of different genes. Three different NP receptors (R) also exist, A, B and C, but their preferred ligands, indicated by arrows, do not coincide with ANP, BNP and CNP. They are all single transmembrane proteins and whilst ANPR-C has a truncated intracellular domain ANPR-A and -B have intracellular domains with guanylate cyclase and protein kinase activity for signal transduction and receptor regulation.

| Drug | Advantages | Disadvantages/side effects |
|---|---|---|
| β-adrenergic receptor antagonist e.g. carvedilol, bisoprolol | Improved survival and reduced hospitalization rates and mortality. Long-term improved LV function | Dose titration and supervision required Contraindications (e.g. asthma) as for any drug in this class. May exacerbate heart failure initially. |
| Angiotensin II antagonist e.g. losartan | Improved LV function | No long term data from clinical end-points |
| Angiotensin converting enzyme inhibitor e.g. ramipril | Improved survival and reduced hospitalization rates and mortality. Improved LV function | Hypotension (~10%), hyperkalemia (~5%), usually in renal impairement, cough (~10%) |
| Aldosterone antagonist e.g. spironolactone | Improved survival and reduced hospitalization rates and mortality. Cheap | Gynecomastia (~10%) impotence in men (~5%), menstrual irregularity (~10%) in women. Hyperkalemia |
| Brain natriuretic peptide e.g. nesiritide | Dose dependent reduction in pulmonary artery pressure. Increased cardiac output. | Intravenous use only. Experimental |
| Endopeptidase inhibitor e.g. candoxatril | Inhibit the breakdown of natriuretic peptides. Improved exercise tolerance | Experimental |
| Endothelin antagonist (ET-$_{1-31}$, BQ123) | Limited studies in the human | Experimental |
| AVP antagonist e.g. VP-985 | Increases free water clearance | Experimental |

nitric oxide and prostacyclin. *Clinical Case 8.2* introduces the roles of these hormones together with that of calcitonin gene-related peptide in vascular homeostasis.

## Clinical Case 8.2:

A previously fit 54-year-old man had suffered a 'cold' for a week before developing a cough, productive of green sputum. He presented to the Emergency Room with increasing shortness of breath such that he was unable to complete sentences. He was an ex-smoker on no medication and with no significant past medical history. He was pyrexial (39.4°C) and cyanosed with capillary blood oxygen saturations of 90% on 6 l/min inspired oxygen via a face-mask. His blood pressure was 120/70 mmHg with a tachycardia of

140/min. His chest contained bilateral crackles on auscultation. His peripheral blood white cell count was raised at $16 \times 10^9$ /l and the chest X-ray markedly abnormal with evidence of a cavitating pneumonia (*Box 8.5*). He deteriorated markedly and required transfer to the Intensive Care Unit where he underwent artificial ventilation.

A pulmonary artery catheter was inserted and investigations showed the cardiac output to be high at 14 l/min with a normal pulmonary artery capillary wedge pressure (15 mmHg). The peripheral resistance was low (SVR 380 dynes s/cm$^5$ – normal 770–1500 dynes s/cm$^5$) and pulmonary vascular resistance PVR 80 dynes s/cm$^5$ – normal <200 dynes s/cm$^5$). At this time, peripheral blood, taken as part of a research study, contained markedly elevated concentrations of calcitonin gene-related peptide (CGRP).

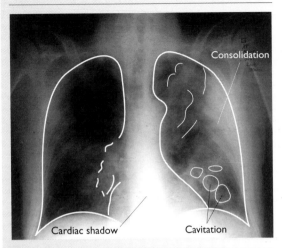

The chest X-ray shows the appearances in the Emergency Room. The left lung shows extensive consolidation with cavitation.

The X-ray shows the appearances in the Intensive Care Unit. The consolidation is now almost confluent in both lungs and the pulmonary artery catheter is visible.

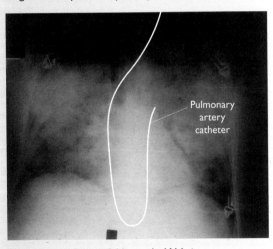

These images are available on the Website.

In sepsis, the presence of endotoxin and early inflammatory cytokines (e.g. TNF, IL-1) results in endothelial cell activation and disruption, disturbing the tonic release of the vasoconstrictor endothelin-1 (ET-1) and the vasodilators nitric oxide (NO) and prostacyclin (PGI$_2$). The activated cells (and also the smooth muscle cells) produce much larger quantities of ET-1, NO and prostaglandins.

The 21 amino acid endothelins, of which there are three isoforms (ET-1, ET-2 and ET-3, *Box 8.6*) are the most potent vasoconstrictors known. They are cleaved from the precursor pro-ET (sometimes referred to as big-endothelin) by a membrane-bound metallopeptidase enzyme. ET-1 is the dominant form in the human vasculature where it occurs mainly in endothelial cells, though it is also found in smooth muscle cells and cardiac myocytes. It is not stored but synthesized *de novo*. ET receptors occur in two forms ET-A and ET-B. ET-A has a high affinity for ET-1 and is expressed on smooth muscle cells. It is considered to mediate the direct vasoconstrictor effects via calcium influx through a non selective ion channel. ET-B receptors are expressed on both endothelial cells and smooth muscle cells in some vascular beds. ET-B stimulation leads to the release of NO (vasodilator) and the prostaglandins thromboxane (vasoconstrictor) and PGI$_2$ (vasodilator). The exact roles of the ET peptides in sepsis are not certain and, experimentally, the use of ET receptor antagonists produces variable results.

Locally produced NO is synthesized from arginine by the action of the constitutively expressed form of endothelial nitric oxide synthase (eNOS). It induces relaxation of smooth muscle cells via paracrine activation of soluble guanylate cyclase that converts GTP to cGMP (*Box 8.7*). In sepsis, the increased NO production is the result of expression of the inducible isoform of NO synthase (iNOS) stimulated by exposure to endotoxin and cytokines. The lung is a major site of iNOS expression in sepsis and increases circulating concentrations of NO. At the same time the physiological action of eNOS is downregulated.

Prostaglandins (PGs) are important regulators of endothelial and kidney functions. A number of PGs is released by endothelial cells. PGI$_2$, like NO, induces vasodilatation whilst thromboxane A$_2$ is a potent vasoconstrictor. The kidney also produces PGs and PGA$_2$ and PGE$_2$ can antagonize the hyper-

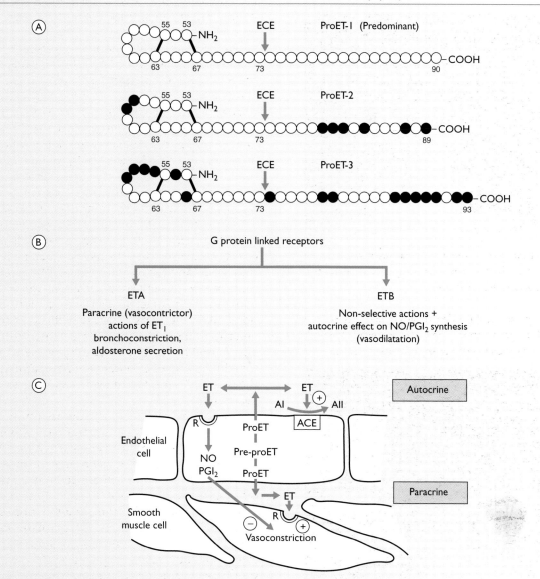

(A) Three isoforms of pro-endothelin (Pro-ET) and their sites of cleavage by endothelin converting enzyme (ECE) to active endothelins. They are products of different genes, but Pro-ET-1 is the predominant isoform. Filled circles represent amino acid differences compared with Pro-ET-1

(B) Several G-protein linked endothelin receptors have been identified but they are generally grouped into ETA and ETB according to their main functions.

(C) The autocrine (vasodilatator, via NO, $PGI_2$) and paracrine (vasoconstrictor) effects of ET-1 on vascular smooth muscle cells. ET-1 is also thought to activate angiotensin converting enzyme (ACE) that converts angiotensin I (AI) to AII.

Abbreviations: NO, nitric oxide; $PGI_2$, prostacyclin; R, ET receptor.

Synthesis of nitric oxide (NO) and its vasodilatory effects on vascular smooth muscle cells

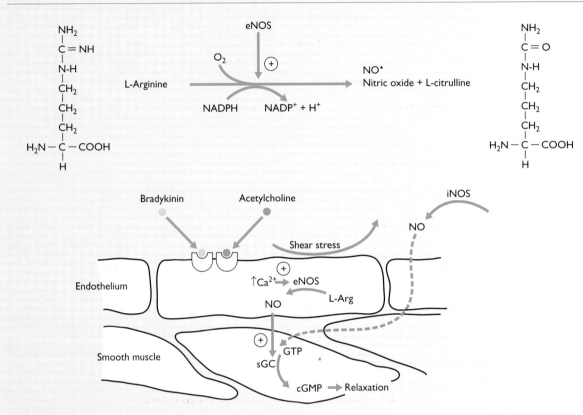

A rise in intracellular $Ca^{2+}$, induced by chemicals or shear stress on the endothelial lining, activates endothelial nitric oxide synthase (eNOS) that converts L-arginine to citrulline and NO. NO diffuses into smooth muscle cells to activate soluble guanylate cyclase (sGC) and the rise in cGMP causes muscle relaxation. In infections, e.g. sepsis, circulating concentrations of NO can rise as a result of inducible iNOS activity and this can have the same vasodilator effect as locally produced NO.

tension induced by the retention of salt and water.

PGs are synthesized by the cyclooxygenase enzyme(s) (COX) and, as with NOS, there is a constitutively expressed isoform, COX-1, and an inducible form, COX-2 (*Box 8.8*). The latter is rapidly induced at sites of inflammation to produce large quantities of prostaglandin and thromboxane. In sepsis, COX-2 is induced by endotoxin and cytokines whilst anti-inflammatory cytokines (e.g. IL-4 and IL-10) and glucocorticoids inhibit COX-2 expression.

As was seen in *Clinical Case 8.2*, septic shock is characterized by a markedly reduced peripheral resistance due to the effects of immune activation on local control of vasomotor tone. It has a mortality of about 50–70% and current treatments have little, if any, effect on the endotoxin and cytokine activated pathways discussed above. Selective COX-2 inhibitors, ET-1 antagonists and iNOS inhibitors are under active development but have not reached the stage of clinical use.

*Clinical Case 8.2* had an acute cavitating pneumonia with secondary septicemia. When trans-

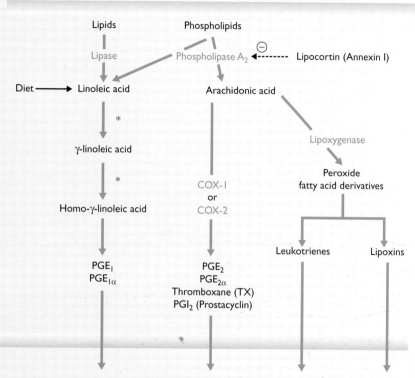

*These are the only two biosynthetic processes that occur in the microsomes of the cell. The rest take place within the plasma membrane.

ferred to the Intensive Care Unit he had a high cardiac output with low peripheral resistance. CGRP, the most potent vasodilator peptide known, has been thought to play a role in the etiology of such pathological states, probably as a result of its release from peripheral nerve endings.

CGRP is a 37-amino-acid peptide, occurring in two forms (α and β) and derived, as its name suggests, from the calcitonin gene by tissue-specific alternative processing (see *Box 5.38*). It belongs to a family of peptides including amylin and adrenomedullin. It is widely distributed with its receptors (of which there are also two types), particularly in the brain and the cardiovascular sys-

tem, but also the thyroid gland and gut. Target cells for CGRP have a cell surface endopeptidase that can cleave the peptide. The $t_{1/2}$ of the peptide in plasma is about 10 min and there is doubt as to whether it functions as a hormone or whether the blood concentration changes merely reflect 'spillage' of the peptide into the circulation. Its widespread distribution throughout the nervous and cardiovascular systems indicates a number of physiological roles. These include altering regional blood flow, direct chronotropic and inotropic effects on the heart, modulation of inflammation and pyrexia, reducing insulin and gastric acid secretion, modulation of sensory transmission. The use of CGRP analogs in a variety of vascular diseases is under active research.

## Hormones and blood cell production – erythropoietin

The regulatory processes that control the production and differentiation of blood cells (hematopoiesis) comprise classical hormones, growth factors and cytokines that can act on bone, blood and, additionally, the liver and spleen. The actions of growth factors and cytokines are generally mediated by paracrine or autocrine mechanisms. Erythropoietin (Epo), secreted by the kidney is a classical hormone and stimulates the production of erythrocytes. A human must produce over a million of these red blood cells each minute to sustain a steady state in which production equals loss, allowing oxygen delivery to tissues and blood pH to be maintained. *Clinical Case 8.3* introduces the endocrinology of erythropoietin.

### Clinical Case 8.3:

A 46-year-old woman presented to the Emergency Room complaining of shortness of breath. There was no evidence for asthma or heart failure but her electrocardiogram was abnormal with evidence of pulmonary hypertension. She was a non-smoker and took no regular medication. There was no family history of serious illness. Echocardiography confirmed the pulmonary hypertension. Her hemoglobin was noted to be markedly elevated at 24 g/dl (NR 11.5–14.5 g/dl) with a hematocrit of 0.60 (NR 0.37–0.47). Analysis of arterial blood gas showed that she was not hypoxic. Chest X-ray showed a prominent pulmonary artery compatible with pulmonary hypertension (*Box 8.9*). CT scan of the lungs (see Website) confirmed pulmonary emboli.

In *Clinical Case 3.1*, thrombus formed in the cardiac atria, as a result of atrial fibrillation and the resulting embolus was arterial to the brain. In *Clinical Case 8.3*, it was probable that the thrombi were venous and embolization was to the lungs. It is apparent from her elevated hemoglobin that this

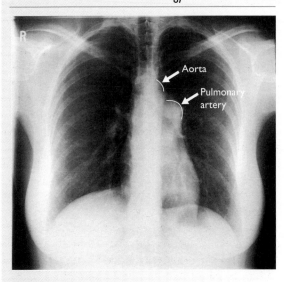

Chest X-ray

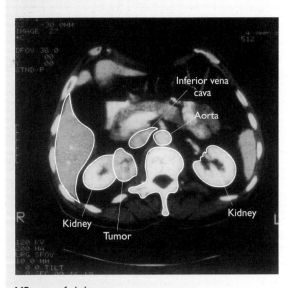

MR scan of abdomen
These images are available on the website.

patient had a marked increase in the number of circulating red blood cells (termed erythrocytosis) that led to an increased blood viscosity and the production of thrombus. Formation of thrombi within, or embolization to, the lungs led to the clinical presentation with dyspnea and pulmonary hypertension.

Erythropoiesis in bone marrow is regulated by the circulating concentration of Epo via the Epo receptor that belongs to the cytokine family of receptors. Signaling is via a number of kinases including JAK/STAT and Ras/MAP kinase pathways. Epo, a glycoprotein with a molecular weight of 34 000, has four effects on erythrocyte progenitor cells. It maintains their viability, promotes cell division, increases hemoglobin synthesis and stimulates morphological maturation. Mutations leading to truncation of the carboxyl terminus (thus removing a negative regulatory element) lead to inherited forms of erythrocytosis.

Epo has been used therapeutically prior to the removal of blood for autologous blood transfusion and illegally by athletes to improve oxygen carriage and, thus, performance. A mutation within the carboxyl terminus of the receptor that increases the sensitivity to Epo and results in a high hemoglobin concentration has been reported in a gold medallist in cross-country skiing in the Winter Olympics.

The cells making Epo are predominantly in peritubular interstitial sites in the kidney although other sites of synthesis (such as the liver and brain) are recognized. Epo synthesis is regulated by oxygen concentration via a poorly understood mechanism involving a heme-containing protein, probably resembling cytochrome b and the nuclear transcription factor HIF-1 leading to an increase in Epo gene expression.

It is clear that an increase in Epo secretion will occur in all forms of hypoxia whether these are physiological (e.g. altitude) or pathological (e.g. an abnormal hemoglobin or lung disease). It will also be apparent that renal failure will lead to Epo deficiency and anemia (*Box 8.10*).

In *Clinical Case 8.3*, the excess of Epo (her venous Epo concentration was 65 mU/l, NR 10–20 mU/l) resulted from production by a renal tumor (*Box 8.10*). Other tumors causing erythrocytosis include those of the liver and cerebellar hemangioblastomas. Primary erythrocytosis termed polycythemia vera is caused by a clonal expansion of cells with an increased sensitivity to Epo though circulating Epo concentrations are low or normal.

---

**Box 8.10:**
**Causes of an increase or decrease in Epo concentrations**

**Increase in Epo**

- Physiological – hypoxia of altitude

- Pulmonary disease – e.g. emphysema

- Cardiovascular disease – e.g. congenital abnormalities resulting in right to left shunts

- Hemoglobin variants – e.g. high $O_2$-affinity

- Tumors – e.g. renal, hepatomas, cerebellar hemangioblastoma, uterine fibroids

**Decrease in Epo**

- Renal disease – e.g. renal failure (of any kind)

- Chronic diseases – e.g. AIDS, malignancy, chronic inflammatory diseases (such as rheumatoid arthritis)

---

The exact mechanism underlying the increased sensitivity in polycythemia vera is not understood.

*Clinical Case 8.3* required a nephrectomy to remove the source of the Epo excess. This was done after initial therapy to reduce the hematocrit (by isovolemic venesection) and the use of intravenous heparin. Patients with secondary erythrocytosis may need regular venesection whilst patients deficient in Epo benefit from adminstration of human recombinant Epo by subcutaneous injection.

## Carcinoid

Episodic, short-lasting changes in vasomotor tone in the cardiovascular system are seen in endocrine deficiencies and excesses. For example, estrogen deficiency may lead to episodic vasodilatation ('hot flushes') whilst release of catecholamines and other peptides from tumors of the adrenal medulla (pheochromocytomas) can stimulate episodic symptoms of hypertension and tachycardia or hypotension (Clinical Case 4.7). The final clinical case demonstrates the effects of the paroxysmal release of a different amine, in this case 5-hydroxytryptamine or serotonin, from what are known as carcinoid tumors.

## Clinical Case 8.4:

A 47-year-old man was referred to the Endocrine out-patients clinic because he had been suffering intermittent episodes of flushing up to six times daily, each lasting approximately a minute associated with wheezing and loud bowel sounds (termed borborygmi). There was no history of skin problems or diarrhea. When seen, the only abnormality was a palpably enlarged liver. His blood pressure was normal. During a spontaneous attack in the clinic, he was noted to develop a 'blush' over the face, neck and upper chest; the trunk and legs were unaffected.

Carcinoid tumors are common and can be seen in 1:150 people at post-mortem and 1:300 appendectomies. The appendix is the commonest site for these tumors followed by the rectum, ileum, lungs, and stomach. Clinical presentations, however, are much less common (incidence ~5 per 100 000 per year) and they occur equally in both sexes with a mean age of about 50 years.

The cells of origin of carcinoids (and, thus, their biochemistry and clinical presentation) differ according to site of origin of the tumor (*Box 8.11*). Rarely, the production of peptides by the tumors leads to clinical presentation as acromegaly or Cushing's syndrome; these may cause great diagnostic difficulty. Classical carcinoid syndrome results from the effects of serotonin together with other contents of tumor secretory granules (including bradykinin, tachykinin, prostaglandins and histamine, depending on the cell of origin) that may be involved in the flushing. In approximately 60% of patients, fibrous plaques develop in the right side of the heart often affecting the tricuspid and pulmonary valves.

The classical symptoms of the 'carcinoid syndrome' – flushing, diarrhea and wheeze – as seen in *Clinical Case 8.4* arise when metastases to the liver result in the release of the amine into the general circulation. Only a minority of patients with carcinoid tumors suffer from the syndrome. The ability of many cells within the body to take *a*mine *p*recursors *u*p and to *d*ecarboxylate them to form

bioactive agents rise to the concept of the *apud* system. It was proposed that these cells shared a common embryonic origin in neuronal ectoderm. Related cells are found in a number of other tissues including the adrenal medulla and sympathetic ganglia. There are histological similarities between carcinoid tumors, medullary cell carcinoma of the thyroid and islet cell tumors. This, together with the observation that carcinoid tumors may occur in patients with other endocrine tumors and that carcinoid tumors may produce a number of other peptides, are compatible with this hypothesis.

Diagnosis of carcinoid syndrome depends in the main on measurement of serotonin metabolites in urine (*Box 8.12*), though measurement of other secreted products such as chromogranin A has also been advocated. When *Clinical Case 8.4* was first seen, the 24 h urinary 5HIAA was 120 µmol/d (NR <30 µmol/d). Ultrasound confirmed widespread liver metastases and biopsy confirmed metastatic carcinoid (*Box 8.13*). The site of the primary tumor was not detected and he was followed in the out-patient clinic. He continued to work full-time and enjoyed his cricket. Some 4 years later, the 24 h urinary 5HIAA was 220 µmol/d. He remained in full-time employment. The 24 h urinary 5HIAA was 990 µmol/d after 21 years and he felt his symptoms warranted treatment. A radiolabeled octreotide scan was performed (*Box 8.13*). This showed marked uptake by the tumor and his symptoms were completely relieved by regular octreotide. He continued to play sport some 22 years after the original diagnosis.

The benign clinical course of *Clinical Case 8.4* illustrates why the term carcin*oid* was coined for this condition as the tumor generally behaves in a much more benign way than metastatic carcin*oma*. The relative rarity of the tumor, together with the variation in clinical behavior, indicates why comparative data on treatment outcomes (*Box 8.14*) are sparse. It also emphasizes the need for properly controlled therapeutic trials with adequate numbers of patients. Had *Clinical Case 8.4* received *any* form of treatment when the tumor was first detected with distant metastases, it would have been regarded as a considerable success 22 years later.

| Site | Type | Clinical characteristics |
| --- | --- | --- |
| Lung/bronchus (2 types) | Well-differentiated (typical carcinoid) | Indolent. Carcinoid syndrome <5%. May present with acromegaly or Cushing's syndrome. 5 year survival >90% |
| | Atypical histology (atypical carcinoid) | Tend to occur in older patients; larger tumors with more aggressive course. 5 year survival ~50% |
| Stomach (3 types) | Associated with atrophic gastritis | More commonly women, often with pernicious anemia, with multifocal tumors and surrounding cellular hyperplasia (a result of the stimulus of hypergastrinemia). Not associated with carcinoid syndrome. Indolent (5 year survival >95%) |
| | Associated with Zollinger-Ellison syndrome | Usually patients with multiple endocrine neoplasia type 1. Not associated with carcinoid syndrome. Indolent (5 year survival >95%) |
| | Sporadic | More common in men and much more aggressive. Clinically may present with atypical carcinoid syndrome (i.e. predominantly flushing) |
| Small bowel | | Often multiple tumors in older patients and associated with carcinoid syndrome. Metastases not related to size of primary tumor. Survival depends on presence (5 year ~30%) or absence (5 year ~60%) of distant metastases |
| Appendix | | More common in younger females. Size of tumor is good predictor of metastases and prognosis. 5 year survival <2 cm diameter and no metastases ~95%, >2 cm with metastases ~30% |
| Colon | | More common in older patients. Carcinoid syndrome in <5%. Tends to present with large primary tumors and metastases (5 year survival ~20%) |
| Rectum | | More common in older patients. Carcinoid syndrome rare. Tumors tend to contain glucagon and glicentin molecules. Size of tumor correlates with likelihood of metastasis and, thus, prognosis that is about the same as for colonic tumors (5 year survival with local disease ~80%, but ~20% with metastases) |

**Box 8.12:**
Synthesis and metabolism of 5-hydroxytryptamine (serotonin)

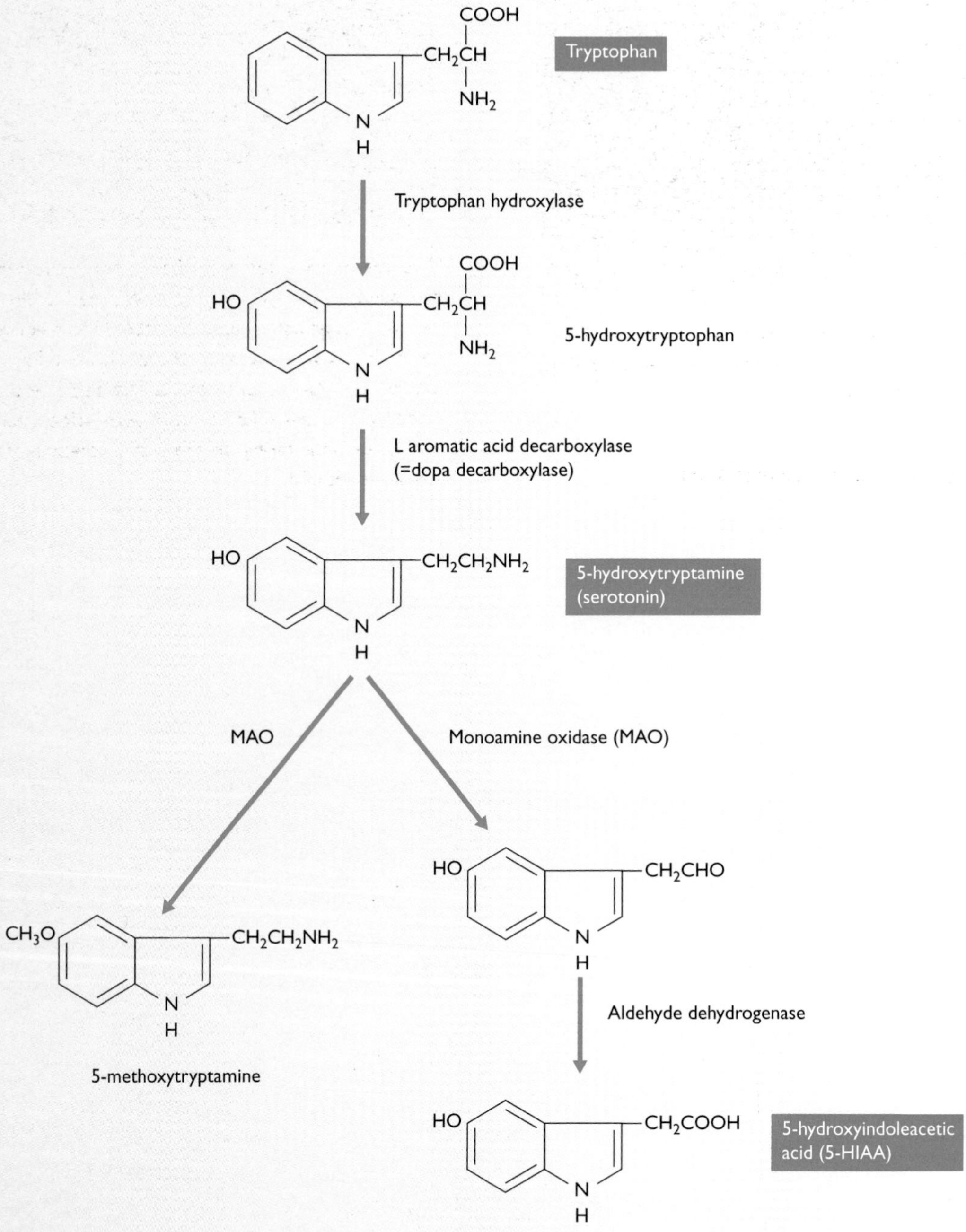
COOH
CH$_2$CH
NH$_2$
N
H
Tryptophan
Tryptophan hydroxylase
COOH
HO
CH$_2$CH
NH$_2$
5-hydroxytryptophan
N
H
L aromatic acid decarboxylase
(=dopa decarboxylase)
HO
CH$_2$CH$_2$NH$_2$
5-hydroxytryptamine
(serotonin)
N
H
MAO
Monoamine oxidase (MAO)
HO
CH$_2$CHO
CH$_3$O
CH$_2$CH$_2$NH$_2$
N
H
Aldehyde dehydrogenase
5-methoxytryptamine
HO
CH$_2$COOH
5-hydroxyindoleacetic
acid (5-HIAA)

Box 8.13:
Liver biopsy and $^{99m}$TC-labeled octreotide scan results of *Clinical Case 8.4*

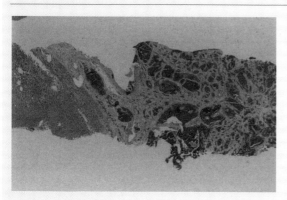

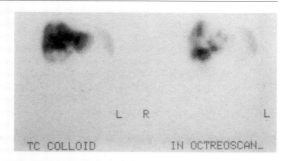

The core of tissue taken from the liver shows the replacement of normal liver with multiple areas of dark cells of carcinoid tissue.

These images are available on the Website.

Two radionucleotide scans have been performed. The left-hand panel shows a $^{99m}$Tc-labelled colloid scan demonstrating patchy uptake of colloid into normal liver cells. The right hand scan shows the uptake of $^{111}$In-octreotide. Note that each is the reciprocal of the other; areas that take up most octreotide take up no colloid demonstrating the areas of carcinoid metastastic replacement of liver.

## Medical

| Drug | Use | Advantages | Disadvantages/side effects |
|---|---|---|---|
| Antihistamines e.g. chlorpheniramine | Symptom relief e.g. gastric carcinoids | Decreases flushing in those cases in which histamine is involved | $H_1$ antagonists may sedate. More recent agents better. |
| Serotonin antagonist e.g. cyproheptadine | Symptom relief e.g. for diarrhea | Effective in symptom relief. | Drowsiness and weight gain |
| Somatostatin analog e.g. octreotide, lanreotide | Symptom relief | $^{111}$In-octreotide scans may be used to screen tumors expressing somatostatin receptors. Effective symptom relief. Has replaced most other agents in medical treatment | Gastrointestinal upset, gallstones. Expensive. Given by injection. |
| Niacin | Prevention of pellagra[*] | Effective prevention in low doses | None in low doses |
| Chemotherapy[†] | Palliation | Used in aggressive metastatic disease | None really effective (~25% response) substantial toxicity |

## Surgical

| Drug | Use | Advantages | Disadvantages/side effects |
|---|---|---|---|
| Surgical excision | To remove primary | Potentially curative. Procedure depends on site and size of tumor and degree of invasion. Local excision may be possible | All depend on site of tumor and its size |
| Hepatic resection | To debulk secondaries | Best option for palliation though the liver is usually diffusely involved and this option is often not possible | Mortality ~5%. Complications (hemorrhage, liver failure) ~30%, 5 year survival ~70%, |
| Hepatic transplant | | | 5 year survival ~50% |
| Hepatic devascularization e.g. embolization | To debulk secondaries | Less invasive and more selective than hepatic artery ligation. Requires medical pretreatment (see above) to prevent 'carcinoid crisis' | Hepatorenal failure and death (~5%) |

## Radiotherapeutic

| Drug | Use | Advantages | Disadvantages/side effects |
|---|---|---|---|
| $^{131}$I-octreotide | Palliation | Non-invasive and less toxic than other palliative therapies | Limited data on efficacy |

## None[‡]

[*]Pellagra may occur if carcinoid tumor use of tryptophan leads to a deficiency.
[†]There is no really effective chemotherapeutic regimen. Those agents used include streptozotocin, 5-flurouracil or cyclophosphamide and more recently cisplatin and etoposide or interferon-$\alpha$.
[‡]A reminder that intervention to treat a patient with a naturally indolent condition (see Clinical Case 8.4) is not necessarily needed.

# CLINICAL CASE QUESTIONS

The following are examples of applied pathophysiology and these clinically based questions can be answered with the information provided in this chapter. Answers and additional material are available on the website.

---

### Clinical Case Study Q8.1:

A 56-year-old man with type 2 diabetes of 23 years duration was seen in the clinic. He was noted to have hypertension (blood pressure 160/100 mmHg) and microalbuminuria and his serum creatinine was 120 μmol/l (NR 50–110 mmol/l). He was prescribed a small daily dose of the angiotensin-converting enzyme inhibitor ramipril. Three days later, he was seen in the Emergency Room having become acutely short of breath. His blood pressure was 110/70 with a tachycardia of 110/min and he had bilateral basal crackles on auscultation of his chest. The chest X-ray indicated that he had developed pulmonary edema. The serum creatinine had risen markedly to 410 μmol/l.

---

Question 1: What pathophysiological process does the course of events suggest?

Question 2: Which investigation would you perform next?

## Clinical Case Study Q8.2:

A 73-year-old woman was seen in the Emergency Room. She had become increasingly short of breath over the previous 12 h. She was taking hydrochlorthiazide 5 mg with amiloride 5 mg daily. When seen she had a blood pressure of 130/70 with a sinus tachycardia of 120/min. The jugular venous pressure was raised 5 cm and the electrocardiogram and chest X-ray obtained are shown in *Box Q8.2*. Her serum sodium was reported to be 119 mmol/l (NR 135–145 mmol/l) with a potassium of 4.0 mmol/l (NR 3.5–4.7 mmol/l) and a urea of 8.0 mmol/l (NR 2.5–8.0 mmol/l). The electrocardiogram and chest X-ray are shown in *Box Q8.2*.

Electrocardiogram and chest X-ray of *Clinical Case Study Q8.2*

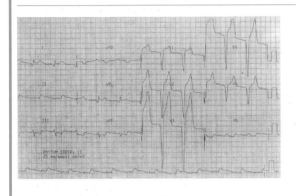
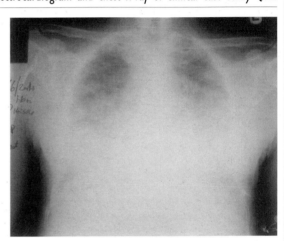

**Question 1:** What is the diagnosis?

**Question 2:** What is the cause of her hyponatremia?

**Question 3:** How would you treat her?

Page numbers in bold refer to boxes

# Index

# Index